Practicals in
Pediatric Allergy

Practicals in Pediatric Allergy

Editor-in-Chief

Krishna Mohan R
DNB DAA ICPP MNAMS
Consultant Pediatrician and Pediatric Allergist
Department of Health Services
Kozhikode, Kerala, India
National Chairperson, Allergy and Applied Immunology Chapter, IAP 2024

Co-Editors

Soundarya M
MD (Pediatrics) ACME DPAA
Consultant Pediatric Allergist
Division of Pediatric Allergy
Department of Pediatrics
KMC Hospital
Mangaluru, Karnataka, India

Hima Mathews P
DCH DNB DPAA FAAP ICPP
Senior Consultant and Allergist
Department of Pediatrics
Lisie Medicity
Kochi, Kerala, India

Foreword

Neeraj Gupta

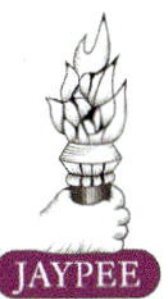

JAYPEE BROTHERS MEDICAL PUBLISHERS
The Health Sciences Publisher
New Delhi | London

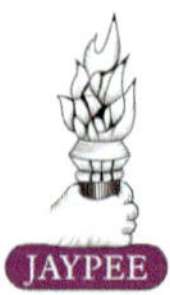

Jaypee Brothers Medical Publishers (P) Ltd

Headquarters
EMCA House, 23/23-B
Ansari Road, Daryaganj
New Delhi 110 002, India
Landline: +91-11-23272143, +91-11-23272703
+91-11-23282021, +91-11-23245672
e-mail: jaypee@jaypeebrothers.com

Corporate Office
4838/24, Ansari Road, Daryaganj
New Delhi 110 002, India
Phone: +91-11-43574357
Fax: +91-11-43574314
e-mail: jaypee@jaypeebrothers.com

Overseas Office
JP Medical Ltd
83 Victoria Street, London
SW1H 0HW (UK)
Phone: +44-20 3170 8910
e-mail: info@jpmedpub.com

EU GPSR Authorised Representative
Logos Europe, 9 rue Nicolas Poussin
17000, La Rochelle, France
Phone: +33 (0) 6 67 93 73 78
e-mail: contact@logoseurope.eu

Website: www.jaypeebrothers.com
Website: www.jaypeedigital.com

Inquiries for bulk sales may be solicited at: jaypee@jaypeebrothers.com

Practicals in Pediatric Allergy

First Edition: 2026, Reprint: **2026**

ISBN: 978-93-6616-712-1

Printed in India

Dedicated to

Our respected teachers, who lit the path of knowledge and inspired us to pursue this field
Our brave little patients, who face their challenges with courage and grace
Our families—for their steadfast love and support

Contributors

Abdul Rauf KK
MD DNB FNB (Ped Crit Care) MRCPCH
Consultant Pediatric Intensivist
Department of Pediatrics
Baby Memorial Hospital
Kozhikode, Kerala, India

Afaq Jalali MD
Consultant Internist
Department of Medicine
Jawahar Lal Nehru Memorial Hospital
Srinagar, Jammu & Kashmir, India

Akshay Holla DCH DNB
Senior Registrar
Department of Pediatrics
Cloud 9 Hospital
Bengaluru, Karnataka, India

Althea Valeen Pinto MD (DVL) DNB
Consultant Dermatologist and Assistant Professor
KMC Hospital
Mangaluru, Karnataka, India

Andrew Bush
MBBS (Hons) MA MD FHEA FRCP FRCPCH FERS FAPSR ATSF
Professor
Department of Pediatrics and
Pediatric Respirology
National Heart and Lung Institute
Imperial College, and Imperial Centre for
Paediatrics and Child Health, London
Consultant Pediatric Chest Physician
Royal Brompton Hospital
London, UK

Anita Krishnan
DLO (AFMC) DNB DAA (CMC, Vellore) PGDMLE
Consultant
Department of Otorhinolaryngology
Bangalore ENT Care Centre and
Apollo Spectra Hospital
Bengaluru, Karnataka, India

Arjun V DO DNB FCRS (AEH)
Consultant and Head
Department of Cornea and Ocular Surface
Comtrust Charitable Eye Hospital
Kozhikode, Kerala, India

Arunima Ashok DCH DNB
Assistant Surgeon and Pediatrician
Department of Health Services
Women and Child Hospital
Kozhikode, Kerala, India

Asef A Wani MS
Professor and Head
Department of Ear, Nose, and Throat
SKIMS Medical College and Hospital
Srinagar, Jammu & Kashmir, India

Asif Ahmed MD
Assistant Professor
Department of Pediatrics
SKIMS Medical College and Hospital
Srinagar, Jammu & Kashmir, India

Ayaz Gull MSc PhD
Research Associate
Department of Immunology
Sher-i-Kashmir Institute of Medical Sciences
Srinagar, Jammu & Kashmir, India

Charu Chandwani MD (Pediatrics) DPAA
Associate Consultant
Department of Pediatrics
Shree Aggarsain International Hospital
New Delhi, India

Dhanesh Volvoikar DCH DPH FACI
Consultant Pediatrician and Allergist
Department of Pediatrics
Healthway Hospital
Goa, India

Dipti Pujari
MRCPCH (UK) MD (Pediatrics) DNB DCH FACI
European Board (EAACI) Certified in Allergology and Immunology
Allergy Consultant and Pediatrician
Deenanath Mangeshkar Hospital and Research Center
Pune, Maharashtra, India

Divya Verma
MSc (Botany) PhD (Botany) MSc (Bioinformatics, University of Edinburgh)
Professor
Department of Botany
Kalindi College (University of Delhi)
New Delhi, India

Francis Kurian MBBS DCH PGPN DAAI
Director
Allergy Asthma Foundation Clinic
Palakkad, Kerala, India

Gouthami P DNB DPAA PGPN
Associate Professor
Department of Pediatrics
RVM Institute of Medical Sciences
Telangana, Hyderabad, India

Hadeeqa Aejaz MBBS
Resident
Jamia Hamdard Medical College
New Delhi, India

Hima Mathews P DCH DNB DPAA FAAP ICPP
Senior Consultant and Allergist
Department of Pediatrics
Lisie Medicity
Kochi, Kerala, India

Imtiyaz A Bhat MSc PhD
Lab Head
Unipath Speciality Labs
Srinagar, Jammu & Kashmir, India

Jyothi Janardhanan MD (Pediatrics)
Fellow
Department of Pediatric Immunology and Rheumatology
Aster CMI Hospital
Bengaluru, Karnataka, India

Krishna Mohan R
DNB DAA ICPP MNAMS
Consultant Pediatrician and Pediatric Allergist
Department of Health Services
Kozhikode, Kerala, India
National Chairperson, Allergy and Applied Immunology Chapter, IAP 2024

Kushalinii Hillson MBChB MRCPCH
Clinical Research Fellow
National Heart and Lung Institute
Imperial College, London
Pediatric Respiratory Registrar
Royal Brompton Hospital
London, UK

Mohammad Naveed MBBS
Medical Officer
Department of Medicine
Jawahar Lal Nehru Memorial Hospital
Srinagar, Jammu & Kashmir, India

Mosam Kamlesh Maroo MD DNB (Pediatrics) FAAP
Consultant
Department of Pediatrics and Allergy
Dr Mosam Maroo's Allergy and Asthma Centre
MRR Children's Hospital
Mumbai, Maharashtra, India

Muzima Jeelani MSc AAAC
Allergy Counselor
Allergy Clinic
Jawahar Lal Nehru Memorial Hospital
Srinagar, Jammu & Kashmir, India

Narayan Prasad Modi MD (Pediatrics) DAA
Professor and Head
Department of Pediatrics
MKCG Medical College
Berhampur, Odisha, India

Narmada S
DNB PhD MRCPCH FRCPCH FIAP DAA PGDDN MBA (Hospital Admin)
Consultant Pediatrician and Director
Nalam Medical Centre and Hospital
Vellore, Tamil Nadu, India

Neeraj Gupta
DCH DNB FRCPCH DAA FAAAAI IDPCCM DPSM
Allergist, Pediatric Intensivist, and
Sleep Medicine Specialist
Department of Pediatrics
Sir Ganga Ram Hospital
New Delhi, India

Nihala Tarannum H
DCH DPSM AASC Fellowship in Allergy and Asthma Procedures ICPP (Pediatric Pulmonology) Certified Pediatric Pulmonology
Consultant Pediatrician, Allergy Asthma and
Pediatric Sleep Specialist
Vellore Speciality Centre
(ENT, Pediatric, Allergy and Asthma Centre)
Vellore, Tamil Nadu, India

Payal Mittal DNB (Pediatric)
Associate Professor
Department of Pediatrics
FH Medical college
Agra, Uttar Pradesh, India

Peter P Vazhayil DCH DNB (Pediatrics) MRCPCH (UK)
Associate Professor
Department of Pediatrics
Government Medical College
Ernakulam, Kerala, India

Priya Sreenivasan
MD DCH MPhil (Clinical Epidemiology)
Professor
Department of Pediatrics
Government Medical College
Thiruvananthapuram, Kerala, India

R Prasanna
DCH DNB MRCPCH (UK) MRCP (Edinburgh) Diploma in Pediatric Allergy and Asthma
Professor
Department of Pediatrics and Neonatology
SRM Medical College Hospital and
Research Centre
Chennai, Tamil Nadu, India

Rahima Saleem DVD MD DNB FRCP
Associate Professor
Department of Dermatology
Government Medical College
Kozhikode, Kerala, India

Reyaz A Malik MD DPAA
Professor and Head
Department of Pediatrics
SKIMS Medical College and Hospital
Srinagar, Jammu & Kashmir, India

S Elayaraja
DCH DNB (Pediatrics) MRCPCH DPAA Fellowship Pediatric Pulmonology
European Diplomate in Pediatric
Respiratory Medicine
Division of Pediatric Pulmonology
Department of Pediatrics
Sri Ramachandra Institute of Higher Education
and Research
Chennai, Tamil Nadu, India

Sagar Bhattad
MD DM (Pediatric Clinical Immunology and Rheumatology)
Consultant
Department of Pediatric Immunology and
Rheumatology
Aster CMI Hospital
Bengaluru, Karnataka, India

Shambo S Samajdar
MD DM (Clinical Pharmacology) DAAI (BV University)
FIPS Fellow Diabetes India
Fellowship in Respiratory and Critical Care (WBUHS) PG
Dip Endo and Diabetes (RCP)
Consultant Physician
Allergy Asthma Treatment Centre
Kolkata, West Bengal, India

Shamsa Tariq MBBS
Resident
Jamia Hamdard Medical College
New Delhi, India

Shebna A Khader MD (Pediatrics) DPAA FAAP
Pediatrician and Allergist
ALLERGO KIDZ Paediatric Allergy Clinic
Kochi, Kerala, India

Sheena P Kochumon
DCH MD (Pediatrics)
Fellowship in Pediatric Genetics and Clinical Genetics
Hmx Pro in Cancer Genomics and Gene Therapy
Assistant Professor
Department of Pediatrics
Amrita Institute of Medical Sciences and
Research Centre
Kochi, Kerala, India

Shilpa Nayak
DCH DAA (CMC, Vellore) DPAA (SGRH, New Delhi)
Asthma Allergy Centre
Mumbai, Maharashtra, India

Sinchana Bhat DCH DNB DAA (CMC, Vellore)
Consultant Pediatrician and Allergy Specialist
Dr Sinchana's Allergy and Asthma Clinic
Mangaluru, Karnataka, India

Sonia Bhatt MD (Pediatrics) DAA PGCAP
Professor and Head
Department of Pediatrics
FH Medical College
Agra, Uttar Pradesh, India

Soundarya M MD (Pediatrics) ACME DPAA
Consultant Pediatric Allergist
Division of Pediatric Allergy
Department of Pediatrics
KMC Hospital
Mangaluru, Karnataka, India

Sowmya Arudi Nagarajan
DCH DAA EAACI Certificate of Excellence in Allergy FAAAI
Consultant Pediatrician and Allergist
Sanjeevini Specialist Clinic and Mallige Hospitals
Bengaluru, Karnataka, India

Surgeon Commander Jayakrishnan VY
MBA (HHM) DNB (Pediatrics) DPAA DPSM
Classified Specialist
Department of Pediatrics
Armed Forces Medical Services
Mumbai, Maharashtra, India

Sushma C DCH FNNF
Consultant Pediatrician and Neonatologist
Department of Pediatrics
Chinmaya Mission Hospital
Bengaluru, Karnataka, India

Swati Kalra MD DNB DPAA
Senior Consultant
Department of Pediatrics
Medanta—The Medicity
Gurugram, Haryana, India

Tabasum Shafi MSc PhD
Research Associate
Sher-i-Kashmir Institute of Medical Sciences
Srinagar, Jammu & Kashmir, India

Taha Ashraf Qureshi MBBS PhD FAAI DAA DPAA
Senior Allergologist
Allergy Clinic
Jawahar Lal Nehru Memorial Hospital
Srinagar, Jammu & Kashmir, India

Tina N Goel DNB (Pediatrics) DPAA
Senior Consultant and Allergist
Department of Pediatrics
Kare N Kure Child Allergy Centre
Aakash Hospital, Cloud Nine Hospital
New Delhi, India

Vikram Patra
MD DCH FACI EAACI Certificate of Excellence in Allergy
Consultant
Department of Pediatric Allergy
Apollo Hospital and MGM New Bombay Hospital
Navi Mumbai, Maharashtra, India

Vivek Oommen Varghese
MS (Ophthalmology) FCRS (AEH)
Assistant Professor
Department of Ophthalmology
Sree Gokulam Medical College and
Research Foundation
Thiruvananthapuram, Kerala, India

Viveka Santhosh Reddy C
MD (Pediatrics, MAHE) PDF in Pediatric Neurology (IGICH)
Pediatric Neurologist
Vihaa Skin Pediatric CNDC
Bengaluru, Karnataka, India

Foreword

In the ever-evolving landscape of pediatric health care, allergic diseases have emerged as a growing challenge—both in prevalence and in complexity. From food allergies and eczema to allergic rhinitis and asthma, the burden on children and their families has deepened, calling for a more nuanced and practical understanding of allergic disorders among pediatricians. It is in this context that *Practicals in Pediatric Allergy* finds its profound relevance. This book is more than a compilation of protocols and procedures—it is a reflection of clinical wisdom, grounded in evidence-based practice and tailored to the realities of pediatric care in India and beyond. It bridges the critical gap between theory and practice, equipping clinicians with the tools, insights, and confidence to diagnose and manage allergic conditions more effectively. As Chairperson of the Indian Academy of Pediatrics (IAP) Allergy and Applied Immunology Chapter, I am particularly heartened to see this initiative led by passionate and skilled professionals. Dr Krishna Mohan R, Editor-in-Chief, brings not only his expertise but also a visionary approach to pediatric allergy education. Ably supported by Dr Soundarya M and Dr Hima Mathews P as Co-Editors, the editorial team has curated a resource that is concise, clinically oriented, and immensely practical.

This book aligns closely with our chapter's mission—to empower pediatricians across the country with knowledge that transforms practice. With clear illustrations, procedural guidance, and real-world applicability, *Practicals in Pediatric Allergy* stands as an essential addition to every pediatrician's library.

I congratulate the Editor-in-Chief, Co-Editors and all the contributors for their dedication to this vital work. May this book serve as a trusted companion in our collective pursuit to improve the lives of children with allergic diseases.

Neeraj Gupta
Chairperson (2025)
IAP Allergy and Applied Immunology Chapter

Preface

Pediatric allergy is a rapidly growing field where scientific progress and clinical challenges go hand in hand. While textbooks and monographs on allergy generally provide extensive theoretical knowledge, pediatricians, trainees, and even specialists frequently face a gap when it comes to the practical aspects. This book, *Practicals in Pediatric Allergy*, has been conceived and developed to bridge precisely this gap.

This book is the first-of-its-kind, dedicated exclusively to the procedures, investigations, and therapeutic techniques that define modern pediatric allergy care. It brings together the collective knowledge and experience of many national and international experts, who have contributed chapters with a strong focus on the "how to" of practice—stepwise methods, precautions, interpretation, and management tips. Each section is written with clarity and simplicity, designed to serve medical students, trainees, pediatricians, and specialists alike.

We hope this volume will serve as both a guidebook and a companion, supporting clinicians at the bedside, in clinics, and during training. It reflects our shared commitment to making pediatric allergy care more structured, safe, and accessible. Above all, it is our hope that *Practicals in Pediatric Allergy* will inspire more pediatricians to engage with this fascinating field and, in doing so, improve the lives of children living with allergies around the world.

Krishna Mohan R
Soundarya M
Hima Mathews P

Acknowledgments

Practicals in Pediatric Allergy is a first-of-its-kind book devoted to the practical aspects of pediatric allergy, focusing on procedures, investigations, and therapeutic interventions that guide day-to-day clinical care. Conceived as a hands-on resource for students, trainees, and practicing clinicians, this book brings together expertise from across the globe and aims to fill an important gap in the literature. We are deeply indebted to all the national and international authors whose invaluable contributions form the backbone of this work, each chapter reflecting their knowledge, experience, and commitment to advancing pediatric allergy. We gratefully acknowledge our teachers, mentors, and colleagues, whose constant guidance and encouragement have inspired us to undertake this endeavor. Our heartfelt thanks go to our families for their unwavering support, patience, and understanding throughout the journey of preparing this book. We also extend our sincere appreciation to Shri Jitendar P Vij (Group Chairman), Mr Ankit Vij (Managing Director), Mr MS Mani (Group President), Mr Sabyasachi Hazra (Director—PG and PNR Content), Ms Pooja Bhandari (Director Production—Books and Journals), Mr Vikas Solanki (Development Editor), and all other team members of M/s Jaypee Brothers Medical Publishers (P) Ltd, New Delhi, India for their professionalism, dedication, and help in bringing this work to print. It is our earnest hope that this volume proves to be a useful companion for practitioners, students, and clinicians engaged in the care of children with allergic diseases.

Contents

CHAPTER 1

Clinical Assessment of Allergy

Krishna Mohan R, Sinchana Bhat

INTRODUCTION

Allergies are one of the major health problems and now rank the third most frequent reason people seek medical care. Their prevalence has dramatically risen over the last decade. Allergic disorders have diverse manifestations and can have multisystemic involvement in an individual. But unfortunately, pediatric allergic diseases are still understudied. A detailed history and physical examination are essential and the most vital part in managing a patient. It can help in identifying the offending allergen, triggers, and lifestyle factors contributing toward the allergies and differentiate between allergy and allergy mimics. Though we have an array of advanced diagnostic techniques in the field of allergy, they should always be utilized after a clinical diagnosis.

HISTORY TAKING IN PEDIATRIC ALLERGY

A questionnaire-based history taking will be appropriate.

Medical History

The history of the onset, duration, and progress of the symptoms is important to elicit at the beginning. A detailed past medical history, including drug history, personal and family history, and social and occupational history, should be taken. After a good history, the physician should be able to conclude the following considerations, as given in **Box 1.1**.

BOX 1.1: Key considerations in assessing pediatric allergic conditions.

- Is the presenting symptom related to an allergic or nonallergic condition?
- Whether there is an identifiable trigger/cofactors?
- How is the progression and the severity of the illness?
- Is it affecting the sleep, play, activity, school, and growth of the child?
- Past medical history/treatment taken, family history/personal history of atopy, environmental history

Is it an Allergic/Nonallergic Condition?

Allergic conditions (IgE-mediated disorders) manifest symptoms immediately or within a maximum of 2 hours of an allergen exposure (temporal association). Occasionally, they result in anaphylaxis as well. Lack of consistency in symptoms and temporal association can rule out an IgE-mediated reaction. Non-IgE mediated disorders have a delayed presentation and rarely cause anaphylaxis. Some of the symptoms of allergic diseases are given in **Table 1.1**.

The severity of an allergic reaction can be graded as given in **Table 1.2**.

TABLE 1.1: Symptoms and probable diagnosis of common allergic conditions.	
Symptoms	***Probable diagnosis***
Nasal	
• Sneezing, itching of the nose, nasal congestion, and rhinorrhea	• Allergic rhinitis
• Absence of pruritus	• Points toward nonallergic rhinitis
• Postnasal drip, facial pain, mucopurulent discharge, anosmia	• Rhinosinusitis
Respiratory	
• Cough, wheezing, chest tightness, dyspnea	• Asthma
• Dry cough lasting for >10 days, more in the early morning, increasing with emotions (crying/laughing), wheezing	• Cough variant asthma/in under five wheezers, high probability of asthma
Skin and mucosa	
• Well-demarcated, raised, and erythematous papules with pale center and associated with intense itching (hives/wheals)	• Urticaria—simple urticaria usually resolves completely within 24 hours without any residual scarring
• Hives which are painful and burning and leave bruising, scarring, or hyperpigmentation	• Urticarial vasculitis
• Deep tissue swelling affecting the mucocutaneous junction. It can persist for a few days once it gets established	• Angioedema
• Intensely pruritic papular/vesicular lesions usually on extensor surfaces, face (infants and young children), and flexural areas at any age. Spares groin and axillary areas	• Atopic dermatitis
Eye	
• Erythema, watering, and itching of eyes	• Allergic/vernal conjunctivitis
Gastrointestinal	
• Perioral and throat itching and tightness, vomiting, diarrhea	• Systemic manifestations of anaphylaxis
Systemic	
• Palpitations, dizziness due to hypotension, collapse or loss of consciousness, impending sense of doom	• Anaphylaxis should always be suspected

TABLE 1.2: Muller's grading of IgE-mediated allergic reaction.	
Grading	***Clinical features***
Grade I	Generalized urticaria, itching, malaise, anxiety
Grade II	Any of the above plus two or more of the following: Angioedema, chest constriction, nausea, vomiting, diarrhea, abdominal pain, and dizziness
Grade III	Any of the above plus two or more of the following: Dyspnea, wheezing, stridor, dysarthria, hoarseness, weakness, confusion, and feeling of impending disaster
Grade IV	Any of the above plus two or more of the following: Fall in blood pressure, collapse, loss of consciousness, incontinence, cyanosis

Whether there is an Identifiable Trigger or Cofactor?

Trigger: Infections; exposure to smoke, dust, and pollen; seasonal changes; and exercise are the known triggers in respiratory allergies. Exacerbation of symptoms following history exposure to a trigger should be elicited.

Cofactors: They can amplify an allergic/anaphylactic reaction by reducing the threshold of the allergen dose needed to produce anaphylaxis. Exercise, stress, consumption of alcohol, menstruation, and drugs such as nonsteroidal anti-inflammatory drugs (NSAIDs) are the most common cofactors. Taking this history is important in food-dependent exercise-induced anaphylaxis (FDEIA), which occurs only when the consumption of food (usually wheat products) occurs 1–4 hours before or after exercise or in the presence of any of these cofactors.

How is the Progression of the Illness?

Assessment of progression of illness since its onset, frequency of the symptoms (seasonal or perennial), treatment response, and symptom control with medications is important to plan the treatment for a patient. For example, treatment can be stepped up or down based on the symptom control in asthma.

Is it Affecting the Daily Activities of the Affected Individual?

Severity of the illness in children can be assessed by the extent to which it affects daily activities such as school, play, and sleep. Comorbid conditions such as adenoid hypertrophy or obstructive sleep apnea can affect school performance due to daytime sleepiness.

Past Medical History

Atopic march describes the sequential progression of atopic disorders from atopic dermatitis in infants to allergic rhinitis and asthma in later childhood. Hence, it is important to know the presence of these allergic conditions in the past. The details of their progression and treatment are also important to plan further management. Prevalence of allergic rhinitis is higher among children with asthma than the general population and ranges from 60 to 80%. About 40–50% of children with allergic rhinitis also have asthma. A history of recurrent infections in a child going to daycare [one upper respiratory infection (URI) per month or 12 per year] may in fact be normal. Children who received repeated nebulization and are treated as pneumonia patients should be evaluated for asthma if previous chest X-rays are normal.

Treatment History

Review of records may be very helpful, especially for a patient with a history of recurrent infection or drug allergy. In individuals with suspected drug allergy, the patient or caregiver may not be able to recollect details of drugs given during an illness. Erroneous labeling of drug allergy for all the medications administered before a drug reaction is also a possibility.

History of intake of herbal/complementary medicines and drugs such as NSAIDs and angiotensin-converting enzyme inhibitors (ACEIs) should be asked. The frequency of need for relievers and dose of controller medications being taken in asthma is important to plan further treatment.

Family History

Allergic disorders are multifactorial disorders or polygenic disorders with a strong interplay of genetics, epigenetics, and environmental factors. Hence, they have a complex inheritance pattern and wide phenotype variability. A family history of allergic disease is common and is one of the most important factors predisposing a child to the development of allergies.

The risk of recurrence in an individual with a relative with asthma is given in **Table 1.3**.

Conditions such as hereditary angioedema and periodic fever syndromes are genetic diseases and follow the Mendelian inheritance pattern. Hence, it is useful to make a pedigree chart in the case sheet of all allergy patients.

TABLE 1.3: Recurrence risk of asthma based on family history.

Relative with asthma	*Recurrence risk*
No relative	5%
Uncle, nephew/niece	10%
Sibling	25%
One parent	25%
Dizygotic twin	35%
Two parents	50%
Monozygotic twin	75%

Environmental History

Home: The distance from the main road, material used to build the house (e.g., wood, brick, mud), ventilation, damp walls or places in the house, recent painting or refurbishing done, the chemicals used for cleaning, the way food is cooked (stoves/biomass fuel), tobacco smoke exposure at home, pets (dogs, cats, birds), cockroach or rat infestation, usage of pesticides/insecticides are important.

The hobbies, sports, or other activities the child participates in are also important to know.

EXAMINATION

Examination includes general examination, assessment of growth by doing anthropometry, head-to-foot examination **(Table 1.4)** to look for signs of allergy, and disease-focused system examination. A systematic head-to-toe examination usually can give a clue to diagnosis. However, a normal examination does not rule out allergy.

Assessment of growth: Measuring the height and weight, plotting on the age-appropriate growth charts, and interpretation of anthro-

TABLE 1.4: Salient findings in allergic conditions based on organ system.

Organ	*Salient findings*
Eyes	• *Dennie-Morgan folds (Dennie lines)*—prominent infraorbital skin folds that extend in an arc from the inner canthus beneath and parallel to the lower lid margin—a feature in AD • *Allergic shiners*—blue-gray to purple discolorations beneath lower eyelids, due to venous stasis—just a sign which suggests an allergic disease, not diagnostic • *Stringy or ropy eye discharge/conjunctival congestion and edema*—in AC • *Chemosis*—conjunctival edema seen in severe cases of AC • *Cobble stoning of tarsal conjunctiva*—in VKC • *Keratoconus*—seen in VKC and periorbital AD (due to persistent rubbing of eyes) • *Posterior subcapsular cataracts*—may be seen in those treated with high-dose or chronic corticosteroids
Nose	• *Deviated nasal septum* • *Transverse nasal crease*—dark and horizontal line due to repeated rubbing of the nose and pushing it upward • *Mucosa*—pale to purple • Inferior turbinate hypertrophy

Contd...

Contd...

Organ	***Salient findings***
	• *Polyps*—have to rule out cystic fibrosis. • *Allergic nasal secretions*—thin and clear • *Sinus tenderness*—in sinusitis
Ear	• Eczematous changes in postauricular area and base of the ear lobe in AD • *Otoscopy*—otitis media with effusion common in AR
Lips	Cheilitis/lip licker's dermatitis—drying of lips due to mouth breathing or continuous licking of lips
Facies	Adenoid facies—dull face, pinched nostrils, open mouth, protruding teeth, high-arched palate
Posterior pharynx	• Postnasal drip • Cobble stoning—chronic postnasal drip and exposure to allergic mediators causing posterior pharyngeal lymphoid hyperplasia • Tonsillar and adenoid hypertrophy
Chest	• Tachypnea, use of accessory muscles, wheeze/rhonchi—during flare-up of asthma
Skin	• Dry skin, hyperlinear palms and soles • Keratosis pilaris seen on cheeks and extensor aspects of limbs in AD • Urticaria, angioedema, dermatographism

(AC: allergic conjunctivitis; AD: atopic dermatitis; AR: allergic rhinitis; VKC: vernal keratoconjunctivitis)

pometry are essential in children with allergies. Height velocity should be monitored in children with chronic asthma as they may have decreased height velocity in the initial years of treatment due to frequent use of oral steroids or high doses of inhaled corticosteroids (ICS). Children with food allergy often have growth failure and nutrient deficiencies due to avoidance of multiple foods. Failure to thrive in a child with chronic cough or recurrent wheezing suggests gastroesophageal reflux disease (GERD) and cystic fibrosis.

Overweight and obesity are important comorbidities that should be addressed during the management of allergic disorders.

SUMMARY

- An accurate and systematic history taking is essential in the diagnosis of allergic diseases.
- A normal examination does not rule out an allergic disorder.
- Disorders that closely mimic allergies should also be borne in mind during evaluation.
- Identification of the allergens by history aids in avoidance measures and management plans.

SUGGESTED READING

1. Thomsen S. Genetics of asthma: an introduction for the clinician. Eur Clin Respir J. 2015; 2(1):24643.
2. Wong GK, Krishna MT. History taking: evaluation of allergic disorders. In: Vedanthan PK (Ed). Textbook of Allergy for the Clinician, 2nd edition. Boca Raton: CRC Press;2021.
3. Woodbury K, Berrilyn J. Ferguson BJ. Physical findings in allergy. Otolaryngol Clin North Am. 2011;44(3):603-10.

CHAPTER 2

Environmental History-taking Tips

Swati Kalra

INTRODUCTION

Childhood asthma is a chronic inflammatory disease of the respiratory system resulting from reversible obstruction of airways following exposure to certain triggers. The triggers leading to airway obstruction may enter the body either through the airways in the form of aeroallergens or through the mouth in the form of food allergens. There is increasing evidence that allergy to environmental allergens, including both indoor and outdoor allergens, is associated with asthma symptoms. Environment plays a significant role in patients having symptoms of allergies. The environment in which children live and spend time exposes them to different allergens, which may serve as triggers for disease initiation and flare-ups. The triggers either can be present in the outside environment/physical environment or can be a part of their indoor/biological environment. Apart from these well-studied factors, the psychosocial environment plays a very crucial role in flare-ups of asthma. **Table 2.1** summarizes some of the important factors attributing to allergic diseases.

BIOLOGICAL/INDOOR ENVIRONMENT

For nearly three decades, there has been mounting evidence that perennial allergens play a causative role in the development of asthma. Perennial allergies happen following exposure to indoor aeroallergens in genetically predisposed individuals. Hence, the indoor environment comprising home, school, and workplace plays a *very crucial role in* asthma and allergic predisposition and flare-ups. There are studies with a proven cause–effect relationship between exposure

TABLE 2.1: Important factors in environmental history predisposing to asthma and allergic diseases.

Indoor environment	*Outdoor environment*	*Psychosocial environment*
Presence of furry pets in the home (especially in the bedroom and/or bed)	Air pollution	Neighborhood
Presence of wall-to-wall carpets	Pollens	Socioeconomic status
Moisture, dampness, and humidifier use	Change in symptoms with a change in climate	Parental stress
Molds and musty odors in any part of the home		Family relationships
Cockroaches in the home		
School, daycare, or work environment		

to house dust mites (HDMs) in the initial 1 year of life and increased risk of asthma in later life. Sensitization to indoor allergens correlates well with indoor allergen exposure in young and school-age children. In many cases, exposure and sensitivity follow a dose-response relationship. Exposure to cockroaches and molds further increases the flare-ups in known asthmatics. Therefore, it is very important to take a detailed history pertaining to all indoor aeroallergens while assessing a child having allergies. HDM, pets such as cats and dogs, cockroaches, rats, and molds such as *Aspergillus fumigatus* are some of the known indoor aeroallergens that have been well studied over the last few decades and have been well associated with an increased risk of allergies and flare-ups in genetically predisposed individuals. Out of these, HDM has been found to be having the strongest association with the development of asthma after exposure during the initial 1 year of life.

House Dust Mite

Dust mites are one of the most prevalent sources of indoor allergens and the most studied allergens in asthma development worldwide. Sensitization to HDM has been consistently found to be one of the strongest associates of asthma in children, adolescents, and adults. The most common dust mite species are Der f 1 (*Dermatophagoides farinae*) and Der p 2 (*Dermatophagoides pteronyssinus*). Dust mite allergens activate the adaptive and innate immune systems, and Der f 1 induces inflammatory cell death in bronchial epithelial cells. There is enough evidence to suggest that symptoms of asthma correlate well with mite allergen levels at home in children as well as adults. It has been a well-studied fact that symptoms of dust mite allergy in asthmatic children as well as adults who are mite sensitive have poor pulmonary function, and aberrant bronchial reactivity correlates with the mite allergen levels in their home. Not only this, but also symptomatology of asthma changes with seasonal changes in exposure to dust mite allergens. Hence, taking a detailed indoor environmental history to identify all possible sources of domestic HDM exposure is very important to identify the degree of allergen exposure. Dust mite allergens can be detected in most dust reservoirs, including beds, carpets, sofas, drapes, soft toys, and clothing.

Pets

Cats and dogs are the most common indoor furry pets, and sensitization is known to be associated with severe asthma in childhood. The review of the literature suggests that patients with higher pet allergen levels are associated with greater asthma severity. It is also attributed to be responsible for difficult-to-control asthma. Around 12% of the general population and 25–65% of children with persistent asthma are sensitized to cat or dog allergens. Fel d 1 and Can f 1 are the major allergens for cats and dogs, respectively, and are present in saliva, hair follicles, and skin. Pet allergens are predominantly carried on small particles (<10–20 mm), allowing them to remain airborne for long periods of time and adhere to clothing and surfaces. Therefore, pet allergens are carried long distances and are passively transferred to environments where no pets are present, leading to indirect exposure. Exposure to pet allergens further increases if pets are allowed to come into the bedrooms and sleeping beds of children with asthma.

Molds

Molds are significant triggers for asthma and allergies, with sensitization rates varying between 15 and 60%. Qualitative indicators of mold exposure, such as visible mold or mildew odors, have been linked to an increased risk of allergic rhinitis and asthma. Studies show that children sensitized to mold during their first few months of life are more likely to experience recurrent wheezing by their first birthday. Mold-sensitized children also tend to have lower lung function and heightened airway hyperresponsiveness compared to their nonsensitized peers. Children can encounter molds in both indoor and outdoor environments. Common indoor molds include *Aspergillus* and *Penicillium*, while outdoor exposure often involves *Alternaria* and *Cladosporium*. Mold spore concentrations are closely tied to indoor dampness and humidity levels. The presence of visible mold, along with a suitable environment (e.g., temperature, substrate, high humidity, or water damage), fosters mold growth, which can exacerbate asthma symptoms. Sensitization to molds such as *A. fumigatus* can lead to conditions such as allergic bronchopulmonary aspergillosis, complicating asthma management. This increases the risk of exacerbations and severe asthma. A recent study highlighted that school and classroom environments can also be sources of mold exposure, with visible mold serving as a predictor of high spore counts. Outdoor exposure to *Alternaria* and *Cladosporium* has been associated with persistent, severe asthma and more frequent exacerbations, underscoring the importance of addressing mold exposure in asthma management strategies.

Microbiome

The microbiome encompasses all the microbes inhabiting our skin and mucosal surfaces, along with their genetic materials and interactions. Its development and stability are influenced by various factors, including the innate immune response, genetics, and environmental elements, such as diet, antibiotic use, and infections. Disruptions in microbiome stability can increase the risk of allergic diseases later in life. Research has linked early-life dysbiosis, or microbial imbalance in the gut microbiota, to a heightened risk of asthma. A study by Arrieta et al. identified the first 100 days of life as a critical period for microbial dysbiosis, influencing the risk of atopic wheezing in young children. This connection is often attributed to the gut–lung axis, which highlights the interplay between gut and lung microbiota. The gut microbiota can impact lung immune responses through the production of bacterial metabolites (such as short-chain fatty acids and histamine) and immune cell modulation. Similarly, the lung microbiota interacts with the airway epithelium and immune cells, affecting both innate and adaptive immune responses. The upper and lower airway microbiome comprises diverse microbial communities that play roles in asthma. Notably, certain phyla have been found to be more prevalent in individuals with asthma. For instance, patients with uncontrolled asthma often exhibit greater microbiota diversity, which correlates positively with bronchial hyperresponsiveness. Understanding these microbial interactions could inform future strategies for asthma prevention and management.

OUTDOOR/PHYSICAL ENVIRONMENT

Air Pollution

Air pollution, comprising pollutants such as particulate matter (PM), carbon monoxide (CO), nitrogen dioxide (NO_2), black carbon, and sulfur dioxide (SO_2), significantly impacts respiratory health, particularly for individuals with asthma. Numerous studies demonstrate that ambient air pollution exacerbates existing asthma conditions. Specifically, exposure to high levels of NO_2, PM2.5, and CO has been linked to changes in the *Foxp3* gene promoter region, which is associated with asthma susceptibility. Various literature reviews have highlighted the fact that there is a strong association between outdoor air pollution and asthma exacerbations, and children are specifically vulnerable to such exposures. Higher concentrations of NO_2, SO_2, and PM2.5 in the surrounding environment correlated well with increased asthma exacerbations. Even short-term exposure to pollutants such as ozone (O_3), NO_2, and SO_2 can trigger worsening symptoms in children. Moreover, research has shown that traffic-related air pollution is linked to higher rates of hospital readmissions for asthma. This is especially concerning for inner-city schools located near highways, heavy traffic, and industrial areas, where air pollution levels tend to be elevated. The close proximity to idling vehicles and dense traffic can exacerbate asthma symptoms in sensitive populations, highlighting the need for targeted interventions and policies to improve air quality in these environments. O_3 exposure is another factor attributing to increased exacerbations, worsening of symptoms, need for rescue medications, and hospital admissions in patients with asthma. This relationship between asthma and airborne traffic-related pollutants has been well studied in urban areas, and the authors have identified the impact of diesel-engine traffic on asthma wheezing and bronchodilator usage, reduction in peak flows, and increased asthma attacks in patients exposed to highway traffic. Hence, taking a detailed history related to proximity of school from residence, time spent in traveling from school to home, distance of residence from the main road, and industrial areas in nearby vicinity becomes really important.

Pollens

Pollen grains are tiny "seeds" dispersed from flowering plants, trees, grass, and weeds. Pollen allergy has been found in 80–90% of children suffering from asthma and in 40–50% of adult-onset asthmatics. Pollens are an important source of outdoor allergens; pollen counts can vary significantly throughout the day and be influenced by weather conditions in short time intervals. The climatic conditions of a particular geographical location have a major impact on pollen counts. Mostly pollination happens during warmer months, but there are few plants that pollinate throughout the year. Changes in climate may cause shifts in precipitation, fewer frost days, warmer air temperatures, and increased atmospheric carbon dioxide (CO_2), and these changes can affect the beginning and ending of the pollen season, number of pollens created, and allergenicity of created pollens. Various surveys have shown that variation in pollen counts is associated with the severity of asthma symptoms, and peak pollen periods have been found to be correlating with asthma exacerbations. It becomes important to monitor the daily pollen count and pollen calendar for those who suffer from allergies so that they can modify their behavior based on these fluctuations. Tree allergens mainly manifest during early spring, while grasses flower during late spring and summer. Likewise, increase in symptoms during summer and fall may suggest sensitization to outdoor molds, and allergic symptom exacerbation during autumn may point toward weed allergens. Therefore, it becomes important to ask for a detailed history of allergic exacerbations during season changes and timing of year as well as have a detailed idea about pollen calendar of various regions for a better understanding of allergic triggers.

PSYCHOSOCIAL ENVIRONMENT

The psychosocial environment is becoming increasingly recognized as a significant contributor to asthma morbidity. It includes a person's neighborhood, socioeconomic status, family relationships, and social networks. It has been observed that asthma disproportionately affects low-income, minority children who live in urban areas and cities; nonadherence to treatment, parental conflicts, more exposure to environmental triggers, low-income households, non-adherence to treatment, exposure to chronic stress, child psychological problems, family functioning, obesity, physical inactivity, and unhealthy diets are some of the factors leading to an increased risk of asthma in these children. Most of the time, caregivers are not able to understand the exact nature of the disease and hence do not follow the treatment advice appropriately. All these factors ultimately lead to an increase in disease-related morbidity.

SUMMARY

Environment has a significant impact on clinical manifestations of allergic disorders. Interplay between genetic predispositions and environmental exposure is instrumental in shaping the immune system, and in utero exposures help in setting up of microbiome of skin, lungs, and intestinal tract. Digging down into a detailed environmental history is of utmost importance to understand the exact causal associations and identify specific triggers of allergies, as it plays a vital role in outlining the appropriate treatment plan of patients with allergies and asthma.

KEY POINTS

- Detailed environmental history is essential for asthma management.
- Indoor allergens especially house dust mite are major asthma triggers
- Outdoor environmental factors including pollens, air pollutants significantly affect asthma symptoms and lead to flare-ups.
- Psychosocial environment influences asthma control, often through indirect effects like treatment nonadherence or increased exposure to triggers.
- Early-life microbiome imbalances increase allergy risk by influencing the immune development and directing the immune system towards allergic pathway.

SUGGESTED READING

1. Deng SZ, Jalaludin BB, Antó JM, Hess JJ, Huang CR. Climate change, air pollution, and allergic respiratory diseases: a call to action for health professionals. Chin Med J (Engl). 2020;133(13):1552-60.
2. Kitinoja MA, Hugg TT, Siddika N, Rodriguez Yanez D, Jaakkola MS, Jaakkola JJK. Short-term exposure to pollen and the risk of allergic and asthmatic manifestations: a systematic review and meta-analysis. BMJ Open. 2020;10(1):e029069.
3. Louisias M, Ramadan A, Naja AS, Phipatanakul W. The effects of the environment on asthma disease activity. Immunol Allergy Clin North Am. 2019;39(2):163-75.
4. Oland AA, Booster GD, Bender BG. Psychological and lifestyle risk factors for asthma exacerbations and morbidity in children. World Allergy Organ J. 2017;10(1):35.

CHAPTER 3

Pollen Grains as Aeroallergens

Divya Verma

INTRODUCTION

Pollen consists of microscopic grains released by plants during their reproductive processes, serving the essential function of fertilizing other plants. Each grain contains the male gametes necessary for fertilizing female ovules, leading to seed production. When pollen is transferred between flowers, it facilitates fertilization and enables seed development. This transfer can occur through various mechanisms, such as wind (anemophily), insects (entomophily), birds, bats, or other animals. Although only about 10% of the more than 250,000 pollen-producing plant species rely on wind for pollination, this method is the primary source of pollen-related allergies. Wind-pollinated plants have evolved to produce vast quantities of dry, smooth, and relatively small pollen grains (typically 20–60 μm) that can easily become airborne. Common plants such as grasses, ragweed, and trees such as birch and oak produce large quantities of these grains, as wind is an unpredictable carrier, necessitating a higher volume of pollen to increase the likelihood of successful fertilization. In contrast, entomophilous (insect-pollinated) plants produce larger, stickier pollen grains, adapted for transport by insects such as bees and butterflies. Flowers such as lilies and daisies rely on insects for pollination, producing less airborne pollen, and are thus less likely to trigger allergies. However, some insect-pollinated plants, such as linden (Tilia), generate excess pollen, which can become airborne. Such plants that can be both insect- and wind-pollinated are classified as amphiphilous.

POLLEN GRAINS AND ALLERGY

While essential for plant reproduction, pollen grains are a common trigger for allergies in humans. Trees, grasses, and weeds release billions of pollen grains into the air, especially during certain seasons. Once airborne, these grains can travel considerable distances, becoming one of the most widespread aeroallergens. Although pollen is harmless for many, in some individuals it can provoke allergic reactions, commonly referred to as "hay fever" or allergic rhinitis. Pollen-induced allergies arise when the immune system mistakenly identifies harmless pollen proteins as harmful, leading to an inflammatory response.

Allergic reactions tend to peak during periods of high pollen production, which vary by plant species. For example, tree pollen allergies are most common in the spring, grass pollen in late spring and early summer, and weed pollen in late summer through early autumn. Symptoms of pollen allergies include sneezing, itchy or watery eyes, nasal congestion, coughing, and, in some cases, exacerbations of asthma. The severity of these symptoms can vary based on individual sensitivity and the concentration of pollen in the environment.

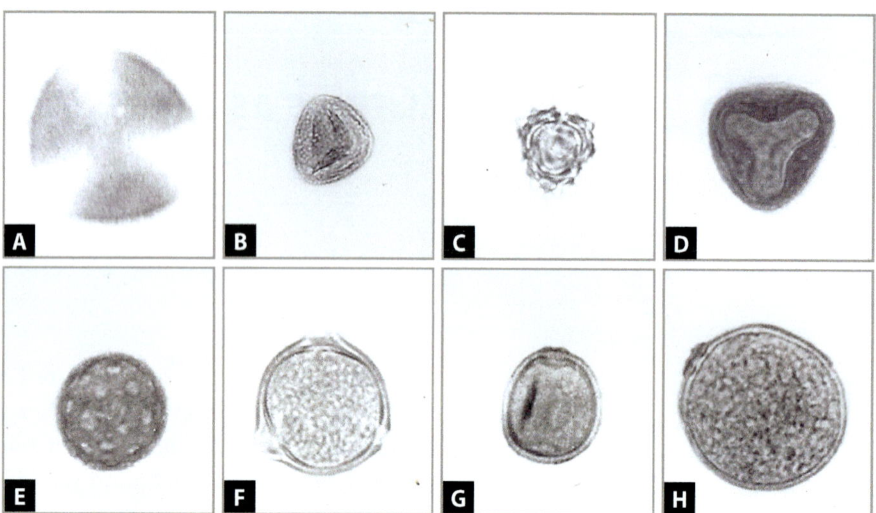

Figs. 3.1A to H: Pollen. (A) *Argemone mexicana*; (B) *Prosopis juliflora*; (C) *Parthenium hysterophorous*; (D) *Xanthium strumarium*; (E) *Chenopodium album*; (F) *Ricinus communis*; (G) *Cynodon dactylon*; (H) *Pennisetum typhoides*.

Pollen grains vary in size, shape, and structure depending on the species producing them. Typically microscopic, pollen grains range from 10 to 100 μm in diameter and are highly resilient due to their outer protective layer, called the exine. This tough, decay-resistant layer allows pollen grains to remain well preserved in soil and sediments for long periods. The exine often exhibits distinct patterns or textures that aid in identifying pollen species **(Figs. 3.1A to H)**. Beneath the exine lies the intine, an inner layer made of cellulose, which is less resistant to environmental stress. Inside the intine is the pollen's cytoplasm, which contains the male reproductive cells responsible for fertilizing the female ovule. Beyond their reproductive function, pollen grains also contribute to allergenicity, as the outer layer contains proteins that can trigger allergic reactions in sensitive individuals.

Allergenicity of Pollen Grains

Pollen allergens are proteins or glycoproteins that become biologically active when dissolved in water, leading to immunoglobulin E (IgE) antibody-mediated allergic reactions within seconds. Two mechanisms have been proposed to explain how allergenic particles are released from pollen cytoplasm. In the first mechanism, allergens quickly diffuse when pollen grains come into contact with mucous membranes in an isotonic medium, causing immediate allergic symptoms on the conjunctiva or nasal surfaces. In the second mechanism, a hypotonic medium such as rainwater causes the pollen grains to rapidly hydrate, releasing smaller inhalable allergenic particles that can reach the lower airways and potentially trigger asthma. Thus, the release of allergens from pollen grains is a prerequisite for their effect on sensitized individuals. The release of pollen allergens can occur either on the mucosal surfaces of the upper airways after exposure to pollen or directly into the external environment. Several environmental factors, such as high relative humidity, heavy rain, and pollutants, can prompt the release of pollen allergens into the air. During periods of high humidity, for example, pollen allergens are released in a process similar to pollination.

In rare instances, such as during thunderstorms, pollen grains may rupture due to osmotic shock, dispersing allergenic particles into the atmosphere. This phenomenon explains the increased incidence of asthma attacks during heavy rainfall.

Diesel engine exhaust particles have emerged as significant environmental pollutants that contribute to the release of pollen allergens. These particles contain minerals such as silica, iron, and aluminum, which can bind multiple allergens to a single particle. In addition to humidity or hydration, pollen allergens can also be released in response to changes in pH, time, and temperature. Under these conditions, pollen grains secrete eicosanoid-like substances that cross-react with leukotriene B4 and prostaglandin E2, leading to the activation of airway mucosa epithelial cells and the release of proinflammatory mediators. Once hydrated, pollen grains may also release various enzymes, including proteases. These proteases are significant because they can damage epithelial tissue, bypassing the body's natural protease inhibitors. This damage can weaken epithelial junctions, facilitating the transport of proteins and making it easier for allergens to reach antigen-presenting subepithelial dendritic cells, ultimately increasing the risk of sensitization in vulnerable individuals.

Monitoring of Pollen Grains

Effective monitoring of pollen grains is crucial for understanding pollen distribution patterns, predicting allergy seasons, and helping allergy sufferers prepare for peak pollen times. Monitoring includes various methods, which are given in the following text.

Ecofloristic Survey

Ecofloristic survey involves identifying and mapping the distribution of allergenic plants in a specific area. By studying the types of plants present in different ecosystems, researchers can predict which pollens are likely to dominate in the air during certain seasons.

Phenology

The study of the timing of biological events, such as the flowering period of plants, is known as phenology. Understanding when plants release pollen helps in predicting peak allergy periods. For example, monitoring the flowering time of birch trees can provide insights into when their pollen will be most abundant.

Pollen Sampling

Pollen sampling is done using devices such as Burkard traps and Hirst spore traps, which collect airborne particles over a given period. These samples are analyzed to determine the concentration and types of pollen in the air. This information is crucial for developing pollen calendars and issuing pollen count reports.

Pollination Calendar and Pollen Calendar

A pollination calendar tracks the flowering and pollination periods of various plant species in a specific region, identifying when certain plants are likely to release pollen. This calendar serves as a predictive tool for anticipating the presence of allergens in the air and is highly valuable for allergy sufferers, researchers, and healthcare professionals.

In contrast, a pollen calendar provides more detailed information on the presence and concentration of different pollen types in the atmosphere throughout the year. It integrates data from phenological studies and pollen sampling to create a comprehensive timeline of allergenic pollen levels, often presented as daily or weekly pollen counts. Pollen calendars are region-specific, as factors such as climate and vegetation significantly influence pollen release patterns.

Both pollination and pollen calendars are essential for helping individuals with pollen allergies manage their symptoms by enabling them to anticipate periods of high allergen exposure. For instance, in temperate climates, tree pollen is typically most abundant in early spring, grass pollen in late spring and summer, and weed pollen in late summer and fall. These calendars empower allergy sufferers to prepare for peak pollen seasons, making them crucial tools for health management.

India is a subcontinent characterized by variable climatic conditions and a remarkable diversity of geography. Its landscapes encompass plateaus, evergreen forests, hills, snow-capped mountain ranges, deserts, and plains. Due to its reliance on monsoon rains, the distribution of precipitation is uneven across the country, contributing to a rich diversity in floristic composition. Considering the climatic, topographical, and ecological variations, India is classified into five biozones: Eastern, western, northern, southern, and central regions. The airborne pollen composition varies significantly across these ecozones and throughout different seasons.

Numerous researchers have conducted extensive atmospheric surveys to create pollen and pollination calendars for various zones across India. A significant initiative, the All India Coordinated Project (AICP) on Aeroallergens and Human Health, sponsored by the Ministry of Environment and Forests of the Government of India, has been successfully completed by Singh et al. This project involved identifying, quantifying, and characterizing important pollen and fungal allergens from 18 different locations, elucidating their allergenic properties.

In north India, the dominant types of pollen recorded include those from the Poaceae (grasses), Chenopodiaceae/Amaranthaceae, and Asteraceae families, which are present throughout the year. Other significant airborne pollen sources comprise species such as *Ailanthus*, *Ricinus*, *Morus*, *Xanthium*, *Cannabis*, *Artemisia*, *Holoptelea*, *Eucalyptus*, *Casuarina*, *Putranjiva*, *Cassia*, *Quercus*, *Pinus*, and *Cedrus*. The peak pollen season for Asteraceae extends from March to October, with the highest concentrations occurring in April, while Poaceae pollen reaches its peak concentration in September.

In central India, the predominant types of pollen identified were from the Poaceae, Chenopodiaceae/Amaranthaceae, Asteraceae, and Apocynaceae families. Aerobiological surveys indicated that the most significant pollen sources include *Rosa*, *Cicer*, *Ricinus*, *Ailanthus*, *Holoptelea*, *Cyperus*, *Argemone*, *Cocos nucifera*, and *Hibiscus*. A survey conducted in Pune highlighted *Parthenium* as the largest contributor to the pollen load, exhibiting two peak seasons: from September to November and from January to April. Additionally, pollen from *Cocos* and *Cassia* was observed throughout the year, with *Cocos* pollen recorded in particularly high concentrations during April–May and November–December.

In eastern India, grass pollen emerged as the major contributors to the total airborne pollen load, accounting for 39%. Pollen from the Asteraceae and Chenopodiaceae/Amaranthaceae families peaked in June. Other significant pollen sources included *Asteraceae*, *Pongamia*, *Areca catechu*, *Xanthium*, and *Cocos*. Additional dominant pollen types recorded were from *Azadirachta*, *Caesalpinia*, *Carica papaya*, *Mangifera indica*, *Eucalyptus*, and *Putranjiva*. Notably, *Trema orientalis* pollen reached high concentrations from May to July. In the Eastern Himalayas, the predominant tree

TABLE 3.1: Pollen calendar for the most prevailing pollen allergens from the five ecozones of India.

Ecozones	*Plant*	*Family*	*Habit*	*Season*
North India	Asteraceae*	Asteraceae	Weed	Throughout the year, with peak in the months of February–April and August–October
	Cheno/Amaranth*,†	Chenopodiaceae/ Amaranthaceae	Weed	Throughout the year, with peaks in the months of February–March and October–November
	Poaceae*	Poaceae	Grass	Throughout the year
	Holoptelea integrifolia	Ulmaceae	Tree	February–April
	Ailanthus excelsa	Simaroubaceae	Tree	January–March
	Eucalyptus spp.	Myrtaceae	Tree	January–April
	Ricinus communis	Euphorbiaceae	Shrub	November–April
	Casuarina equisetifolia	Casuarinaceae	Tree	January–May
	Putranjiva roxburghii	Putranjivaceae	Tree	March–May
	Cassia spp.	Caesalpiniaceae	Tree/Weed	April–June
	Quercus spp.	Fagaceae	Tree	August–October
	Pinus spp.	Pinaceae	Tree	March–July
	Cedrus deodara	Pinaceae	Tree	August–December
	Platanus orientalis	Platanaceae	Tree	March–May
	Narcissus spp.	Amaryllidaceae	Weed	February–May
	Salix spp.	Salicaceae	Tree	March–June
Eastern India	Cheno/Amaranth*,†	Chenopodiaceae/ Amaranthaceae	Weed	Throughout the year, with peak in the months of February–March and October–November
	Poaceae*	Poaceae	Grass	Throughout the year
	Asteraceae*	Asteraceae	Weed	Throughout the year, with peak in the months of February–April and August–October
	Trema orientalis	Cannabaceae	Tree	February–May and September–November
	Areca catechu	Arecaceae	Tree	Throughout the year, with peak from February to April and August to October

Contd...

Contd...

Ecozones	Plant	Family	Habit	Season
	Cocos nucifera	Arecaceae	Tree	Throughout the year, with peak from February to April and August to October
	Borassus flabellifer	Arecaceae	Tree	March–May
	Phoenix sylvestris	Arecaceae	Tree	January–April
	Azadirachta indica	Meliaceae	Tree	March–June
	Acacia auriculiformis	Fabaceae	Tree	February–June and September–November
	Cassia spp.	Fabaceae	Tree/Weed	February–October
	Cycas circinalis	Cycadaceae	Tree	April–July
	Madhuca indica	Sapotaceae	Tree	March–April
	Pongamia pinnata	Fabaceae	Tree	April–June
	Peltophorum pterocarpum	Fabaceae	Tree	March–May and September–November
	Delonix regia	Fabaceae	Tree	April–June
	Solanum sisymbriifolium	Solanaceae	Weed	Throughout the year
	Xanthium strumarium	Asteraceae	Weed	August–September
South India	Cheno/Amaranth*,†	Chenopodiaceae/ Amaranthaceae	Weed	Throughout the year, with peak in the months of February–March and October–November
	Cyperaceae*	Cyperaceae	Sedge	Throughout the year
	Poaceae*	Poaceae	Grass	Throughout the year
	Casuarina	Casuarinaceae	Tree	February–June
	Parthenium hysterophorus	Asteraceae	Weed	Throughout the year
	Spathodea campanulata	Bignoniaceae	Tree	August–February
	Cocos nucifera	Arecaceae	Tree	Throughout the year, with peak from February to April and August to October
	Eucalyptus spp.	Myrtaceae	Tree	January–April
	Peltophorum	Fabaceae	Tree	March to May and September–November
Western India	Poaceae*	Poaceae	Grass	Throughout the year
	Cheno/Amaranth*,†	Chenopodiaceae/ Amaranthaceae	Weed	Throughout the year, with peak in the months of February–October

Contd...

Contd...

Ecozones	Plant	Family	Habit	Season
	Azadirachta indica	Meliaceae	Tree	March–June
	Parthenium hysterophorus	Asteraceae	Weed	Throughout the year
	Moringa oleifera	Moringaceae	Tree	December–January
	Prosopis juliflora	Fabaceae	Tree	February–May
	Casuarina equisetifolia	Casuarinaceae	Tree	February–June
	Eucalyptus spp.	Myrtaceae	Tree	January–April
	Syzygium spp.	Myrtaceae	Tree	March–April
	Ricinus communis	Euphorbiaceae	Shrub	November–April
Central India	Poaceae*	Poaceae	Grass	Throughout the year
	Asteraceae*	Asteraceae	Weed	Throughout the year, with peak from February to April and August to October
	Cyperaceae*	Cyperaceae	Sedge	Throughout the year
	Cheno/Amaranth*,†	Chenopodiaceae/ Amaranthaceae	Weed	Throughout the year, with peak in the months of February–October
	Rosa spp.	Rosaceae	Shrub	Throughout the year
	Ricinus communis	Euphorbiaceae	Shrub	November–April
	Ailanthus excelsa	Simaroubaceae	Tree	January–March
	Holoptelea integrifolia	Ulmaceae	Tree	February–April
	Argemone mexicana	Papaveraceae	Weed	November–May
	Cocos nucifera	Arecaceae	Tree	February–April and August–October
	Hibiscus spp.	Malvaceae	Shrub	July–September

*Families are listed in cases where the pollen in isolated form was difficult to identify at the genus/species level.
†Pollen of the families Chenopodiaceae and Amaranthaceae are morphologically alike and are difficult to distinguish from one another; they are grouped together as Cheno/Amaranth.

pollen types identified were from *Acer*, *Alnus nepalensis*, *Betula*, *Bucklandia populnea*, *Eucalyptus*, and *Pinus*.

In southern India, pollen from the Poaceae family was the most abundant type recorded. Other dominant pollen sources included *Casuarina*, *Parthenium*, *Spathodea*, *Chenopodiaceae/Amaranthaceae*, *Cyperaceae*, *Cocos*, *Peltophorum*, and *Eucalyptus*.

In western India, pollen from several stenopalynous families, such as Poaceae, Chenopodiaceae, Amaranthaceae, and Cyperaceae, was represented throughout the year, with grass pollen being the predominant type in the total pollen flora. Other significant pollen sources included *Azadirachta*, *Asteraceae*, *Brassica*, *Cassia* spp., *Holoptelea*, and *Parthenium*. Two major pollen seasons were identified: August to October and March to April, with the highest pollen concentrations occurring in August. The lowest pollen occurrence was recorded during May and June, coinciding with high temperatures and low relative humidity. Additionally, frequent sandstorms in June leads to the accumulation of sand on slides, complicating pollen identification. The lowest pollen count of June is due to these sandstorms.

Clinical studies focusing on pollen allergens have been conducted at various medical centers across all five biozones of India as part of the AICP on Aeroallergens and Human Health, sponsored by the Ministry of Environment and Forests, Government of India. These investigations have identified significant allergenic pollen types from various regions of the country.

Table 3.1 provides a pollen calendar for the most prevailing pollen allergens from the five ecozones of India. It will provide useful data to physicians treating allergy patients for selecting pollen allergens during calendar months of the year that will help to get proper diagnosis and treatment. This would also aid the pollen allergy patients so that they can plan their travel accordingly and can escape from the incidence of allergy.

CONCLUSION

Pollen grains, essential for plant reproduction, play a significant role as aeroallergens for a large portion of the population. Their structure, primarily the proteins on the outer layer, contributes to their allergenicity. Monitoring pollen grains through ecofloristic surveys, phenology, and pollen sampling is vital for managing allergies and understanding the impact of different pollen species on public health. Tools such as the pollination and pollen calendars are invaluable for predicting allergy seasons and helping those affected by pollen allergies manage their symptoms effectively.

KEY POINTS

- Pollen grains are essential for plant reproduction but act as major aeroallergens, especially those from wind-pollinated plants.
- Allergic rhinitis and asthma are triggered when pollen proteins are recognized as harmful by the immune system, leading to IgE-mediated responses.
- Environmental factors such as humidity, rainfall, thunderstorms, and air pollution (e.g., diesel exhaust) can increase pollen allergen release and severity of allergic reactions.
- Pollen monitoring techniques—such as ecofloristic surveys, phenology studies, pollen sampling, and pollen calendars—are vital for predicting allergy seasons.
- Region-specific pollen calendars developed for India highlight variations across ecozones, with grasses, weeds, and trees as the main allergenic sources.
- Understanding pollen distribution patterns supports public health by enabling better diagnosis, treatment, and preventive strategies for allergy sufferers.

SUGGESTED READING

1. All India Coordinated Project on Aeroallergens and Human Health. Report. New Delhi: Ministry of Environment and Forests.
2. D'Amato G. Airborne paucimicronic allergen-carrying particles and seasonal respiratory allergy. Allergy. 2001;56(12):1109-11.
3. Sedghy F, Varasteh AR, Sankian M, Moghadam M. Interaction between air pollutants and pollen grains: the role on the rising trend in allergy. Rep Biochem Mol Biol. 2018;6(2):219-24.
4. Singh AB, Kumar P. Aerial pollen diversity in India and their clinical significance in allergic diseases. Indian J Clin Biochem. 2004;19(2):190-201.

CHAPTER 4

Pollen Sampling Techniques

Divya Verma

INTRODUCTION

Pollen grains are tiny particles released by trees, grasses, and weeds for the purpose of fertilizing other plants of the same species. When inhaled by people who are allergic, these particles can trigger an immune system response, leading to allergic rhinitis, commonly known as hay fever. Pollen grains contain specific proteins that can act as allergens. In individuals prone to allergies, their immune system treats these proteins as threats. These proteins are designed to promote plant reproduction, but in humans, they can lead to an overreaction of the immune system.

Airborne pollen concentrations in a specific area are influenced by the local vegetation. However, pollen can be transported by wind and dispersed by turbulences within the lowest atmospheric layer, from where it can be uplifted to free atmosphere by convection and enter air masses moved by synoptic systems. This way, pollen can undergo long distance dispersal, traveling dozens of kilometers.

Airborne pollen monitoring is the most reliable and feasible method to evaluate allergic hazard for pollinosis sufferers. Monitoring stations are generally located in urbanized, densely populated areas. They collect atmospheric pollen through air samplers placed on the rooftop, between 15 and 20 m from the ground level, raised at least 1 m off the floor, and distant from any airflow barrier. This placement, along with a vegetation and geoclimatic evaluation of the monitored area, is important to reduce sampling biases, and should be kept similar among stations to enhance comparability of results. Since the beginning of aeropalynology, many pollen samplers have been proposed. Samplers commonly employed for airborne pollen monitoring are addressed in this chapter. No single sampler is appropriate for all applications, and investigators must select the sampler type and method of analysis carefully, based on the type of data to be collected.

PASSIVE SEDIMENTATION SAMPLERS

The oldest and simplest pollen monitoring devices are the passive sedimentation samplers, in which pollen naturally settles on the collecting surface due to gravity (gravimetric air sampler). This method often consists of exposing a coated microscope slide or open Petri dish containing agar (often called a settle plate) to the outdoor atmosphere or indoor air for a set period of time. Gravity sampling is nonquantitative for atmospheric concentrations of aeroallergens and is affected by particle size, shape, and air movement. Gravity samplers are biased

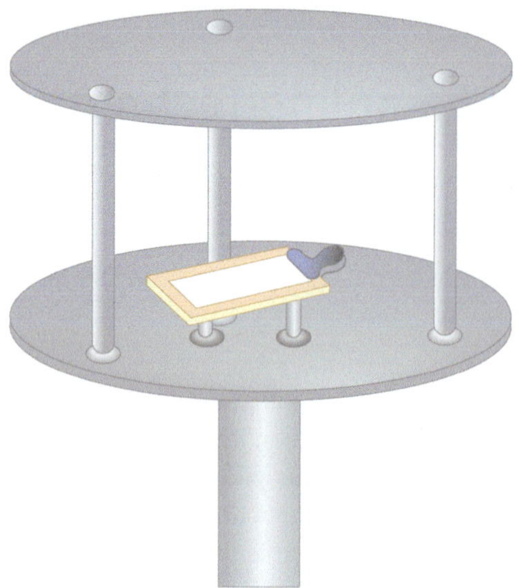

Fig. 4.1: Durham collector.
Source: https://www.ishikawa-gp-cl.com.

toward larger and, therefore, heavier pollen and spore types. Examples of sedimentation samplers are Durham and SIGMA-2-like samplers that can collect daily or weekly pollen samples. Sedimentation samplers have been progressively abandoned in aerobiology, except for specific applications **(Fig. 4.1)**.

ACTIVE SAMPLING DEVICES

There are several active sampling devices, including impingers, cyclones, and impactors. However, all active bioaerosol sampling systems consist of five fundamental elements, which are necessary to undertake accurate sampling:

1. Inlet to the sampling device
2. Transport of the air sample through the device
3. Particle size selection (not always present)
4. Collecting medium
5. Pump and calibrated flow monitoring

IMPACTION SAMPLERS

Impactor samplers are the preferred method for particle sampling due to their cost-effectiveness, portability, and the availability of various commercial systems. These devices operate by utilizing the inertia of particles to separate them from the air stream, leading to the deposition of particles onto a solid or agar surface as the air stream diverts around the surface. This air stream deflection occurs in both suction impactors and rotating arm impactors. A diverse range of impaction samplers is available for applications in both outdoor and indoor environments.

HIRST-TYPE VOLUMETRIC SPORE TRAP

The Hirst-type volumetric spore trap is the most widely used air sampler for pollen monitoring globally. This device, developed by Dr Hirst in 1952, has become the gold standard in aerobiology due to its effectiveness and reliability in capturing airborne particles such as pollen and spores. It pulls a constant and known volume of air through a small inlet, ensuring that the amount of airborne pollen collected is proportional to the concentration in the atmosphere. The device operates continuously, usually over a 24-hour period, with particles deposited onto a sticky surface, often a rotating drum or microscope slide. This provides time-segmented data that helps track fluctuations in pollen levels throughout the day. Its design allows for the collection of small, wind-borne particles such as pollen and fungal spores, making it highly effective for monitoring airborne allergens. The Hirst-type trap is widely used by meteorological agencies, allergy research institutions, and environmental monitoring stations across the world for its accuracy in tracking pollen levels and predicting pollen seasons.

BURKARD 7-DAY RECORDING VOLUMETRIC SPORE TRAP

The Burkard 7-day recording volumetric spore trap is a widely used air sampler designed for the continuous collection of airborne particles for up to 7 days without needing manual intervention. The Burkard trap draws a known and constant volume of air through a narrow orifice, ensuring that the concentration of collected particles is proportional to the airborne particle concentration. The device typically samples air at a rate of about 10 L/min. The trap uses a sticky collection surface (a drum or tape) that rotates slowly, with each section corresponding to a particular time frame. This setup provides a continuous record of airborne particles, which can be analyzed under a microscope for both quantity and type. The Burkard spore trap is capable of capturing particles as small as 3 µm, making it highly sensitive and effective for detecting both small and large bioaerosols such as pollen grains, fungal spores, and bacteria. Designed for outdoor environments, the Burkard trap is weather-resistant and can operate in various climates and weather conditions, making it ideal for long-term environmental monitoring **(Fig. 4.2)**.

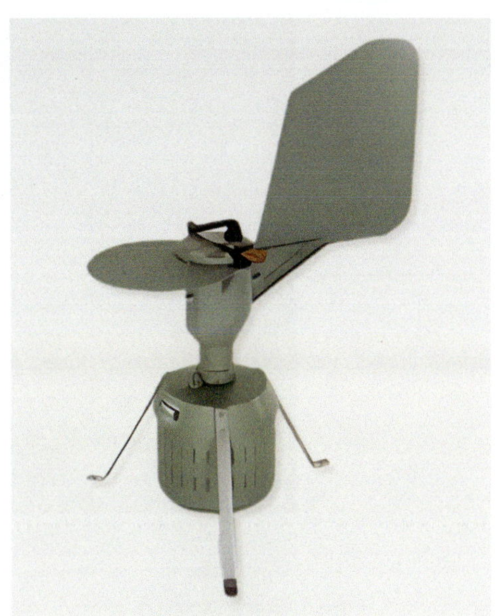

Fig. 4.2: Burkard spore trap.
Source: burkard.co.uk.

ROTOROD SAMPLER

The Rotorod sampler is an efficient air sampling device widely used in the fields of aerobiology, allergy monitoring, and environmental research due to its simplicity, portability, and effectiveness in capturing particles for short-term monitoring. It consists of two or more thin rods (plastic or metal) coated with a sticky substance (e.g., silicone grease) that rotate at a set speed. As the rods spin, they pass through the surrounding air, trapping airborne particles such as pollen grains and spores on their sticky surface. The Rotorod sampler is small, lightweight, and battery-operated, making it ideal for both outdoor and indoor use in various environmental conditions. After sampling, the rods are removed, and the collected particles are analyzed under a microscope. Sampling duration can vary, from short intervals (minutes to hours) to more extended periods (up to 24 hours), depending on the application. The speed of the rotating rods can be adjusted to control the volume of air sampled, which is useful for different environmental conditions and particle concentrations. Its portability allows it to be easily deployed in multiple locations for real-time air sampling. The device is easy to use, typically requiring minimal setup and maintenance **(Figs. 4.3A to C)**.

ANDERSEN CASCADE IMPACTOR

The Andersen cascade impactor is a multistage air sampling device designed to collect

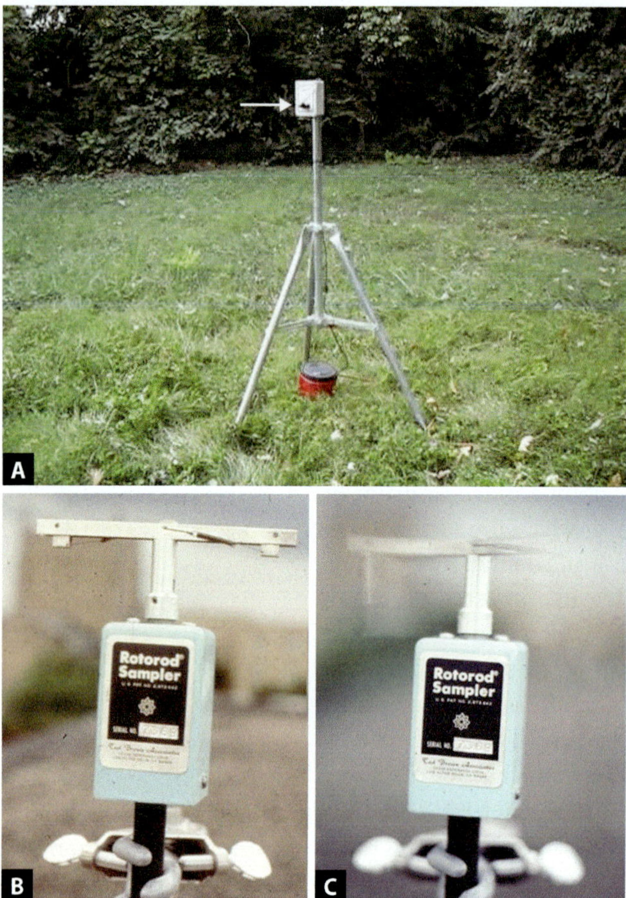

Figs. 4.3A to C: (A) Rotorod sampler installed on ground; (B) The two sampling arms are folded onto a support bar; (C) When the device starts rotating, the sampling arms open vertically downward and expose the impaction rods.
Source: https://www.slideshare.net/.

airborne particles based on their size through inertial impaction. The Andersen cascade impactor consists of several stages, each with progressively smaller nozzles. As air is drawn through the device, larger particles are captured on the upper stages, while smaller particles move deeper into the impactor and are collected on subsequent stages. This design allows for size-selective sampling, providing data on the size distribution of airborne particles. The device operates based on the principle of inertial impaction, where particles with sufficient mass do not follow the airstream's changes in direction and collide with the impactor surfaces, leading to their collection. The velocity of the airflow and the design of the nozzles are optimized to enhance particle capture efficiency. The Andersen impactor is designed to operate at specific flow rates, typically around 28.3 L/min (1 cubic foot/min). This allows for consistent sampling across different applications and environments. Each stage of the impactor has a collection surface, which can be coated

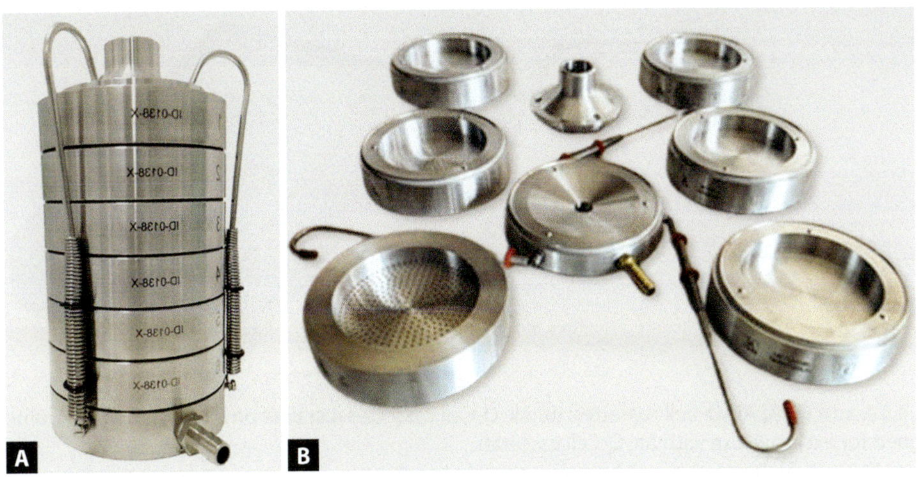

Figs. 4.4A and B: Andersen six-stage cascade impactor. (A) Assembled; (B) Dismantled.
Source: http://www.labautomate.net/.

with an adhesive or a culture medium (such as agar plates) for biological analysis. This allows researchers to identify and quantify the collected particles. The Andersen cascade impactor is a sophisticated and versatile air sampling device which requires careful setup and calibration, often needing trained personnel, and can be more expensive than simpler samplers due to initial and maintenance costs. Additionally, analyzing samples typically involves labor-intensive laboratory work, including microscopic examination and particle quantification **(Figs. 4.4A and B)**.

PORTABLE AND PERSONAL SAMPLERS

Portable and personal samplers are essential tools in air quality monitoring. These devices are designed for individual use or can be easily transported, allowing for flexible sampling in various environments. Personal samplers are used to determine more precise levels of exposure to aeroallergens or other airborne particles. The air intake velocity of the instrument tends to mimic the human breath rate.

Burkard Personal Sampler

The Burkard personal sampler is lightweight and compact, making it easy for individuals to carry and use throughout their daily activities. It is part of the Burkard line of spore traps, and its portable design allows for monitoring in various settings, whether indoors or outdoors. The sampler operates on battery power, enabling it to be used without the need for an external power source. The device typically includes an adjustable airflow mechanism that allows users to set the sampling rate according to the specific environmental conditions. It typically uses a sticky collection medium, such as an adhesive slide or tape, to trap particles as air is drawn into the device. The device may allow for time-segmented sampling, where samples can be collected over specific time intervals, providing a more detailed profile of exposure during different activities or environmental conditions **(Figs. 4.5A and B)**.

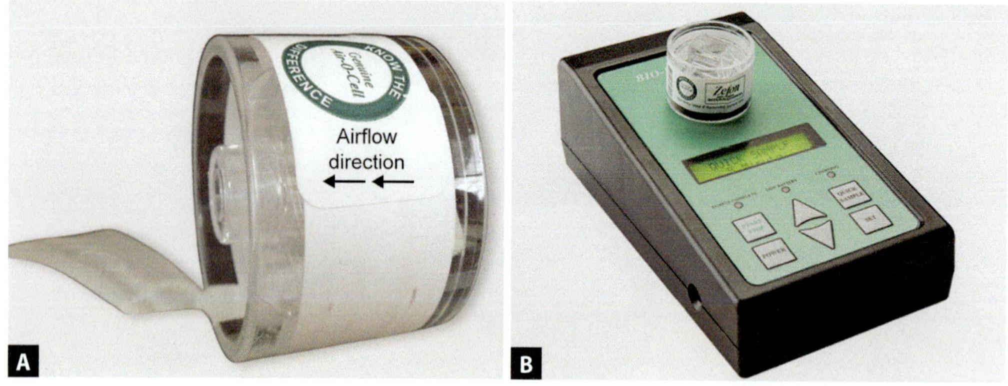

Figs. 4.5A and B: (A) Air-O-Cell cassettes; (B) Air-O-Cell cassettes installed on battery-powered pumps designed for exclusive use with Air-O-Cell cassettes.
Sources: https://lcslaboratory.com/; http://envcoglobal.com/

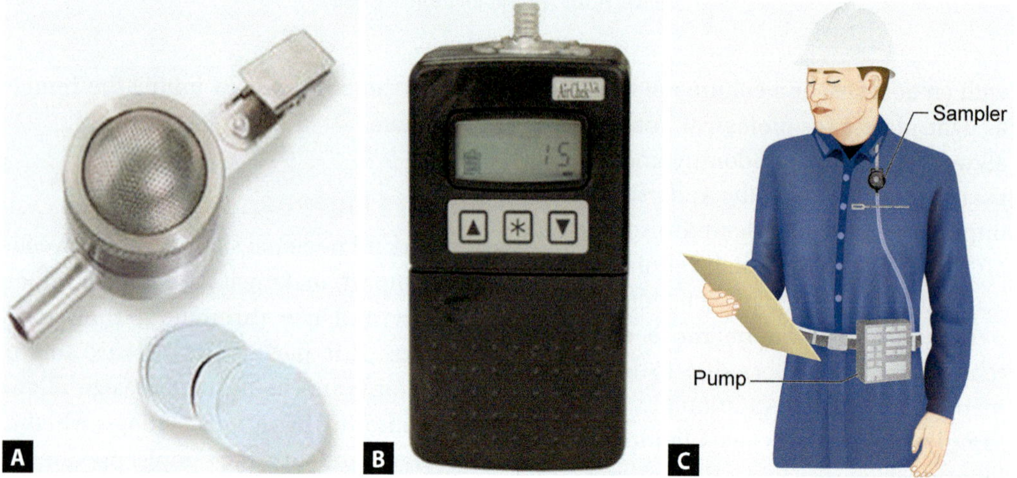

Figs. 4.6A to C: (A) Button sampler; (B) AirChek XR5000 pump; (C) Usage of button sampler with pump.
Source: www.mdpi.com/.

Button Aerosol Sampler

The Button aerosol sampler is a reusable filter sampler featuring a porous, curved inlet designed to enhance particle collection across the filter surface. Its spherical inlet design renders the sampler largely insensitive to wind conditions, making it suitable for a range of applications in both indoor and outdoor environments. The device consists of a disposable filter cassette that is typically worn in the breathing zone, often attached to a lapel, and is connected to a lightweight, battery-powered pump worn at the waist. The typical flow rate is approximately 2 L/min, and the sampler can be utilized for extended periods **(Figs. 4.6A to C)**.

Nasal Air Sampler

A nasal air sampler has been developed to achieve more precise personal exposure measurements than traditional filters. This innovative personal sampler functions as an impaction sampler that is worn just inside the nostrils, requiring no external power source, as it relies on normal human respiration to impact airborne particles onto a pressure-sensitive adhesive tape. It effectively collects particles measuring 5 µm and larger with minimal discomfort to subjects. The nasal air sampler has been employed to assess inhaled pollen, spores, dust mite allergens, and other allergens, with subsequent analysis conducted through microscopy or immunochemistry.

Although the reliability of personal samplers has been debated, they are regarded as a valuable complement to standard diagnostic allergy tests. However, significant challenges to their application in large-scale epidemiological studies arise from their relatively high costs, the user engagement they necessitate, and the extensive data analysis required following their use.

POLLEN ANALYSIS

Manual Pollen Counts

Once collected by air samplers, pollen can be analyzed using various methods, depending on the research objectives. The primary purpose of pollen sampling is to provide information regarding atmospheric pollen concentrations. Pollen counts represent the most prevalent form of analysis. Identification of allergenic pollen is performed by trained personnel using light microscopy at a magnification of 400×, focusing on the overall morphology of the pollen grains, including features such as the exine, intine, and cytoplasm. This technique rarely permits species-level identification; instead, airborne pollen grains are typically categorized at the family or genus level or classified into a nonphylogenetic group known as "pollen type," which encompasses different plant species that possess morphologically indistinguishable pollen grains.

Automatic Pollen Counts

Automatic pollen counting involves the use of technology and automated systems to monitor and quantify airborne pollen concentrations in real time. It is a significant advancement in environmental monitoring, providing real-time, accurate data on airborne pollen concentrations. Their application in public health, research, and agriculture makes them valuable tools for managing and understanding the impact of pollen on health and the environment.

These systems continuously monitor the air for pollen and provide immediate results, allowing for timely alerts and responses. Automatic pollen counters use various sampling methods (e.g., impaction, filtration) to collect airborne pollen grains without the need for manual intervention. Advanced algorithms and software analyze the collected samples, identifying and quantifying different types of pollen based on their size and morphology. These devices use laser technology to detect and count particles in the air based on their size. They can differentiate between pollen types by analyzing the scattering of light as particles pass through a laser beam. Many systems offer remote access to data, allowing users to view real-time pollen counts via online platforms or mobile applications. Some systems can integrate meteorological data (temperature, humidity, wind speed) to provide a more comprehensive understanding of pollen dispersal patterns. Users can receive alerts when pollen counts exceed certain thresholds, helping those with allergies prepare and avoid high-exposure situations.

Molecular Pollen Analysis

Molecular pollen analysis involves the use of molecular techniques, primarily DNA-based methods such as polymerase chain reaction (PCR), real-time PCR (qPCR), and DNA barcoding to identify and quantify pollen types in environmental samples. This approach offers several advantages over traditional morphological methods, which rely on the visual identification of pollen grains under a microscope. Molecular techniques provide higher resolution, increased sensitivity, and the ability to analyze a broader range of species, including those that may be challenging to distinguish morphologically. Even though this field is still at an early stage, its future prospects are promising.

POLLEN ALLERGENS SAMPLING

Conventional monitoring of allergenic pollen does not provide a comprehensive assessment of pollen allergenicity. In fact, the allergen content can vary both quantitatively and qualitatively within a single pollen type. Consequently, a more functional classification of pollen allergens is based on cross-reactivity rather than botanical origin. This approach acknowledges that atmospheric patterns of cross-reactive allergens may be more clinically significant than mere combinations of airborne pollen types. Additionally, pollen allergens can be transported by particles considerably smaller than pollen grains, necessitating the use of samplers that feature high intake velocities and low diameter cutoff specifications.

Two devices commonly employed for monitoring allergens are cyclone samplers **(Fig. 4.7)** and cascade impactors **(Figs. 4.4A and B)**, which are typically positioned on rooftops following criteria similar to those used for pollen traps. The cyclone sampler operates as a volumetric air sampler that directs air into a rotating stream within a cylindrical or conical tube, causing airborne particles to adhere to the walls due to centrifugal force. This technology enables the sorting of particles based on their mass, shape, and size, thereby enhancing the accuracy of allergen monitoring.

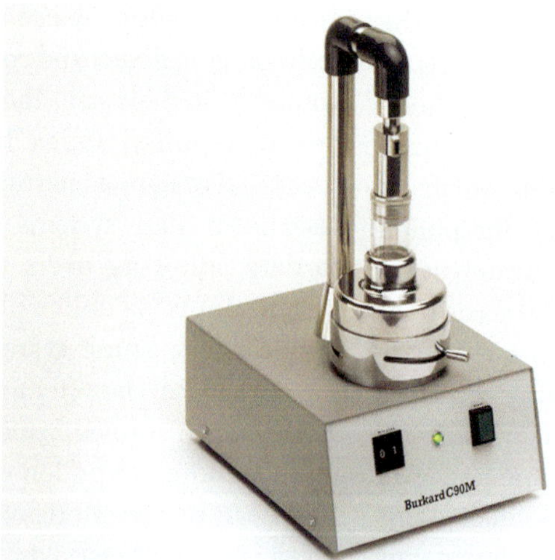

Fig. 4.7: Cyclone sampler
Source: https://burkard.co.uk/

In conclusion, pollen sampling techniques have evolved significantly, from basic passive sedimentation samplers to advanced active devices and molecular analysis methods. While traditional methods, such as manual pollen counting, provide foundational insights, the development of automated systems and personal samplers has enhanced the accuracy, convenience, and real-time monitoring of airborne pollen and allergens. These advancements contribute to a better understanding of pollen dispersal patterns and allergenicity, providing valuable data for environmental monitoring, public health, and allergy management. The future of pollen sampling lies in further refining these techniques, particularly through molecular analysis, automated technologies, and the integration of artificial intelligence, to offer more precise and comprehensive information.

SUMMARY

- Passive sedimentation samplers collect pollen through natural settling, while active devices such as impingers, cyclones, and impactors actively pull air through to collect particles, offering more accurate data.
- The Hirst-type volumetric spore trap and Burkard 7-day recording spore trap are globally used for continuous, time-segmented pollen monitoring due to their precision and effectiveness.
- Devices such as the Rotorod sampler, Burkard personal sampler, and Button aerosol sampler allow individual exposure tracking and portable sampling, suitable for diverse environments.
- Traditional manual pollen counting is done using microscopes, but new technologies, such as automatic pollen counting, provide real-time monitoring and data on pollen concentrations.
- Molecular pollen analysis using DNA-based methods, along with allergen-specific sampling, offers a more detailed and functional understanding of pollen allergens beyond visual identification.

KEY POINTS

- Pollen sampling techniques range from simple passive sedimentation samplers to advanced active and molecular devices.
- Active samplers such as impingers, impactors, and cyclones provide more accurate data than gravity-based methods.
- Widely used devices like the Hirst-type volumetric spore trap and Burkard 7-day recording trap enable continuous, time-segmented monitoring of airborne pollen.
- Portable samplers (Rotorod, Burkard personal sampler, Button aerosol sampler) allow individual exposure tracking in diverse environments.
- Traditional manual microscopy is being complemented by automatic pollen counting, molecular analysis, and allergen-specific sampling.
- Integration of molecular methods and artificial intelligence represents the future of high-resolution pollen monitoring for health and environmental applications.

SUGGESTED READING

1. Mainelis G. Bioaerosol sampling: classical approaches, advances, and perspectives. Aerosol Sci Technol. 2020;54(5):496-519.
2. Muilenberg ML. Sampling devices. Immunol Allergy Clin North Am. 2003;23(3):337-55.
3. Suanno C, Aloisi I, Fernández-González D, Del Duca S. Monitoring techniques for pollen allergy risk assessment. Environ Res. 2021;197:111109.

CHAPTER 5

Cross-reactivity Concepts for a Practitioner

Surgeon Commander Jayakrishnan VY

INTRODUCTION

Cross-reactivity is a crucial concept in allergy diagnostics and management. In pediatric allergy, understanding cross-reactivity between allergens can significantly influence both diagnostic approaches and therapeutic decisions. Cross-reactivity occurs when the immune system recognizes and reacts to similar protein structures shared between different allergens, leading to a clinical reaction to substances that were not initially identified as allergens. This chapter will cover the basic principles of cross-reactivity, its clinical relevance, and practical considerations for the practitioner.

BASIC MECHANISMS OF CROSS-REACTIVITY

Cross-reactivity occurs when immune recognition sites, known as epitopes, are shared across different allergen sources, causing IgE antibodies to react to multiple-related proteins. This phenomenon commonly occurs between botanically and zoologically-related species and is especially relevant in the context of pediatric allergy **(Fig. 5.1)**.

Pathogenesis-related 10 Proteins

PR-10 proteins (pathogenesis-related proteins) play a critical role in plant defense mechanisms and are conserved across various plant species. In allergies, PR-10 proteins are known to be cross-reactive due to their structural homology, commonly resulting in reactions to fruits and vegetables in individuals sensitized to birch pollen. The birch pollen PR-10 protein, Bet v 1, has homologues in apples (Mal d 1), cherries (Pru av 1), and carrots (Dau c 1), often causing pollen-food syndrome. PR-10 proteins are labile, sensitive to heat and digestion, and mainly associated with oral symptoms such as itching and swelling, especially when the foods are consumed raw.

Profilins

Profilins are small, highly conserved proteins involved in cellular structure, found widely across plants, animals, and fungi. In allergology, profilins act as panallergens because they are widely distributed across plant species. Sensitization to profilins can cause cross-reactivity between pollen and foods, particularly in individuals with grass or weed pollen allergies. Profilins are typically unstable (heat- and digestion-sensitive), causing mild, localized symptoms. Bet v 2 in birch pollen, Api g 4 in celery, and Cuc m 2 in melons are well-known examples, often resulting in reactions to melons, tomatoes, and other foods.

Lipid Transfer Proteins

Lipid transfer proteins (LTPs) are highly stable proteins, resistant to heat and

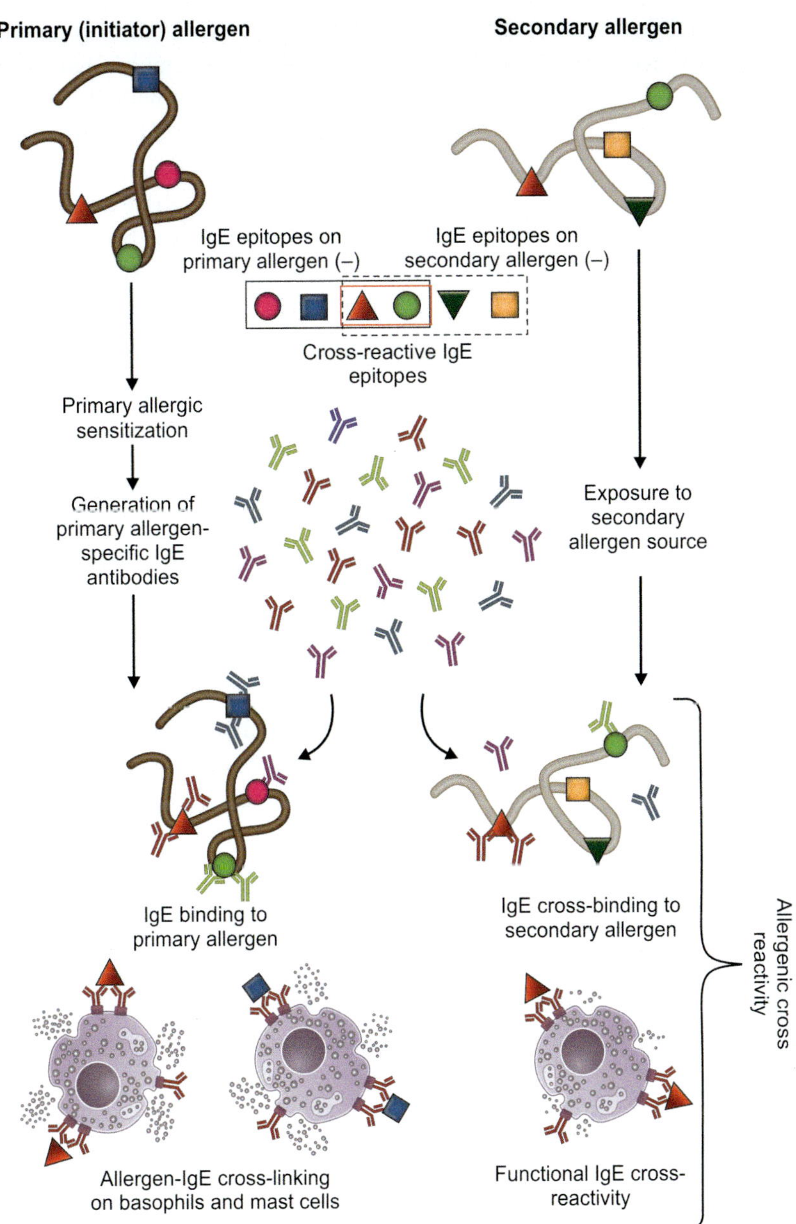

Fig. 5.1: Pathophysiology of cross-reactivity.

digestion, found in many plant foods. Their structural resilience allows LTPs to trigger systemic reactions, including anaphylaxis. This stability makes LTPs particularly significant in cross-reactivity, especially in Mediterranean populations, where severe allergic responses to fruits such as peaches and apricots are common. For example, Pru p 3, an LTP in peaches, is cross-reactive with the LTP Cup s 3 in cypress pollen, leading to significant food-pollen cross-reactivity and an increased risk of severe reactions.

Tropomyosins

Tropomyosins are muscle proteins found in invertebrates, including crustaceans, house dust mites, and mollusks. Due to their high structural similarity, tropomyosins act as panallergens, causing cross-reactivity between dust mites, shrimp, and other shellfish. Tropomyosins are stable to heat and digestion, often causing severe allergic reactions even after cooking. For instance, Der p 10 in house dust mites and tropomyosins in shrimp highlight how cross-reactivity extends between inhalant and food allergens, making it essential for clinicians to recognize the risks associated with these stable proteins.

CLINICAL IMPLICATIONS OF CROSS-REACTIVITY

Understanding cross-reactivity's clinical implications is essential for practitioners, especially when distinguishing between sensitization and true allergy **(Table 5.1)**. Cross-reactivity may result in widespread sensitization to multiple biologically-related allergens, though not all cases lead to clinically significant reactions. The implications of cross-reactivity are influenced by factors such as the type of allergen (degree of protein homology, stability), the patient's immune response, and environmental or cofactors that can enhance the clinical severity of reactions.

Pollen-food Syndrome

Also known as oral allergy syndrome, *pollen-food syndrome* (PFS) is the most recognized form of cross-reactivity. It occurs primarily in individuals sensitized to specific pollens, leading to mild symptoms, typically localized to the oral cavity, when consuming certain raw fruits or vegetables. For example, birch pollen-allergic individuals often experience itching or swelling in the mouth when consuming foods such as apples, cherries, or carrots, which share homologous proteins (PR-10 family) with birch pollen's Bet v 1. Studies indicate that PFS affects a significant portion of the population in regions with high birch pollen exposure, with the prevalence varying between 20 and 50% in different geographic areas.

House Dust Mite and Shellfish Cross-reactivity

Tropomyosins, structural proteins highly conserved across invertebrates, are responsible for cross-reactivity between house dust mites and shellfish. Patients sensitized to dust mites may develop allergic reactions to crustaceans such as shrimp, lobster, and crabs. The stability of tropomyosins to heat and digestion often results in systemic reactions, including anaphylaxis. For example, tropomyosin Der p 10 in house dust mites and Pen m 1 in shrimp highlight the cross-reactive potential that poses a clinical challenge. Such cross-reactive reactions are more prevalent in regions with high house dust mite exposure and seafood consumption.

Latex–fruit Syndrome

This syndrome involves cross-reactivity between latex and certain fruits such as bananas, avocados, and kiwis. Latex contains proteins such as Hev b 6.02, which shares structural similarity to proteins in these fruits. This cross-reactivity is particularly relevant in clinical settings, where individuals repeatedly exposed to latex, including healthcare workers and patients with frequent medical procedures, are at a higher risk. For example,

TABLE 5.1: Common cross-reactivities.

Primary allergen	***Source***	***Cross-reactive foods/ allergens***	***Typical symptoms***	***Notes***
Birch pollen (Bet v 1)	Trees (Birch)	Apples, pears, carrots, celery, almonds, cherries	Oral itching, tingling, swelling of mouth/throat	Common in birch pollen allergy regions; related to PR-10 proteins
Grass pollen	Grasses (e.g., Timothy)	Melons (watermelon, cantaloupe), tomatoes, oranges	Oral allergy symptoms, sometimes mild GI discomfort	Patients with grass pollen allergies often react to fruits/vegetables related to profilins
House dust mite	*Dermatophagoides* species	Shrimp, lobster, crab	Systemic reactions, including potential for anaphylaxis	Tropomyosin cross-reactivity; reactions can be severe, especially in adults
Latex	Natural rubber latex	Bananas, avocados, kiwis, chestnuts, passion fruit	Oral itching, swelling, potential for systemic reactions	Latex–fruit syndrome; significant in healthcare settings due to latex exposure
Ragweed pollen	Weeds (Ragweed)	Melons (watermelon, cantaloupe), bananas, cucumbers, zucchini	Oral allergy symptoms, itchy mouth/throat	Often seen in regions with high ragweed pollen; related to profilin proteins
Mugwort pollen	Weeds (Mugwort)	Celery, carrots, spices (e.g., parsley, coriander)	Oral itching, GI symptoms, occasionally systemic symptoms	Known as the Mugwort–Celery–Spice syndrome, also related to profilins
Cypress pollen	Trees (Cypress)	Peaches, oranges, apples, kiwi	Oral itching, swelling, GI symptoms	LTP cross-reactivity, common in Mediterranean populations

Contd...

Contd...

Primary allergen	***Source***	***Cross-reactive foods/ allergens***	***Typical symptoms***	***Notes***
Cat dander	Cat fur, dander	Pork (rare cross-reactivity)	GI discomfort, potential for systemic reactions	Rare cross-reactivity known as "pork–cat syndrome"
Peanut	Legumes (Peanut)	Tree nuts (almonds, hazelnuts, cashews), soybeans	Oral itching, swelling, anaphylaxis (severe cases)	Significant in children; cross-reactivity due to similar storage proteins
Ficus	Ficus plants	Latex, bananas, avocados	Oral itching, respiratory symptoms	People with fig (Ficus) allergies may also react to latex-related foods
Ash pollen	Trees (Ash)	Olives	Oral itching, swelling, mild respiratory symptoms	Related to olive pollen cross-reactivity in Mediterranean regions
Sunflower seed	Sunflower plants	Melons (watermelon, cantaloupe), other seeds	Oral itching, mild GI symptoms	Related to seed allergies, often appears with other pollen allergies
Buckwheat	Buckwheat	Other cereals (rare cross-reactivity with rice, wheat)	GI symptoms, respiratory symptoms, occasionally severe	Not common, more likely in regions with high buckwheat consumption

(GI: gastrointestinal; LTP: lipid transfer protein; PR: pathogenesis-related) children with spina bifida, who often undergo multiple surgeries, are especially vulnerable to latex sensitization and subsequent cross-reactive responses to certain foods.

Legume Allergy

Legumes, such as peanuts, soybeans, and chickpeas, frequently exhibit cross-reactive allergic responses due to shared proteins. Peanut allergy, a common legume allergy, is often linked with cross-reactivity to other legumes and tree nuts. This adds complexity in clinical management, as sensitization to peanuts does not necessarily mean a clinical reaction to all legumes, underscoring the need for individualized testing and dietary recommendations.

Tree Nut Allergy

Cross-reactivity is prevalent within tree nuts, including walnuts, almonds, cashews, and hazelnuts, due to shared protein structures. Management of tree nut allergies is complex since reactions to one type of tree nut can sometimes indicate cross-sensitization without a true clinical reaction to all nuts, requiring a nuanced approach to dietary restrictions.

Fish Allergy

Fish allergies are frequently related to the parvalbumin protein, which is consistent across many fish species such as salmon, tuna, and cod. This homology often results in cross-reactive responses to multiple fish types, though it does not extend to shellfish, allowing for specific dietary recommendations based on fish-only sensitization.

Hen's Egg Allergy

Commonly seen in children, hen's egg allergy is associated with proteins such as ovomucoid and ovalbumin. While some children outgrow this allergy, others remain sensitized to both raw and cooked egg proteins. Limited cross-reactivity may occur with eggs from other birds, but this is not universal, enabling targeted management strategies.

Cow's Milk Allergy

Cow's milk allergy, particularly common in infants, can present with cross-reactive sensitization to milk from other mammals, such as goat and sheep, due to similar casein and whey proteins. This allergy often manifests with gastrointestinal and respiratory symptoms, and although some children outgrow it, others require long-term avoidance of all mammalian milks.

CO-ALLERGY CONSIDERATIONS AND RELATED RISKS

Co-allergies are frequently observed among patients with multiple food or environmental sensitivities, such as peanut and tree nut allergies or sensitivities to tree pollens and certain fruits. These co-allergies complicate diagnostic processes, as overlapping symptoms may mask true allergenic sources. Component-resolved diagnostics (CRD) and oral food challenges play a critical role in differentiating primary allergens from clinically irrelevant cross-reactive sensitizations.

Diagnostic and Management Considerations

Given the prevalence and variable clinical impact of cross-reactivity, a structured approach is essential **(Table 5.2)**.

Component-resolved Diagnostics

The use of molecular allergology, or CRD, allows for precise identification of the

TABLE 5.2: Comparison of various diagnostic tools in cross reactivity.

Diagnostic tool	***Purpose***	***Sensitivity***	***Specificity***	***Use cases***
Skin prick testing (SPT)	Detect sensitization to allergens	High for inhalants	Moderate for foods	Initial allergy diagnosis, screening
Component-resolved diagnostics (CRD)	Identify specific allergenic proteins	High (component-level)	High	Differentiating primary vs. cross-reactivity
Oral food challenge (OFC)	Confirm clinical allergy	Gold standard	High	Confirmation of food allergy in cross-reactivity

specific allergen components responsible for sensitization. This diagnostic technique helps differentiate between primary sensitization to an allergen and cross-reactive responses that might not result in clinical symptoms. CRD enables the detection of IgE antibodies specific to particular allergenic proteins, such as Bet v 1 in birch pollen allergy, which can indicate a potential cross-reactivity with foods such as apples and carrots. By pinpointing the exact proteins involved, CRD reduces the likelihood of overdiagnosing allergies based on cross-reactive sensitizations, helping practitioners focus on clinically relevant allergens.

Oral Food Challenges

In situations where CRD suggests potential cross-reactivity, but the clinical significance remains uncertain, oral food challenges (OFCs) serve as the gold standard to confirm or rule out actual food allergies. During an OFC, the patient is gradually exposed to the suspected food allergen under controlled conditions to observe any allergic reactions. This method is particularly valuable for children sensitized to multiple related foods, as it minimizes unnecessary dietary restrictions by identifying only those allergens that cause significant symptoms upon ingestion.

Immunotherapy Options

Allergen immunotherapy (AIT) can be a useful intervention for managing cross-reactive allergies, especially in cases where inhalant allergens, such as pollen, also lead to food-related symptoms. For instance, immunotherapy for birch pollen has been shown to alleviate symptoms associated with cross-reactive foods in patients with PFS. However, due to the complexity of cross-protective effects, immunotherapy decisions should be carefully considered. Stable allergens, such as LTPs and tropomyosins, which can trigger severe reactions, may require cautious assessment before immunotherapy is initiated, weighing the potential benefits against risks.

SUMMARY

Cross-reactivity represents a substantial consideration in pediatric allergy, influencing diagnostic and management strategies. By understanding protein families such as PR-10, profilins, LTPs, and tropomyosins, and integrating advanced diagnostics and tailored management plans, practitioners can effectively address the challenges posed by cross-reactive allergies and enhance patient outcomes.

KEY POINTS

- Cross-reactivity occurs when IgE antibodies recognize structurally similar proteins across different allergen sources, significantly influencing pediatric allergy diagnosis and management.
- Major protein families include *PR-10 proteins, profilins, lipid transfer proteins (LTPs),* and *tropomyosins,* each differing in stability and clinical relevance.
- *Common syndromes: Pollen–food syndrome, house dust mite–shellfish cross-reactivity,* and *latex–fruit syndrome,* ranging from mild oral symptoms to systemic, potentially severe reactions.
- Cross-reactivity also complicates *legume, tree nut, fish, egg, and milk allergies,* making individualized testing and dietary planning essential.
- *Diagnostic tools:* Skin prick test (SPT) for screening, component-resolved diagnostics (CRD) for precision, and oral food challenges (OFC) as the gold standard to confirm true clinical allergy.
- *Management* focuses on accurate diagnosis, avoiding unnecessary dietary restrictions, and selective use of allergen immunotherapy, with special caution for stable allergens such as LTPs and tropomyosins.

SUGGESTED READING

1. Alessandri C, Ferrara R, Bernardi ML, Zennaro D, Tuppo L, Giangrieco I, et al. Molecular approach to a patient's tailored diagnosis of the oral allergy syndrome. Clin Transl Allergy. 2020;10:22.
2. Chafen JJ, Newberry SJ, Riedl MA, Bravata DM, Maglione M, Suttorp MJ, et al. Diagnosing and managing common food allergies: a systematic review. JAMA. 2010;303: 1848-56.
3. Faber MA, Van Gasse AL, Decuyper II, Sabato V, Hagendorens MM, Mertens C, et al. Cross-reactive aeroallergens: which need to cross our mind in food allergy diagnosis? J Allergy Clin Immunol Pract. 2018;6(6):1813-23.
4. Gupta N, Agarwal P, Sachdev A, Gupta D. Allergy testing—an overview. Indian Pediatr. 2019;56:951-7.
5. Gupta N, Moitra S, Nagarajan S. Comprehensive Textbook of Allergy: Striking the Right Balance, 1st edition. New Delhi: Jaypee Brothers Medical Publishers Pvt. Ltd.; 2024.
6. Kamath SD, Bublin M, Kitamura K, Matsui T, Ito K, Lopata AL. Cross-reactive epitopes and their role in food allergy. J Allergy Clin Immunol. 2023;151(5):1178-90.
7. Krishna MT, Mahesh PA, Vedanthan P, Moitra S, Mehta V, Christopher DJ. An appraisal of allergic disorders in India and an urgent call for action. World Allergy Organ J. 2020;13(7):100446.
8. Mari A, Scala E. Cross-reactivity between inhalant and food allergens. Clin Exp Allergy. 2006;36(5):667-75.
9. Popescu FD. Cross-reactivity between aeroallergens and food allergens. World J Methodol. 2015;5(2):31-50.
10. Werfel T, Asero R, Ballmer-Weber BK, Beyer K, Enrique E, Knulst AC, et al. Position paper of the EAACI: food allergy due to immunological cross-reactions with common inhalant allergens. Allergy. 2015;70: 1079-90.

CHAPTER 6

Skin Testing in Pediatric Allergy

Sonia Bhatt, Payal Mittal

INTRODUCTION

Allergy skin testing (AST) is a bioassay that exposes the body to an antigen, revealing the presence of specific immunoglobulin E (IgE) antibodies on the surface of sensitized mast cells. Skin prick testing (SPT) reveals the presence of specific IgE antibodies to protein and peptide allergens. Small doses of allergen are introduced into the epidermis and the superficial, nonvascular dermis, where they interact with specific IgE attached to mast cells in the skin. This interaction triggers the release of histamine and other mediators, resulting in a visible wheal-and-flare reaction that peaks around 15 minutes after exposure.

Allergy skin testing has several applications, primarily used to diagnose IgE-mediated conditions such as allergic rhinitis, allergic conjunctivitis, allergic asthma, atopic dermatitis, food allergies, and drug allergies. AST is also valuable for standardizing allergenic extracts, conducting epidemiological and pharmacological research, and evaluating the effectiveness of antiallergic treatments.

MECHANISM OF ALLERGIC REACTION (FIG. 6.1)

Phases in allergic reaction are (1) sensitization and (2) re-exposure.

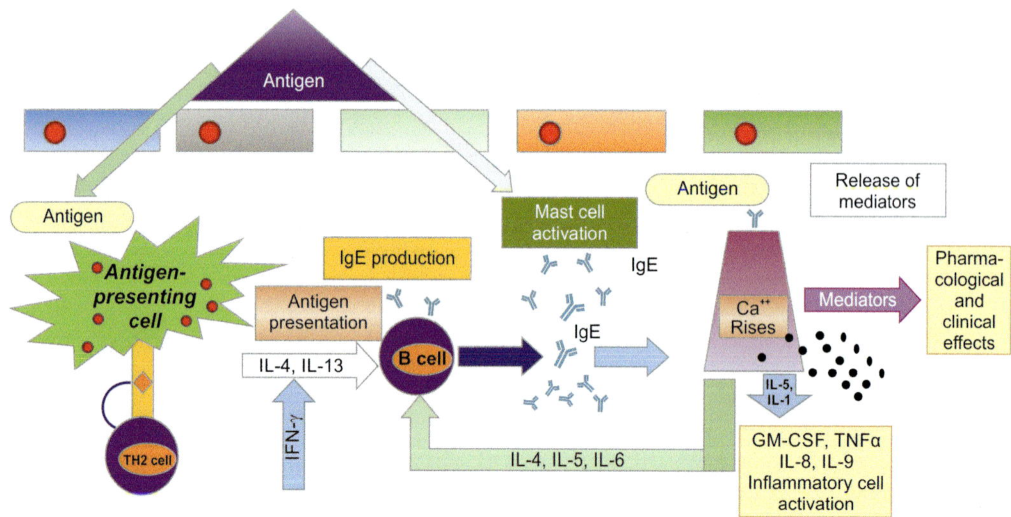

Fig. 6.1: Mechanism of allergic skin reaction. (GM-CSF: granulocyte-macrophage colony-stimulating factor; IFN-γ: interferon-gamma; IgE: immunoglobulin E; IL: interleukin; TNFα: tumor necrosis factor alpha)

Sensitization

In individuals with a genetic predisposition, the initial exposure to an allergen activates T cells, which occurs through antigen presentation by antigen-presenting cells (APCs).

The activated T cells then induce B cells to undergo class switching via interleukin-4 (IL-4) and IL-13, leading to the production of IgE antibodies. The generated IgE circulates freely in the bloodstream and also binds to high-affinity FcεRI receptors on the surface of mast cells and basophils. This phase, where specific IgE is bound to mast cells, is known as sensitization.

During AST, mast cells are exposed to an antigen. If these cells have been sensitized, the antigen triggers cross-linking of cell-bound IgE, causing the release of mediators such as histamine, tryptase, and leukotrienes. These substances induce vasodilation, increase vascular permeability, and promote exudation, resulting in the typical wheal-and-flare reaction.

TYPES OF ALLERGY SKIN TESTING

The following are three primary types of skin testing used in allergy diagnosis:

1. *SPT*: It is also known as prick skin testing (PST). This is the most common method for diagnosing immediate IgE-mediated allergies. It is widely used due to its minimal risk of serious side effects and the high-quality information it provides when performed and interpreted correctly.
2. *Intradermal testing (IDT)*: This technique is used to diagnose both immediate IgE-mediated allergies and delayed-type hypersensitivity. Although IDT can be more sensitive than SPT, it involves a greater risk of adverse reactions and demands substantial technical skill for accurate interpretation.
3. *Patch testing*: It is primarily used to diagnose contact hypersensitivity and other delayed-type hypersensitivity reactions; patch testing is typically conducted by dermatologists and some immunologists. Unlike SPT and IDT, patch testing does not apply to immediate- or IgE-mediated allergies and will not be further covered here.

INDICATIONS FOR SKIN PRICK TESTING

Skin prick testing is generally suitable for diagnosing:

- Allergic rhinitis and rhinoconjunctivitis
- Allergic asthma (though not routinely used for this purpose)
- Atopic dermatitis
- Food reactions that lead to severe responses such as anaphylaxis, immediate acute urticaria, or sudden eczema flare-ups
- Suspected latex allergy
- Less common disorders such as allergic bronchopulmonary aspergillosis, eosinophilic esophagitis, and eosinophilic gastroenteritis

However, SPT is usually *not indicated* for:

- Nonspecific rashes lacking allergic or atopic features
- Food intolerance without clinical features of allergy (e.g., irritable bowel syndrome)
- Reactions to respiratory irritants such as smoke, fumes, or perfumes
- Allergy screening in asymptomatic cases (e.g., family history of allergy)

FACTORS INFLUENCING ALLERGEN SKIN TESTS

Medications

Conventional doses of antihistaminic cause suppression of the skin reactivity **(Table 6.1)**.

TABLE 6.1: Drugs and duration of AST suppression.

Drugs	***Suppression of AST activity (days)***
Antihistamines: Cetrizine, loratidine, and terfenadine	3–5 days
Astemizole	60 days
Ketotifen	5 days
Tricyclic antidepressants	2 weeks

Note: Steroids, LABA, and H2 antagonists do not interfere with SPT interpretation.
(AST: allergy skin testing; LABA: long-acting beta-agonist; SPT: skin prick testing)

Medications that may be contraindicated in skin prick testing: Certain medications can disrupt the body's normal compensatory responses during anaphylaxis, including:

- Beta-blockers
- Angiotensin-converting enzyme (ACE) inhibitors (considered a relative contraindication)

Age

The skin reactivity generally declines in extreme of ages (infants and >60 years).

Area of the Body

The reactivity for the antigen in various body parts is given as follows:

Mid and upper back > Lower back and forearm

The antecubital area is the most reactive part of the upper arm, while the wrist is the least reactive. The radial side of the forearm is about 50% less reactive than the ulnar side. A minimum distance of 2 cm must be maintained between any two adjacent test sites.

CONTRAINDICATIONS

Skin prick testing should not be performed in patients with diffuse dermatological conditions or severe dermatographism.

Relative Contraindications/ Precautions

Skin prick testing should be avoided in non-specialist settings for safety reasons in cases of uncontrolled asthma, pregnancy, babies, and infants.

PATIENT SELECTION CRITERIA

Age

Skin prick testing has no strict age limitations; however, interpreting results can be challenging in very young children and the elderly due to reduced skin reactivity.

SELECTION OF ANTIGEN FOR ALLERGY SKIN TESTING

The selection of antigens for AST is crucial and depends on various factors such as history of the patient and the local aerobiology data (airborne allergens specific to a region). There are no strict guidelines, but a structured approach helps in identifying potential allergens.

MAJOR CATEGORIES OF ALLERGENS

- *Inhalants (airborne allergens):* These are substances that people breathe in and can trigger allergic reactions, especially respiratory issues such as asthma.
    - *Indoor antigens:* House dust mites, cockroaches, pets (animal danders), and molds. They are a significant cause of asthma and allergic rhinitis, especially in children and young adults.
    - *Outdoor antigens:* Pollens, grasses, weeds, and mold spores. Outdoor allergens tend to cause seasonal allergies.
- *Ingestants (food allergens):* These are food-related allergens that can cause gastrointestinal or skin reactions.

- *Injectable allergens (venoms):* These include allergens such as bee or wasp venom, which can cause severe reactions, including anaphylaxis.

In selecting antigens for testing, it is essential to focus on the patient's environment and symptoms. Indoor allergens are particularly important for people with respiratory symptoms such as asthma, as they can play a key role in both diagnosis and treatment.

ALLERGEN TEST PANELS

The patient's clinical condition and exposure history should be taken into account before allergy testing. To manage the patient effectively, the fewest allergens should be chosen for testing. For general practitioners or respiratory labs, a small panel of 8–12 inhalant allergens is typically sufficient. The composition of allergen panels should also reflect local variations in flora and fauna.

FOOD ALLERGENS

Skin prick testing for IgE-mediated food allergies is a valid diagnostic method, but its interpretation is often complex. False positives are common.

MAINTENANCE OF ALLERGEN EXTRACTS

Clear labeling of allergen extract is essential. They must be kept in a temperature-monitored refrigerator and only removed briefly during testing. Since the potency of allergen extracts can decrease over time, it is essential to regularly verify their expiration dates.

POSITIVE AND NEGATIVE CONTROLS

These controls are essential to ensure the reliability and accuracy of skin prick tests, allowing clinicians to distinguish true allergic reactions from nonspecific skin responses.

- *Positive control*: The positive control typically consists of a histamine solution (commonly histamine phosphate at 10 mg/mL), which directly triggers a skin wheal-and-flare response or codeine (generally a 9% solution), which induces wheal and flare indirectly by causing degranulation of cutaneous mast cells. The positive control is used to confirm the skin's ability to react appropriately **(Table 6.2)**.
- *Negative control*: The negative control typically consists of the same solution that the allergens are diluted in, such as a saline buffer or 50% glycerol, but without any allergen. This control helps identify nonspecific reactions, such as dermatographism, where a patient may develop a small flare or wheal simply from the pinprick, regardless of allergen exposure **(Table 6.3)**.

TABLE 6.2: Interpretation of positive reaction.

Response to allergen (wheal size)	***Interpretation***
<3 mm	Uninterpretable or possible antihistamine intake by the patient
≥3 mm larger than the negative saline control	Positive

TABLE 6.3: Interpretation of negative control reaction.

Negative control reaction	***Interpretation***
0–3 mm wheal	Acceptable
Significant (e.g., a wheal >3 mm)	Severe dermatographism, necessitating the rejection of the test as uninterpretable

SKIN PRICK TEST PROCEDURE

Requirements

- *Allergen extracts:* The specific allergens to be tested
- *Positive and negative control solutions:* To validate the test results
- *Sterile lancets:* Used for pricking the skin
- *Sharps container:* For safe disposal of used lancets
- *Marker pen:* To mark the skin and identify the test sites
- *Ruler:* To measure the size of wheal
- *Record document:* To document the test results
- *Gloves (optional):* For hygienic handling of materials

Devices for Allergy Testing

- *Lancet types:* The most common lancet has a single sharp point, but there are variations such as Duotip lancets with two points or multipoint lancets designed to test multiple allergens simultaneously. The lancet may be a single-use device for each allergen or part of a multipoint system.
- *Application methods:* The lancet or device is dipped into the allergen extract before pricking the skin. Alternatively, a small droplet of allergen extract is applied to the skin, and the lancet is then used to prick through the droplet into the skin.

Procedure

The rationale, procedure, precautions, and performance details should be thoroughly explained to the patient and family. The following steps are generally recommended:

The steps to perform SPT are given as follows:

- *Documentation:* Prepare the allergy skin test record sheet.
- *Introduction:* The person conducting the test should introduce himself.
- *Explanation:* Procedure should be clearly explained.
- *Skin preparation:* Clean the area to be tested, using a 70% alcohol swab, and allow it to dry. Hairy skin should be shaved a day before.
- *Marking test sites:* Testing sites should be marked with skin marking pen following an order. Starting with the negative saline control and ending with the positive histamine control.
- *Antigen placement:* Apply small drops of the antigen to the marked sites, ensuring the correct order and numbers correspond to the recording sheet.
- *Pricking the skin:* Swiftly prick the test site through the antigen drop using a skin testing needle, applying light pressure while pulling the needle upward.
- Only 0.3 μL antigen enters the dermis; hence, minimal amounts of antigen for testing must be used.
- Wheal diameter in millimeters should be measured after 15 minutes of inoculation of positive control.

RESULT REPORTING (SKIN PRICK TEST)

- *Reporting forms:* The report form should include the following information, as given in **Table 6.4**.
    - Patient particulars, date of test, and region tested
    - Correct name of each allergen tested, including positive and negative control, should be mentioned, followed by any common name.
    - Any allergens not tested should be clearly crossed out to avoid confusion.
    - The size of the resultant wheal for each allergen should be recorded.

TABLE 6.4: Model of allergy skin testing report.

Name:____________________ Age/sex:__________

Patient ID:_________________ Dr Name:_________________

Date:_________________

Time done:_________________ Time read:_________________

Pediatric routine panel

*Number*__________ *Allergens*__________ *Wheal diameter (in mm)*__________

1. Dust mite mix (D&F)
2. Cockroach
3. *Prosopis juliflora*
4. *Parthenium*
5. *Sorghum halepense*
6. *Alternaria tenuis*
7. Dog danger
8. Cat danger

Foods

1. Chicken
2. Egg white
3. Fish
4. Milk
5. Groundnut
6. Soya
7. Wheat
8. Saline control

Histamine control

Interpretation

- *Standardized quantitative reporting:*
  - The primary result should be wheal's mean diameter in millimeters, measured according to the suggested method and time frame.
- *Method of recording SPT results*:
  - A chart should be maintained, with the wheal (and optionally the flare) size in millimeters recorded next to each allergen name. Numerical recording of wheal diameter is essential for good clinical practice. Avoid using qualitative marks (e.g., +, ++) as the primary result.

SUMMARY

Allergy skin testing is highly effective for identifying sensitization. When combined with patient history, AST plays a crucial role in managing allergies, guiding decisions on allergen immunotherapy, and selecting the appropriate antigens for treatment. It is a safe, reliable, and efficient tool for allergists.

KEY POINTS

- It is recommended to measure allergy skin test in millimeters and avoid a semiquantitative grading system.

- Blotting the test site immediately after pricking does not seem to affect the final reaction size, which is particularly beneficial for pediatric patients.
- AST results can be positive even in individuals who do not show clinical symptoms.
- For testing food items such as fruits and vegetables, fresh material should be used with the "prick and prick" method.
- When reporting AST results, the term *sensitized* should be used instead of *allergic*. Always include both positive and negative controls in the report.

SUGGESTED READING

1. Ansotegui IJ, Melioli G, Canonica GW, Caraballo L, Villa E, Ebisawa M, et al. IgE allergy diagnostics and other relevant tests in allergy, a World Allergy Organization position paper. World Allergy Organ J. 2020; 13(2):100080
2. Barbaud A. Skin testing and patch testing in non-IgE-mediated drug allergy. Curr Allergy Asthma Rep. 2014;14(6):442.
3. Des Roches A, Paradis L, Bougeard YH, Godard P, Bousquet J, Chanez P. Long-term oral corticosteroid therapy does not alter the results of immediate-type allergy skin prick tests. J Allergy Clin Immunol. 1996; 98(3): 522-27.
4. Frati F, Incorvaia C, Cavaliere C, Di Cara G, Marcucci F, Esposito S, et al. The skin prick test. J Biol Regul Homeost Agents. 2018; 32(Suppl 1):19-24.
5. Heinzerling L, Mari A, Bergmann KC, Bresciani M, Burbach G, Darsow U, et al. The skin prick test—European standards. Clin Transl Allergy. 2013;3(1):3.
6. Henzgen M, Ballmer-Weber BK, Erdmann S, Fuchs T, Kleine-Tebbe J, Lepp U, et al. Skin testing with food allergens. Guideline of the German Society of Allergology and Clinical Immunology (DGAKI), the Physicians' Association of German Allergologists (ADA) and the Society of Pediatric Allergology (GPA) together with the Swiss Society of Allergology. J Dtsch Dermatol Ges. 2008; 6(11):983-88.
7. Konstantinou GN, Bousquet PJ, Zuberbier T, Papadopoulos NG. The longest wheal diameter is the optimal measurement for the evaluation of skin prick tests. Int Arch Allergy Immunol. 2010;151(4):343-5.
8. Patel G, Saltoun C. Skin testing in allergy. Allergy Asthma Proc. 2019;40(6):366-8.
9. Platt MP, Wulu JA. Rational approach to allergy testing. Otolaryngol Clin North Am. 2017;50(6):1103-10.
10. Savi E, Peveri S, Cavaliere C, Masieri S, Montagni M. Laboratory tests for allergy diagnosis. J Biol Regul Homeost Agents. 2018;32(Suppl 1):25-8.
11. Tourlas K, Burman D. Allergy testing. Prim Care. 2016;43(3):363-74.
12. van Ree R, Hummelshøj L, Plantinga M, Poulsen LK, Swindle E. Allergic sensitization: host-immune factors. Clin Transl Allergy. 2014;4(1):12.

CHAPTER 7

In Vitro Tests in Pediatric Allergy

Gouthami P

INTRODUCTION

Childhood allergies are increasingly on the rise, posing greater challenges in diagnosis.

In vitro and in vivo modalities of allergy testing play a pivotal role in addressing parental concerns about multiple commonly suspected allergies, such as milk, egg, bananas, brinjal, or pain medications. In vitro tests offer a more practical alternative to traditional in vivo methods, such as skin prick tests. These tests allow the detection of specific immunoglobulin E (IgE) antibodies against common allergens in the blood samples.

The safety profile of these tests helps allergists to rule out unnecessary parental concerns, minimizes dietary restrictions, allows evidence-based management, and improves compliance with treatment, ultimately enhancing the child's well-being and quality of life.

IMMUNOGLOBULIN E AND MEDIATED IN VITRO TESTS

Immunoglobulin E

Immunoglobulin E, the last among the five types of immunoglobulins discovered by Ishizaka and Johansson, stirred up the research community since its discovery.

Immunoglobulin E Differs from Other Immunoglobulins

Immunoglobulin E is a unique molecule, a monomer composed of two epsilon-heavy chains and two light chains. The variable regions of both heavy and light chains form antigen-specific binding sites capable of binding a total of two antigens.

The structure lacks a hinge region increasing the flexibility to adapt and interact with its receptors.

Heavy glycosylation with seven N-linked glycosylations on each heavy chain further makes the molecule different from other immunoglobulins. This facilitates binding to a high-affinity cellular receptor, Fc-epsilon-RI.

IgE receptors and their expression: The role of IgE is accomplished as the Fc portion binds to a receptor on a particular cell type, such as a mast cell and eosinophil. The predominant IgE-binding receptors are Fc-epsilon-RI and Fc-epsilon-RII and CD23.

Fc-epsilon-RI:

- High-affinity receptor
- Located on mast cells, basophils, dendritic cells, macrophages, and eosinophils
- Mediates type 4 hypersensitivity reactions
- Immunity to parasitic infections
- Cytokine production
- Antigen presentation

CD23:

- Low-affinity receptor
- Prominent areas of expression are B-cells, T-cells, and antigen-presenting cells (APCs)

Flowchart 7.1: Immunological basis of IgE production and activation.

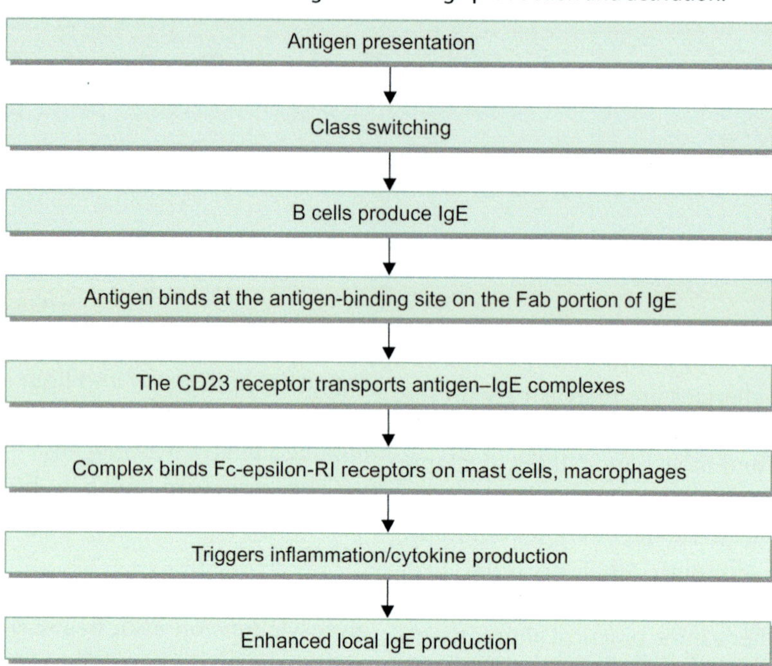

- Plays a role in homeostasis of IgE synthesis and navigation across airway and gut epithelia
- Facilitated antigen presentation.

IgE production, subsequent binding to receptors, and activation of mast cells follow a complex immunological path in atopic individuals **(Flowchart 7.1)**.

Facilitated Antigen Presentation

Instead of T cells, antigen–IgE complexes present the peptide/antigen presentation mediated by CD23 receptors.

B cells present antigenic peptides to T cells with molecular diversity via facilitated antigen presentation (FAP).

Epitope spreading—FAP mediates development of antibody response to different antigens on exposure to a single antigen forming the basis of sensitization to multiple unrelated antigens and hence explains the phenomenon of atopic march.

Serum Specific Immunoglobulin E Testing

The mere presence of specific IgE (sIgE) is not sufficient to diagnose clinical manifestations of allergy in a child; however, it is necessary.

The substrate with the allergen can be represented by a solid-phase allergosorbent or a liquid-phase conjugated allergen. The allergens being adsorbed can be raw allergens or molecules extracted from natural allergens by biochemical purification or with recombinant DNA technology.

Radioallergosorbent test (RAST) was the first assay for sIgE detection, which has technically evolved many fold.

The allergen in RAST is bound to a solid medium, and the patient's blood is exposed to the allergen. The presence of sIgE in the blood is detected by a radioactive anti-IgE antibody.

Enzyme-linked immunosorbent assay (ELISA) is a technique that replaces radioactive substrate with an enzyme linked to the anti-IgE antibody.

ImmunoCAP/fluorescent immunoassay is a novel technology that revolutionized IgE testing.

The technique yields higher sensitivity as the allergens are bound to cellulose-made sponge-like solid material, which increases the surface area, facilitating the binding of more allergens. The quantitative measurements of IgE levels aid in diagnosis, prognosis, and follow-up care. Fluorescent labeling of the enzyme allows better quantification of IgE making the test a gold standard.

Phadiatop is a qualitative screening test for multiple allergens that operates with two panels: Phadiatop and Phadiatop infant. The screening tool works on the basis of immunoCAP technology and offers sensitivity of 84%, specificity of 90%, positive predictive value of 70.8%, and negative predictive value of 91.7%. The result <0.35 kU/L is negative and conveniently rules out IgE-mediated reaction to the particular allergen.

Commonly used symptom-based allergy panels are:

- *Respiratory/rhinitis/wheeze panel:* House dust mite, cat dander, dog dander, Bermuda grass, ragweed, *Aspergillus fumigatus,* and *Alternaria*
- *Eczema panel:* Egg, milk, fish, peanut, soybean, wheat, dog dander, Bermuda grass, and house dust mite.

Multiplex and microarray testing ALEX/ISAC is the latest advancement in the last decade, where over a hundred allergens and allergen components are tested in minimal blood volume on a single chip, making the test more cost-effective. The test is beneficial where multiple cross-sensitizations are suspected.

IMMULITE has avidin solid phase to which biotinylated allergen is coupled.

Roche diagnostics COBAS and Hycor HYTEC are the latest advancements.

The sIgE can be measured by the usage of single reagents *(singleplex)* or with a predefined panel of molecules *(multiplex).*

Liquid phase sIgE assays are not commonly used. Though the allergen suspension in liquid media allows free and faster interaction, the tests lack sensitivity due to background noise, limiting their use for research purposes.

Total Immunoglobulin E

Total IgE levels are elevated in various conditions other than allergy. Lower levels of IgE do not rule out IgE-mediated conditions. Hence, it is not a reliable marker of atopy or allergy. Higher levels of IgE in children are observed in parasitic infestations, multiple myeloma, immune dysregulation polyendocrinopathy enteropathy X-linked syndrome (IPEX), Omenn syndrome, Wiskott–Aldrich syndrome, Comel-Netherton syndrome, hyper-IgE syndrome, and atypical complete DiGeorge syndrome.

The levels of IgE correlate with disease severity in allergic bronchopulmonary aspergillosis (ABPA). Total IgE levels, moreover, act as a dose-determining parameter in omalizumab therapy.

NONIMMUNOGLOBULIN E-MEDIATED TESTS

The clinical features in allergy are not always explained by type I hypersensitivity, but may result from other forms of hypersensitivity. Hence, non-IgE-mediated tests come to diagnostic aid.

Lymphocyte Transformation Test

Lymphocyte transformation test (LTT) test was initially confined to biomedical research but gradually evolved as a diagnostic tool to detect non-IgE-mediated allergy.

Flowchart 7.2: Involved in lymphocyte transformation test (LTT).

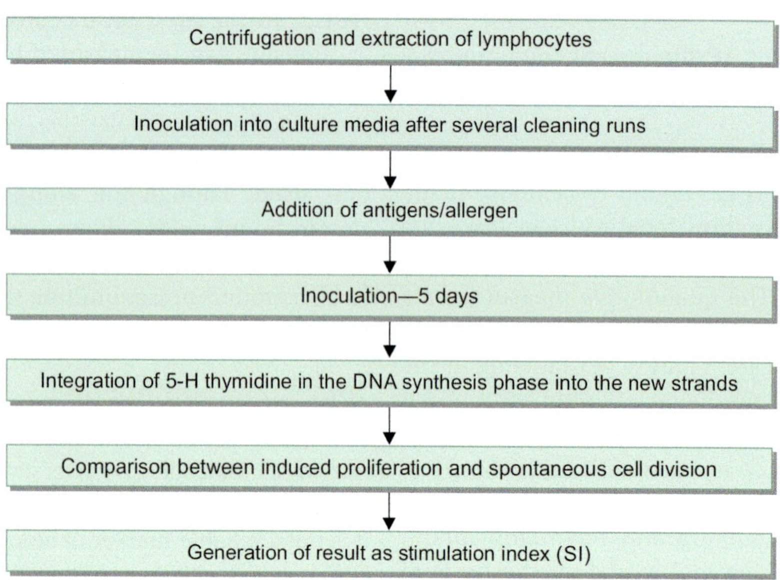

The principle of the test is the cell division of lymphocytes on culture media after appropriate inoculation with the allergen. A complex array of steps is included in performing a LTT **(Flowchart 7.2)**.

The ratio of proliferation rates in stimulated test run versus spontaneous proliferation is called the stimulation index. It is denoted by SI.

Applications: LTT is chiefly implicated in drug allergies where non-IgE-mediated T-cell-mediated reactions are pathognomonic.

Basophil Activation Test

Exposure to an allergen results in degranulation of basophils and release of histamine. Functional assessment of these basophils using flow cytometry forms the basis of the basophil activation test (BAT). CD63, a surface protein, is the most commonly upregulated marker used for BAT. Histamine release is directly and strongly correlated with the expression of CD63.

The result in BAT is denoted graphically as a dose-response curve, with the percentage of CD63-positive cells on the *y*-axis and the allergen concentration on the *x*-axis.

The antigenic affinity, epitope diversity and density, and molecular characteristics of basophils influence the dose-response curve.

Basophil activation test is executed on a fresh whole blood sample, preferably processed within 24 hours, a delay which results in decreased reactivity. The antihistamines and topical steroids do not interfere with the test result; however, oral steroids need to be stopped at least 3 weeks before the test.

The positive and negative predictive values of BAT are 95% and 98%, respectively.

Advantages

Basophil activation test BAT can be effectively considered when:

- False-positive skin prick test (SPT) results

- No extracts of allergens for SPT or sIgE
- No relevance between the patient's history and SPT results
- Before performing provocation tests
- Aids in assessing response to allergen-specific immunotherapy.

BIOMARKER-BASED TESTS

Post an allergic reaction occurs an upsurge of biomarkers irrespective of the allergen triggering the reaction. Eosinophil cationic protein and histamine release test are the two biomarker-based tests used to evaluate the degree of the allergic reaction rather than the specific allergen.

Eosinophilic Cationic Protein

Airway inflammation is associated with a cascade of reactions and release of inflammatory mediators from eosinophilic granules. Eosinophilic cationic proteins (ECP), major basic protein, eosinophil peroxidase, and eosinophil-derived neurotoxin are the major mediators. 6–24 hours after the allergen exposure, ECP is found in serum, sputum, and nasal secretions. Research has shown a significant role of ECP in risk stratification, response to therapy, and anticipating acute exacerbations, especially in asthmatics and allergic rhinitis.

Histamine Release Test

Allergen-induced basophil histamine release assay (A-BHRA) measures the amount of histamine released when an allergen is applied. The test also aids in the diagnosis of anaphylaxis, mastocytosis, and various other allergic manifestations.

Fresh whole blood from the patient or donor blood with basophils sensitized with IgE from the patient's serum can be processed to detect allergen sensitization.

TABLE 7.1: Comparison between in vitro and in vivo tests.

In vitro testing	*In vivo testing*
Involves drawing of blood	Simple and painless
Easy for young children	Difficult for small kids, requires cooperation
Results in a few hours	Results in 15–20 minutes
Number of allergens to be tested is limited	Unlimited, can perform prick-on-prick test
Can be safely done by a technician	Needs expertise to perform
Expensive	Affordable
Results not interfered by drugs	Interfered with drugs such as antihistamines

ADVANTAGES AND DISADVANTAGES OF IN VITRO TESTS OVER IN VIVO TESTS

In vitro allergy testing provides advantages over in vivo tests in diagnosing allergy and suffers certain limitations in comparison with in vivo tests **(Table 7.1)**.

IN VITRO TESTS IN FOOD ALLERGY

In vitro tests serve the objective of the requirement of a food challenge in confirming food allergy. A recent history explaining a chronology of an allergic reaction after intake of food, SPT ≥3 mm, and/or sIgE to the allergen ≥0.35 kU/L is sufficient to confirm the diagnosis without the need for a food challenge. In patients with inconclusive history and inconsistent SPT, sIgE to whole allergen or to components or the BAT may be warranted, to decide upon oral food challenge (OFC).

The approximate positive predictive value (PPV) of sIgE levels of 32 kU/L of cow milk, 7 kU/L of egg, 15 kU/L of peanut, and 20 kU/L of fish is 95%. This research emphasizes the role of in vitro testing in food allergy.

IN VITRO TESTS IN DRUG ALLERGY

The drug challenge test and SPT are the gold standard diagnostic modalities in drug allergy. However, in vitro tests offer a safer alternative in drug hypersensitivity reactions manifesting as severe cutaneous adverse reactions. BAT and LTT reliably serve the diagnostic purpose in such clinical scenarios.

Most commonly used in vitro tests and their role in drug allergy:

- Serum tryptase—confirmation of hypersensitivity and risk stratification
- BAT—identification of culprit drug
- Specific IgE—identification of culprit drug
- Eosinophils—used during the course of the reaction
- Lymphocyte transformation test—after the resolution of the reaction
- Enzyme-linked immunoSpot (ELISpot)—after the resolution of the reaction.

IN VITRO TESTS IN ANAPHYLAXIS

Several mediators which are released in the course of an anaphylactic reaction, such as tryptase, histamine, chymase, carboxypeptidase A3, platelet-activating factor, and other products from mastocytes, can be subsequently assessed to diagnose anaphylaxis. Serum-specific IgE and BAT offer alternatives in the diagnosis of anaphylaxis. BAT further provides an added advantage in patients suspected with anaphylaxis to beta-lactams, nonsteroidal anti-inflammatory drugs, neuromuscular blocking agents, and drugs for which there is no technique to measure sIgE.

SUMMARY

In vitro allergy tests are safer and practical alternatives to in vivo methods, hence have become an essential tool in pediatric allergy diagnosis. These tests guide evidence-based management. Various modalities involved are ImmunoCAP, Phadiatop, multiplex microarrays, basophil activation test (BAT), lymphocyte transformation test (LTT), and biomarker-based assays. In vitro testing plays a pivotal role in food allergy, drug hypersensitivity, and anaphylaxis diagnosis, while also supporting therapeutic decisions such as omalizumab dosing.

KEY POINTS

- *Specific IgE tests* (ImmunoCAP, ELISA, Phadiatop) provide quantification for allergy diagnosis especially food allergy.
- *Non-IgE mediated tests* like LTT and BAT help in drug allergy and T-cell-mediated hypersensitivity.
- *Biomarker tests* (eosinophil cationic protein, histamine release) assess severity rather than allergen specificity.
- *Anaphylaxis diagnosis* can be supported by tryptase, histamine, and BAT when sIgE is not available.
- Total IgE levels are *not reliable for diagnosis* but aid in the diagnosis of ABPA and omalizumab dosing.

SUGGESTED READING

1. Godwin L, Sinawe H, Crane JS. Biochemistry, Immunoglobulin E. Treasure Island (FL): StatPearls Publishing; 2025.
2. Nyfeler B, Pichler WJ. Sensitivity and specificity of the lymphocyte transformation test to drugs. Clin Exp Allergy 1997;27:175-81.
3. Oettgen HC. Fifty years later: emerging functions of IgE antibodies in host defense, immune regulation, and allergic diseases. J Allergy Clin Immunol. 2016;137(6):1631-45.
4. Santos AF, Alpan O, Hoffmann HJ. Basophil activation test: Mechanisms and considerations for use in clinical trials and clinical practice. Allergy. 2021;76(8):2420-32.
5. Santos AF, Brough HA. Making the most of in vitro tests to diagnose food allergy. J Allergy Clin Immunol Pract. 2017;5(2):237-48.
6. Sutton BJ, Davies AM, Bax HJ, Karagiannis SN. IgE antibodies: from structure to function and clinical translation. antibodies (Basel). 2019;8(1):19.

CHAPTER 8

Component-resolved Diagnostics

Hima Mathews P

INTRODUCTION

Allergic diseases are on the rise, and the diagnosis of allergy is always challenging. Knowledge about the appropriate use of allergy testing is an important component of allergic disorder management. Allergy testing can assist in the possible identification of the individual allergen involved and can help to decrease the morbidity and mortality for patients. In vitro allergy tests have a significant role in diagnosing allergy. With the advancement in molecular biology, component-resolved diagnostics (CRD) have become one of the most useful in vitro tests, which detect specific IgE (sIgE) antibodies against individual molecular allergenic components instead of whole allergen extracts and hence allow more precise diagnosis.

PRINCIPLES AND TECHNIQUES OF COMPONENT-RESOLVED DIAGNOSTICS

Progression in the field of molecular biology in the last few years has enabled the detection, cloning, and recombinant production of various allergen protein components, allowing detection and quantification of sIgE antibodies to these allergenic components. The first one to be identified and cloned was the major allergen Der p 1 from house dust mite (*Dermatophagoides pteronyssinus*) in the late 1980s.

Conventional allergy tests use allergen samples from natural sources, which contain crude allergen extracts with allergenic and nonallergenic parts. People who have allergies might be sensitive to many different proteins, but only a small number of them are allergenic and can actually cause symptoms. CRD finds sIgE antibodies that are directed against single allergenic components using recombinant methods. CRD can clearly differentiate between cross-reactive determinants and real clinically important allergic sensitization.

Principle of Component-resolved Diagnostics

Molecular level testing for allergies using CRD is the process of finding specific allergenic protein components in an allergen source. Skin prick tests (SPT) and sIgE tests use crude allergen extracts, which are made up of both allergic and nonallergenic proteins. CRD breaks these complicated mixtures down into their individual parts, which makes it possible to find the exact proteins that cause allergic responses. Usually, methods like microarray analysis are used for this, which can find IgE antibodies against many sensitive parts at the same time **(Fig. 8.1)**.

Allergen Nomenclature Database

The official website for the WHO/IUIS Subcommittee on Allergen Nomenclature is

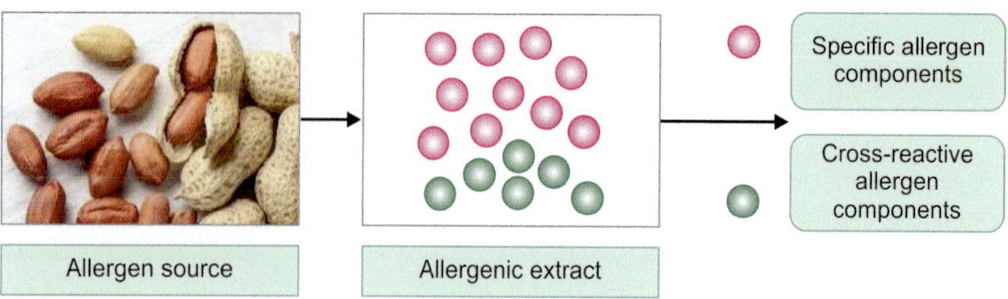

Fig. 8.1: Principle of component-resolved diagnostics (CRD).

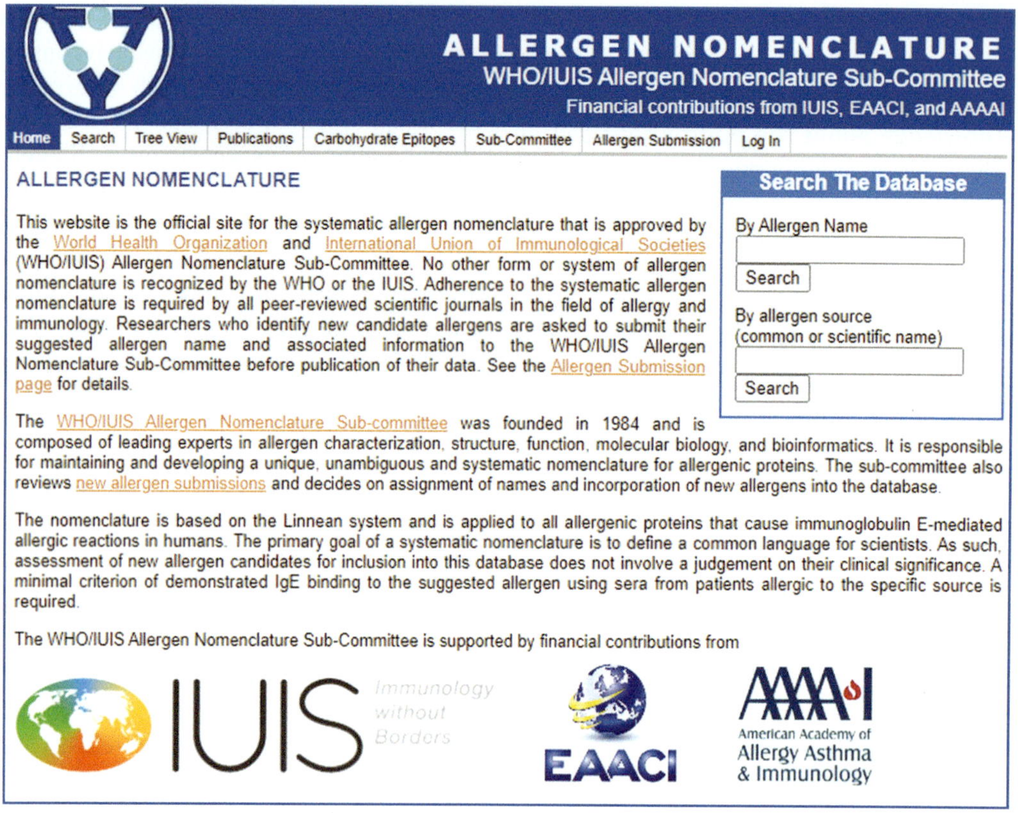

ALLERGEN NOMENCLATURE
WHO/IUIS Allergen Nomenclature Sub-Committee
Financial contributions from IUIS, EAACI, and AAAAI

Home | Search | Tree View | Publications | Carbohydrate Epitopes | Sub-Committee | Allergen Submission | Log In

ALLERGEN NOMENCLATURE

This website is the official site for the systematic allergen nomenclature that is approved by the World Health Organization and International Union of Immunological Societies (WHO/IUIS) Allergen Nomenclature Sub-Committee. No other form or system of allergen nomenclature is recognized by the WHO or the IUIS. Adherence to the systematic allergen nomenclature is required by all peer-reviewed scientific journals in the field of allergy and immunology. Researchers who identify new candidate allergens are asked to submit their suggested allergen name and associated information to the WHO/IUIS Allergen Nomenclature Sub-Committee before publication of their data. See the Allergen Submission page for details.

Search The Database
By Allergen Name
Search
By allergen source (common or scientific name)
Search

The WHO/IUIS Allergen Nomenclature Sub-committee was founded in 1984 and is composed of leading experts in allergen characterization, structure, function, molecular biology, and bioinformatics. It is responsible for maintaining and developing a unique, unambiguous and systematic nomenclature for allergenic proteins. The sub-committee also reviews new allergen submissions and decides on assignment of names and incorporation of new allergens into the database.

The nomenclature is based on the Linnean system and is applied to all allergenic proteins that cause immunoglobulin E-mediated allergic reactions in humans. The primary goal of a systematic nomenclature is to define a common language for scientists. As such, assessment of new allergen candidates for inclusion into this database does not involve a judgement on their clinical significance. A minimal criterion of demonstrated IgE binding to the suggested allergen using sera from patients allergic to the specific source is required.

The WHO/IUIS Allergen Nomenclature Sub-Committee is supported by financial contributions from

IUIS Immunology without Borders
EAACI
AAAAI American Academy of Allergy Asthma & Immunology

Fig. 8.2: WHO/IUIS subcommittee website on allergen nomenclature—www.allergen.org.

www.allergen.org. This site lists all allergens and isoforms that are recognized by the subcommittee and is updated on a regular basis. As defined in the 1994 revision, allergen names consist of the first three letters from the genus, one letter from the species epithet, followed by an Arabic numeral. Allergens from the same source are classified in biochemical groups (designated by an Arabic numeral that contains two digits), usually according to the order in which they were identified (e.g., Der p 1 or Bet v 1). For example, Peanut—*Arachis hypogaea* (Ara h1, Ara h2, etc.). We can avail the details of each allergen from the website **(Fig. 8.2)**.

TABLE 8.1: German cockroach allergens.

Species	Allergen	Biochemical name	MW (SDS-PAGE)	Route of allergen exposure
Blattella germanica (German cockroach)				
	Bla g 1	Nitrile specifier, microvilli-like protein with unknown function	46 kDa	Airway
	Bla g 2	Inactive aspartic protease	36 kDa	Airway
	Bla g 3	Hemocyanin, Arylphorins/TO Arthropod hemocyanins	78.9 kDa (by mass spectrometry)	Airway
	Bla g 4	Calycin, lipocalin	21 kDa	Airway
	Bla g 5	Glutathione S-transferase (GST) class sigma	23 kDa	Airway
	Bla g 6	Troponin C	21 kDa	Airway
	Bla g 7	Tropomyosin	33 kDa	Airway
	Bla g 8	Myosin, light chain	21 kDa	Airway
	Bla g 9	Arginine kinase	40 kDa	Airway
	Bla g 11	Alpha-amylase	57 kDa	Airway
	Bla g 12	Chitinase	58 kDa	Airway

Source: WHO/IUIS allergen nomenclature database. www.allergen.org.

The data regarding the German cockroach allergens from the WHO/IUIS website are presented in **Table 8.1**.

CHARACTERISTIC FEATURES OF COMPONENT-RESOLVED DIAGNOSTICS

A single test which could be useful for screening, diagnosis, monitoring, and assessing the prognosis: CRD can be used as a screening and diagnostic test, and at the same time can predict the role of immunotherapy and the future course of that particular allergy.

A single test can detect up to 300 allergens: One of the greatest advantages of CRD is that around 300 allergenic components can be detected in a single run. In children, SPT with >20 allergens are extremely difficult, and sIgE tests can detect only one or a few allergens at a time. CRD has a specific role in pediatrics as multiple pricks and samplings could be avoided.

Allergen avoidance measures can be planned more effectively with CRD: If Ara h1 is positive in peanut allergy, roasting at high temperature increases allergenicity. If Ara h1 or Ara h2 is positive, a high risk of severe clinical reactions is anticipated and hence total avoidance and measures such as handling EpiPen for emergency is recommended.

In CMPA, if Bos d4 (alpha-lactalbumin) is positive, it is susceptible to heat denaturation, and hence there is only a very low risk of reaction to baked milk and has a higher chance of outgrowing the allergy. If Bos d8 (casein) is positive, which is resistant to heat denaturation, there is a higher risk of reaction to all forms of milk.

Helps in choosing the right candidate for allergen immunotherapy: CRD enables the development of personalized immunotherapy plans, enhancing efficacy and safety. In case of house dust mite allergy, if Der p 10 is positive and Der p 1 and 2 (major dust mite allergens) are negative, immunotherapy will not be effective as Der p 10 belongs to the tropomyosin group, which cross-reacts with other crustaceans such as shellfish, crab, and cockroaches. The information regarding sensitization to specific components of an allergen may support the decision about immunotherapy of an allergic patient. A patient not sensitized to the major antigenic components will not benefit from specific immunotherapy.

Detection of molecular components helps in risk stratification: The components that are heat-stable and digestion-resistant are associated with the highest risk of serious clinical reactions in the sensitized patient when exposed to the allergen. Therefore, the sensitization to those components has prognostically significant implications.

Examples:
Gal d 1 (ovomucoid), the major egg allergen, causes severe allergic reaction with persistent egg white allergy.

Cow's milk: Bos d 8 (casein) is a major allergic component causing cow's milk allergy, including severe systemic reactions.

Peanut: Ara h 1, Ara h 2, Ara h 3 are storage proteins of peanuts (*Arachis hypogaea*), being the major allergens responsible for sensitization of peanut allergy, and these proteins were identified as potent allergens, causing severe systemic and anaphylactic reactions **(Fig. 8.3)**.

Unanticipated allergen triggers can be identified: During evaluation of allergy, SPT and in vitro tests are planned according to the correlating clinical history. As we do only targeted testing, it is highly likely that we may miss the culprit allergen. In CRD, around 300 allergens are tested simultaneously, and hence a retrospective history focusing on positive results may help us to identify allergens, which are unanticipated.

Use of molecular allergenic components ensures the quality and consistency of the test: SPT and sIgE tests use whole allergen extracts. Storage, handling, and technique can affect the SPT results. Being a molecular level

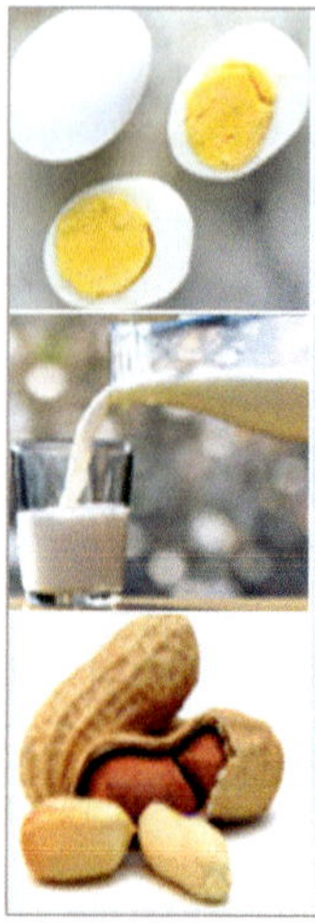

	Allergens	Gal d 1	Gal d 2	Gal d 3	Gal d 4	Gal d 5
	Family	Ovomucoid	Ovalbumin	Ovotransferrin	Lysozyme	Serum albumin
	Severity	+++	++	++	++	++
	Allergens	Bos d 4	Bos d 5	Bos d 8	–	–
	Family	Κ-lactalbumin	Λ-lactoglobulin	Casein	–	–
	Severity	++	++	+++	–	–
	Allergens	Ara h 1	Ara h 2	Ara h 8	Ara h 9	–
	Family	Storage protein	Storage protein	PR-10	LTP	–
	Severity	+++++	+++++	++	++++	–

Fig. 8.3: Summary of the severity of allergic reactions of various components in egg, milk, and peanut.

test, the quality of allergenic components is assured and will be consistently reproducible, which is difficult in SPT.

Persistence or remission in food allergy can be predicted: As we could identify the individual molecular allergenic components it could predict the future course of a particular food allergen, whether that particular allergy will persist or remit.

Example: Among the milk allergens, if Bos d8 (casein) is positive, there is a higher risk of reaction to all forms of milk, and they are unlikely to outgrow milk allergy, especially if sIgE titers are high.

CRD is the future of allergy tests and could aid in research and development in the field of allergy: CRD provides valuable data for researchers, facilitating the discovery of new allergenic components and the development of novel therapeutic approaches.

Identifies true and cross-reactive allergen sensitization and effectively blocks cross-reactive carbohydrate determinants (CCD) interference: SPT positivity to multiple allergens causes a diagnostic dilemma, and in these scenarios, CRD can add information on the genuine primary sensitizers to distinguish them from sensitization due to cross-reactivity **(Fig. 8.4)**. Cross-reactivity in allergic reactions occurs when the proteins in one substance (typically pollen) are similar to the proteins found in another substance (e.g., food). For example, a patient who is allergic to birch tree pollen can have a reaction on eating an apple. Cross-reactivity depends on the presence of conserved antibody-accessible surface structures of proteins. It is observed between members of the same protein family. There is a high degree of cross-reactivity among crustacean shellfish (e.g., shrimp, lobster, crab, crawfish). Usually, cross-reactivity is attributable to labile allergens (e.g., PR-10 and profilins) and associated with mild oral reactions, while heat and proteolysis-resistant allergens that primarily sensitize through the oral route are associated with systemic reactions in addition to local reactions [e.g., seed storage proteins

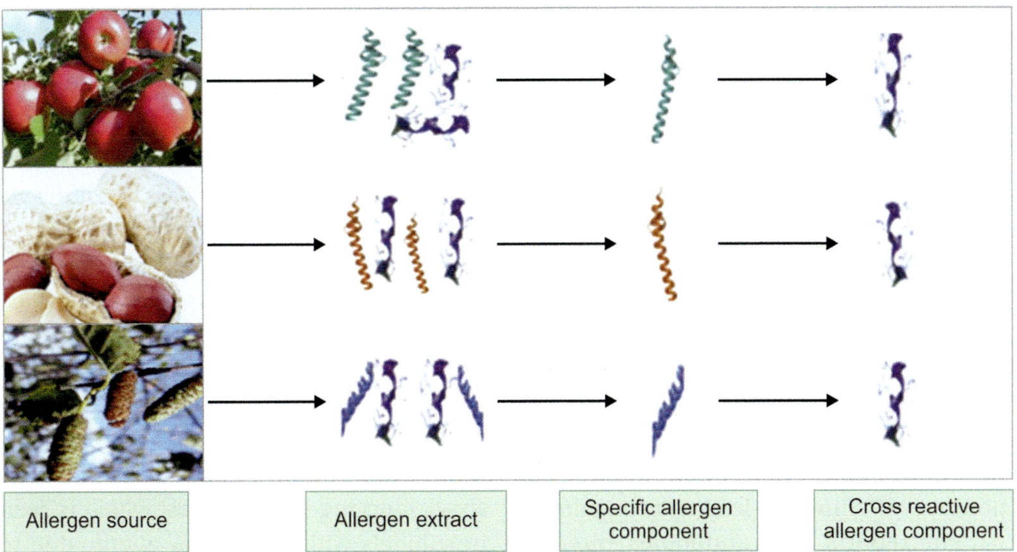

Fig. 8.4: Diagrammatic representation of specific and cross-reactive allergen components.

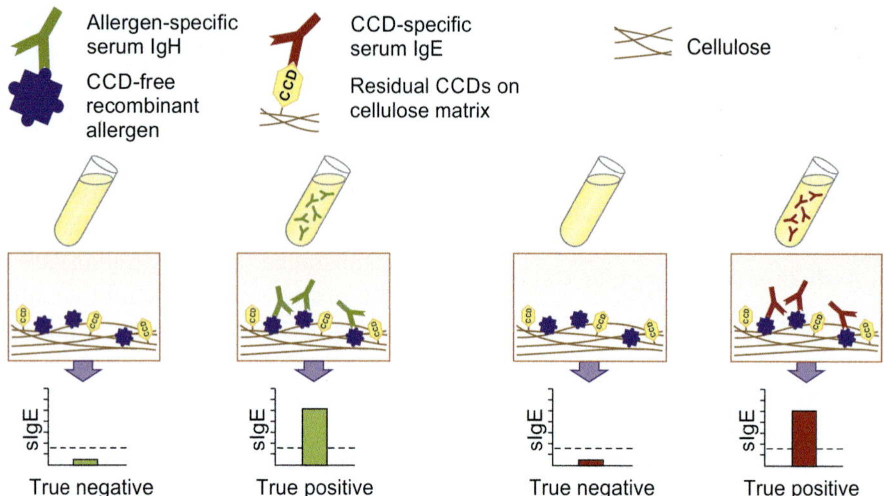

Fig. 8.5: Interference of cross-reactive carbohydrate determinants (CCD) in detection of allergen-sIgE. *Source:* Grosch J, Altmann F, Cross-reactive carbohydrate determinants—history and relevance in allergy diagnostics. Labline Magazine, April 2023.

and nonspecific lipid transfer proteins (nsLTP)]. When patients present a negative history of allergy but positive allergen tests, either the patients have been sensitized by the allergens, but without symptoms of allergy, or some components of allergen extracts of no clinical relevance cause false-positive results, such as "CCD".

Cross-reactive carbohydrate determinant is a carbohydrate residue with a simple structure that exists widely in pollen, food, insect, and latex allergen extracts. CCD can cause false-positive results, leading to erroneous avoidance measures and treatment plans. Therefore, it is crucial to identify CCD-sIgE for the purpose of accurate diagnoses of allergic diseases. Two methods to identify the presence of CCD-sIgE are either to screen CCD-sIgE directly through CRD or to use a CCD inhibitor and then to identify the allergen-sIgE subsequently. The automatic blocking of CCD significantly reduces the number of clinically irrelevant results in patient reports. IgE antibodies directed against CCDs can give a wrong impression of clinically irrelevant polysensitization, leading to inaccurate diagnosis and subsequent nonindicated immunotherapy. CCD blocker is included, which cannot combine with the CCD structures present on the allergens, preventing the binding of CCD-specific antibodies to CCDs on purified allergens **(Fig. 8.5)**.

Common Allergy Cross-reactivity Between Pollen and Foods (Table 8.2)

Complex allergic conditions like cat-pork syndrome can be clearly analyzed: Example—Pork-cat syndrome is caused by immunoglobulin E (IgE)-mediated hypersensitivity to cat serum albumin, which cross-reacts with porcine serum albumin due to antigenic similarity between the two proteins. Its characteristic manifestation is generalized urticaria, angioedema, respiratory disturbance, and anaphylactic shock after ingestion of pork, which is seen in subjects with cat dander allergy due to cross reactivity between cat serum albumin

TABLE 8.2: Cross-reactivity between pollen and food.

Pollen	*Fruits*	*Vegetables*	*Nuts*	*Grains*
Birch	Kiwi, apple, pear, plum, peach, nectarine, apricot, cherry, banana, fig, avocado, strawberry, dried plum, mango	Celery, carrot, parsnip, parsley, dill, cumin, cilantro, fennel, potato, tomato, pepper (green), chicory	Hazelnut, almond, walnut, peanut	Soy, wheat, lentils, peas, beans
Alder	Apple, cherry, peach, pear, strawberry, raspberry	Celery, parsley	Hazelnut, almond, walnut	
Grass	Fig, melon, orange, kiwi, watermelon	Tomato, potato	Peanut	
Mugwort	Mango	Celery, carrot		
Ragweed	Banana, watermelon, melon, honeydew, cantaloupe	Squash, pepper, cucumber, artichoke, hibiscus, zucchini,		Sunflower seeds

and pork serum albumin. CRD can identify the specific allergenic components causing a diagnostic dilemma.

SINGLEPLEX VERSUS MULTIPLEX COMPONENT-RESOLVED DIAGNOSTICS

Component-resolved diagnostics allergens can be either recombinant or naturally purified, and sIgE can be measured either in singleplex or multiplex platforms. With multiplex CRD comprehensive picture of the patient's sensitization profile can be availed, and no preselection of allergens by the physician is required. Depending on the aim of the CRD, the cost and availability in each country, and the complexity of the case, the clinician can choose one or the other. For idiopathic anaphylaxis and suspected food or respiratory allergies with multiple sensitizations, a multiplex CRD should be performed. Multiplex assays allow up to 300 allergen assays in parallel with the use of very low serum quantities and no interference from very high total IgE. Singleplex assays are more sensitive and more suitable for monitoring sensitization.

COMPONENT-RESOLVED DIAGNOSTICS IN FOOD ALLERGY TESTING

The gold standard test for diagnosing food allergy is a double-blind, placebo-controlled food challenge (DBPCFC). DBPCFC is a complicated, time-requiring procedure that carries risk for life-threatening complications such as anaphylaxis. CRD plays a major role in food allergy, and it optimizes the decision of oral food challenge (OFC) in food allergy. In a particular food, different allergenic components have different clinical relevance. *Example:* Identification of primary sensitizer and cross-reactive allergens helps in diagnosing the true culprit allergen. CRD in food allergy could significantly reduce the need for adrenaline autoinjectors and OFC and improve the quality of life.

The major components (pan allergens), widely distributed in natural products and associated with food allergy, include:

- Carbohydrate determinants (CCDs)
- Profilins
- Pathogenesis-related protein 10 (PR-10)
- Nonspecific lipid transfer proteins (nsLTPs)
- Storage proteins

These components differ in terms of heat and digestion stability, cross-reactivity among species, and severity of induced allergic reactions. The detection of sIgE against food components may also explain cross-sensitization between different allergens. The interpretation of CRD test results requires specific knowledge about the properties of the different protein families and their role in the development of specific symptoms, especially in terms of predicting the severity of clinical reactions. IgE against CCDs may cause positive reactions in an immunoassay detecting antibodies against crude extract of an allergen that is not clinically relevant. At the other extreme, patients sensitized to storage proteins are at high risk for anaphylaxis/severe systemic reactions. Severity of the allergic reaction to a component is related to its resistance to heat and digestion in the gastrointestinal tract.

LIMITATIONS OF COMPONENT-RESOLVED DIAGNOSTICS

- As it is costly, affordability is a major limiting factor, especially in developing countries.
- Only an allergy expert with significant knowledge about the allergenic component could interpret CRD.
- Positive tests should be interpreted carefully on the background of history. The presence of sensitization does not always indicate true clinical allergy.
- Overdiagnosis of allergy, especially with the multiplex tests, may lead to unnecessary avoidance and immunotherapy if not properly interpreted.
- More scientific research and data are needed to interpret the CRD results.

SUMMARY

As allergic diseases are on the rise, in vitro diagnostic tests have an important role in clinical medicine. The molecular level allergy testing by CRD is a step forward in allergy diagnosis. It allows for more accurate, personalized, and effective treatment plans for allergic patients. The lack of crude allergen extracts used in SPT and sIgE can be fixed by molecular allergenic component tests. The knowledge about how allergenic components are related to clinical symptoms is important in order to diagnose, treat, and predict the future of food allergies. This will make DBPCFC much less necessary. It will be the future of allergy testing.

KEY POINTS

- In CRD precise diagnosis is possible due to specific allergen component analysis.
- CRD distinguishes between cross reactivity and co-sensitization.
- Even though CRD is a promising investigation it should not be misused and has to be interpreted with caution.
- We require further research to understand the clinical implications of CRD.

SUGGESTED READING

1. Callery EL, Keymer C, Barnes NA, Rowbottom AW. Component-resolved diagnostics in the clinical and laboratory investigation of allergy. Ann Clin Biochem. 2020;57(1):26-35.
2. Dodig S, Čepelak I. The potential of component-resolved diagnosis in laboratory diagnostics of allergy. Biochem Med (Zagreb). 2018;28(2):020501.
3. Emmert V, Lendvai-Emmert D, Eklics K, Prémusz V, Tóth GP. Current practice in pediatric cow's milk protein allergy-immunological features and beyond. Int J Mol Sci. 2023;24(5):5025.

4. Matricardi PM, Kleine-Tebbe J, Hoffmann HJ, Valenta R, Hilger C, Hofmaier S, et al. EAACI molecular allergology user's guide. Pediatr Allergy Immunol. 2016;27 (Suppl 23): 1-250.
5. Treudler R, Simon JC. Overview of component resolved diagnostics. Curr Allergy Asthma Rep. 2013;13(1):110-7.
6. Tuano KS, Davis CM. Utility of component-resolved diagnostics in food allergy. Curr Allergy Asthma Rep. 2015;15(6):32.
7. van Erp FC, Klemans RJ, Meijer Y, van der Ent CK, Knulst AC. Using component-resolved diagnostics in the management of peanut-allergic patients. Curr Treat Options Allergy. 2016;3:169-80.

CHAPTER 9

Rhinolaryngoscopy in Allergy Practice

Anita Krishnan

INTRODUCTION

Rhinolaryngoscopy is a medical procedure that allows the examination of the nose and throat, including the eustachian tubes, adenoids, vocal cords, and more, with the help of fiberoptics. The conventional methods, such as anterior rhinoscopy using Thudichum's speculum, can only look about half an inch into the nose, in which gross pathologies such as deviated nasal septum, polyps, or other space-occupying lesions, the inferior and middle turbinates can be visualized. Conventional posterior rhinoscopy and indirect laryngoscopy using laryngeal mirrors are cumbersome. The conventional methods do not allow good visualization of the recesses, such as eustachian tube ostium, torus tubarius, sphenoethmoidal recess, middle meatus, and sinus ostia. The images are inverted and indirect; hence, the quality of the image is not as good as fiberoptic images.

Endoscopy allows for enhanced visualization and more comprehensive evaluation, improving the diagnostic outcomes. The possibility of manipulation allows for intervention also. There are a range of indications for the use of an endoscope in pediatric otolaryngology, in both emergencies and nonemergencies, including airway obstruction, foreign body removal, evaluation of hoarseness, globus sensation, recurrent epistaxis, evaluation of obstructive sleep apnea, fiberoptic-endoscopic evaluation of swallowing, and assessment and treatment of vocal fold lesions.

INDICATIONS

Rhinolaryngoscopy is an invaluable tool in the diagnosis and management of airway disorders:

- Diagnosing conditions affecting the nose, throat, and voice box
- *Chronic nasal obstruction:* Persistent nasal blockage despite medical therapy (antihistamines, decongestants, etc.)
- In patients with persistent cough, post-nasal drip, hoarseness, or difficulty swallowing, not responding to conservative treatment
- Recurrent or persistent rhinosinusitis where symptoms are unresponsive to standard treatment for sinusitis
- Allergic rhinitis with poor response to treatment where coexisting conditions such as nasal polyps, deviated septum, or adenoidal hypertrophy that could hinder response to allergy treatment are suspected
- Suspected adenoid hypertrophy to assess adenoidal size and obstruction
- Recurrent or chronic otitis media where allergies are the suspected etiology to visualize the nasopharynx and eustachian tube orifice

- Laryngeal symptoms such as chronic hoarseness of voice or phonatory issues
- Unexplained epistaxis (nosebleeds)
- For purposes of documentation, where the images or video may be recorded for further analysis or comparison with future examinations to assess the response to treatment. As there is no radiation involved as in CT scan or X-rays, this is a safe and repeatable investigation.
- *Nasal cytology:* To collect smears from abnormal areas to look for eosinophilic predominance, which is indicative of allergic pathology, or neutrophilic milieu, which is indicative more of infectious pathology.
- Visualizing and removal of impacted foreign bodies of the nose, throat, and upper gastrointestinal (GI) tract.
- *Assessment prior to surgery:* Before adenoidectomy or sinus surgery, to evaluate the anatomy and guide surgical decision-making
- Biopsy of nasal polyps or tumors for preoperative planning

CONTRAINDICATIONS

There are no absolute contraindications for flexible rhinolaryngoscopy (F-RLS):

- Diagnostic endoscopy in acute epiglottitis and croup is a contraindication in pediatric larynx as there is a chance of precipitating laryngospasm, and if absolutely necessary, must be left to an experienced ENT specialist.
- In burns and soft-tissue injury with edema of the laryngopharynx, it is better to avoid instrumentation.
- *Stridor or angioedema:* Stimulation of the laryngopharynx has the potential to further compromise the airway.
- In coagulopathies and craniofacial trauma, rhinolaryngoscopies have to be performed with caution.

EQUIPMENT

Rhinolaryngoscopes are currently available as rigid scopes, eyepiece scopes, videoscopes, and flexible fiberoptic rhinolaryngoscopes.

Rigid rhinolaryngoscopes are primarily used in operation theaters for surgical procedures. The rigid scopes come in various diameters, such as 4 mm (adult) and 2.7 mm (pediatric), and lens angles of 0°, 30°, 45°, and 70° are the ones commonly used in surgical practice.

The flexible fiberoptic rhinolaryngoscope is a small, flexible plastic tube with fiberoptics for viewing the airway. This can be attached to a television camera to provide a permanent record of the examination and to play back and explain to the patient the pathology while discussing their symptoms. In a pediatric allergy practice, it is prudent to invest in a flexible rhinolaryngoscope, due to the ease with which it can be used. The learning curve is faster, the chances of injury due to instrumentation are much less than rigid scopes, and one instrument can handle almost all outpatient requirements.

Flexible rhinolaryngoscopes come in disposable single use or multiple use. The COVID-19 pandemic brought in the need for balancing careful infection control with fiscal and environmental responsibility. This led to the advent of single-use flexible rhinolaryngoscopes. Once used, the disposable devices are transported to specialized facilities where they are disassembled and converted to raw materials and energy.

TECHNIQUE OF EXAMINATION: PREPARATION AND POSITION

During the procedure, the nose is decongested with a nose spray of oxymetazoline or xylometazoline. In certain cases, especially in endoscope-assisted nose and paranasal sinus surgeries, the nose is decongested by packing the nose with adrenaline cotton patties.

This is followed by a local anesthetic nose spray; the commonly used one is 10–15% lignocaine. One could also use 4% lignocaine drops instilled along the septum and lateral walls in a very slow trickle with the patient lying supine with his neck hyperextended, or 4% lignocaine can be delivered to the nose by a standard nasal atomizer. While performing rigid nasal endoscopy, it is easier if the patient is supine with the head end elevated by 15°, whereas F-RLS can be done both in the sitting position and in the supine, lying down position. For scoping a small child, it is more comfortable if the child is sitting slightly reclined on the parent's lap.

TECHNIQUE OF RHINOLARYNGOSCOPY

The patient is given a brief description of the procedure at the very onset to keep them at ease. A thin layer of Savlon antiseptic liquid (cetrimide 3.0% w/v and chlorhexidine digluconate 0.3% w/v) applied to the tip of the scope over the lens provides adequate antifogging. The shaft of the scope can be lubricated with lignocaine jelly to enhance the anesthetic effect.

The examination is conducted in a consistent sequence, with the scope entering the nasal cavity in three passes. The scope is held in the right hand with the thumb being free to move the lever, which tilts the tip of the scope up and down. The left-hand thumb, index, and middle fingers stabilize the tip of the scope to slowly slide it into the nose. In the first pass, the scope is passed between the floor of the nasal cavity and the inferior turbinate, slowly advancing to the nasopharynx to examine the adenoids and eustachian tube orifices and fossa of Rosenmüller on either side. In the second pass, the endoscope is passed between the middle turbinate and inferior turbinate to examine the middle meatus, sinus ostia, sphenoethmoidal recess and sphenoid ostium and superior turbinate. While withdrawing the endoscope, the tip can be rotated laterally for a better view of the middle turbinate, uncinate, ethmoid bulla, and infundibulum. The third pass is done above the middle turbinate, and the tip of the endoscope is tilted 90° upward to inspect the olfactory cleft. While examining the nasal cavity, encourage the patient to breathe through the mouth to prevent fogging of the lens on the tip of the scope by the warm exhaled air. Especially in children who have small nasal passages, certain parts of the nasal examination can get uncomfortable. The presence of deviated nasal septum, polyps, etc., obstructs the free passage of the scope, but with adequate training, it is possible to maneuver the scope down into the nasopharynx and further into the laryngopharynx.

After entering the nasopharynx, the endoscope tip is gently flexed inferiorly. The clinician should ensure that the endoscope stays in the midline along the posterior pharyngeal wall. The patient is encouraged to breathe gently through the nose at this juncture and avoid swallowing to prevent the soft palate from obstructing the view. Swallowing at this point will not be dangerous but could cause an uncomfortable sensation, just as if someone were to touch the back of the throat.

The endoscope is advanced into the oropharynx to check on the base of tongue, the epiglottis, the valleculae, the glosso-epiglottic fold, and the lateral epiglottic folds. The endoscope is then passed over the tip of epiglottis to visualize the arytenoid and cuneiform cartilages, the aryepiglottic folds and true vocal cords, the interarytenoid space and a few upper rings of trachea which can also be seen through the glottic chink. At this point, the patient is asked to say "eeee" or "aha" to assess the mobility of the vocal cords.

ANATOMIC STRUCTURES VISUALIZED AND OBSERVABLE PATHOLOGIES

The parts of the upper aerodigestive tract that are visualized during rhinolaryngoscopy are nasal cavity **(Figs. 9.1A and B)**, nasopharynx, oropharynx, larynx, and hypopharynx in order of appearance while the scope is introduced through the nose.

Nasal Cavity

The nasal cavity is the first area examined and is a complex space with several important structures. The nasal vestibule is the entrance to the nasal cavity and is lined with skin containing hair (vibrissae). Folliculitis and furuncles are the pathologies expected here, along with human papillomavirus (HPV) warts and foreign bodies. The nasal valve is the narrowest part of the nasal airway and is the area at the junction of the upper lateral cartilage, the anterior end of the inferior turbinate, and the nasal septum. A deviated spur of the nasal septum and hypertrophied anterior end of the inferior turbinate can further compromise the nasal valve and cause increased nasal blockage.

Nasal Septum

Nasal septum is the bony cartilaginous partition wall dividing the nasal cavity into left and right sides. The septum is rarely straight in adults and is formed by the quadrangular septal cartilage anteriorly, resting on the groove of the maxillary crest, articulating with the thin perpendicular plate of ethmoid posteriorly and the thicker vomer bone inferiorly.

It may show deviations, perforations, hemangiomatous polyps, or septal spurs. The Little's area is located at the anterior-inferior part of the nasal septum. The vascular network of arteries that form the Kiesselbach's plexus is situated here and could be seen as prominent and congested or raw areas in children suffering from recurrent epistaxis.

Turbinates (also called Concha)

Turbinates are scroll-like structures on the lateral nasal walls, and their examination can reveal inflammation, hypertrophy, or

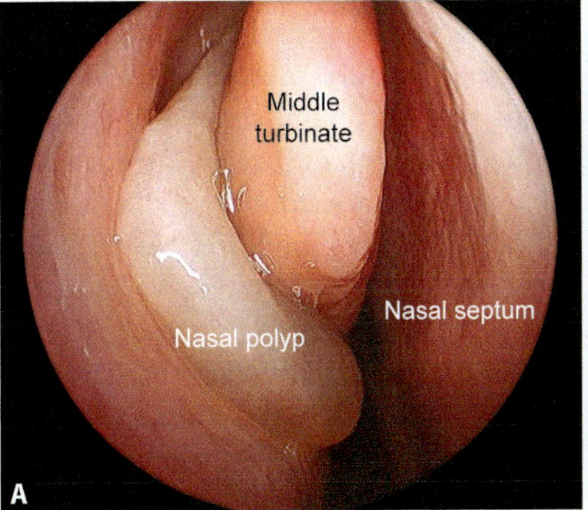

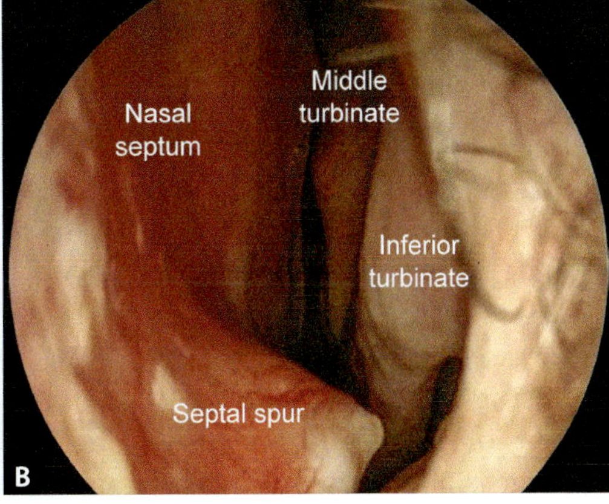

Figs. 9.1A and B: Rhinolaryngoscopic view of nasal cavity.

atrophy. The turbinates provide warming, cooling, and humidification of inspired air. They also provide resistance to airflow, aiding in the filtration of inspired air.

Inferior turbinates are the largest and extend the whole length of the nasal cavity. The different pathologies change the shape and texture of the turbinates. In patients with allergic rhinitis, the turbinates have a characteristic pale bluish color with a boggy, turgid appearance that could be partially or almost totally blocking the nasal cavity and looks extra moist. In nonallergic rhinitis, the inferior turbinates are congested and hypertrophied with a fleshy, beefy appearance. In rhinitis sicca and rhinitis medicamentosa, the turbinates are fleshy, beefy, and crusty.

Middle turbinates are smaller and located above the inferior turbinates. This is a common location to see nasal polyps and thick mucopurulent secretions that signify acute and chronic sinusitis.

Superior turbinates are the smallest and highest in the nasal cavity. In general terms, edema, erythema, secretions, polyps, and bluish boggy swelling of mucosa all indicate inflammation.

Nasal Meatus

The area lying immediately posteroinferior to the turbinates, or between the turbinates and the lateral nasal wall, is termed the nasal meatus.

Inferior meatus is posteroinferior to the inferior turbinate and contains nasolacrimal duct (NLD) opening. In chronic dacryocystitis, the NLD opening could look edematous and congested, with mucopurulent secretions in severe cases.

Middle meatus is situated between the inferior and middle turbinates and is the drainage site for frontal, maxillary, and anterior ethmoid sinuses.

This is a key area that shows the earliest signs of sinonasal diseases such as polyps. Mucopurulent secretions seen here signify sinusitis and bulging signifies pressure in the sinuses and thinning of sinus walls as seen in mucopyoceles or space-occupying lesions.

Superior meatus lies between the middle and superior turbinates and is the drainage site for posterior ethmoid and sphenoid sinuses. Sphenoethmoidal recess is the area above the superior turbinate and contains the opening to the sphenoid sinuses.

Nasopharynx

The area of the pharynx where the choana opens into is the nasopharynx. The important structure to look for is the adenoids. Depending on the amount of space in the nasopharynx occupied by the adenoids, it is graded as:

- *Grade 1:* <25% obstruction of the nasopharynx
- *Grade 2:* 25–50% obstruction of the nasopharynx
- *Grade 3:* 50–75% obstruction of the nasopharynx
- *Grade 4:* >75% obstruction of the nasopharynx

In some cases, mucus or purulent discharge may be visible on the surface of the adenoids, suggesting chronic adenoiditis or coexisting sinusitis. These children complain of postnasal drip and short, dry cough, or frequent clearing of throat. The eustachian tube cushions are important structures on the lateral wall of the nasopharynx, which could be pressed upon by enlarged adenoids. If this is observed, it is important to check the middle ear for secretory otitis media and do tests for eustachian tube dysfunction.

Rhinolaryngoscopy is an important tool in both the diagnosis and management of choanal atresia **(Fig. 9.2)**.

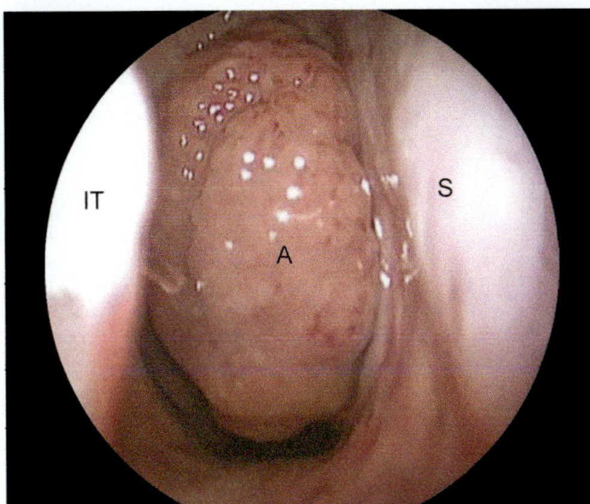

Fig. 9.2: Rhinolaryngoscopic view of nasopharynx. (A: adenoids; IT: inferior turbinate; S: septum)

Oropharynx

The oropharynx extends from the base of the tongue to the pharyngeal wall.

The structures visualized in the oropharynx are the palatine tonsils bilaterally, the tonsillar pillars, the base of tongue where one may sometimes encounter lingual thyroid or lingual tonsils, posterior and lateral pharyngeal walls.

Cobble-stoning of the posterior pharyngeal mucosa is a sign of chronic postnasal drip and irritation, often seen in children with chronic allergies or rhinosinusitis.

Larynx

The larynx is situated just below the pharynx and comprises three paired smaller cartilages (arytenoids, corniculate, cuneiform) and three larger unpaired cartilages (epiglottis, thyroid, cricoid). The epiglottis is situated at the base of the tongue and forms a lid to protect the airway from aspiration of gastric contents and is the first structure visualized in a laryngoscopy. The pediatric epiglottis is more anteriorly slanted overhanging the glottic aperture and covering it partially making the visualization of the glottic chink tricky.

At the base of the tongue, the pocket of cartilage anterior to the epiglottis is the vallecula, and the most commonly observed pathology in the vallecula is a mucous retention cyst.

Posterior to the epiglottis, the glottic chink is visualized where the glistening white paired vocal cords are seen and their texture and movements can be assessed by asking the patient to phonate.

Laryngeal redness or vocal cord edema is suggestive of allergic laryngitis or laryngopharyngeal reflux. Long-standing laryngopharyngeal reflux disorder (LPRD) shows interarytenoid pachydermia.

Juvenile laryngeal papillomas, vocal nodules, vocal cord polyps, cysts of the vocal cords, vocal cord paralyses, etc., are some of the common pathologies observed in children.

Hypopharynx (Fig. 9.3)

The inferior portion of the pharynx, comprising the posterior pharyngeal wall, the postcricoid region, and the paired recesses lateral to the larynx, called the pyriform sinuses, constitutes the hypopharynx.

Pooling of saliva in the pyriform sinus signifies obstruction at postcricoid or impacted foreign body in the upper digestive tract.

SUMMARY

Rhinolaryngoscopy can complement allergy testing and help refine treatment strategies, especially in children with complex or refractory symptoms, with suspected sinus drainage issues, adenoid hypertrophy, or nasal polyps contributing to recurrent infections. It helps in differentiating allergic and nonallergic causes of symptoms along with other laboratory workup and allergic skin

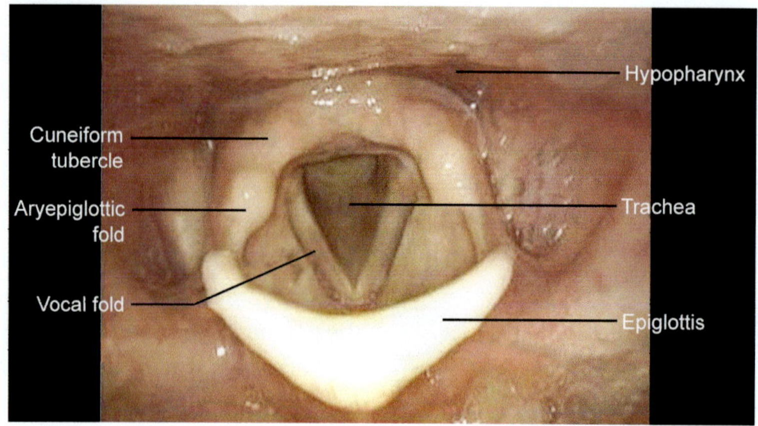

Fig. 9.3: Rhinolaryngoscopic view of hypopharynx.

testing. Rhinolaryngoscopy has its limitations too and is a complementary diagnostic tool in the management of allergic rhinitis. Advances in rhinolaryngoscopic techniques and instrumentation have expanded the role of rhinolaryngoscopy in pediatric allergy management.

Flexible rhinolaryngoscopy is an underused procedure that can provide allergists-immunologists and other physicians with several benefits over the existing imaging techniques.

Direct visualization of the nasal cavity is an easily mastered skill that can facilitate complete evaluation of the nasopharyngeal tract. It is a simple, safe, convenient, and economic procedure. F-RLS is indeed underused in allergy-immunology.

KEY POINTS

- Superior visualization of nasal and laryngeal structures beyond conventional methods.
- Key diagnostic tool in allergy practice for refractory rhinitis, sinus disease, adenoids, and laryngeal symptoms.
- Particularly valuable in children with recurrent infections or coexisting anatomical issues.
- Flexible scopes preferred—safer, easier, less traumatic, and versatile for outpatient use.
- Safe and repeatable—radiation-free, allows documentation, biopsy, foreign body removal, and cytology.
- Underused yet highly useful—deserves wider application in allergy–immunology practice.
- Photographs in this chapter are courtesy

ACKNOWLEDGMENT

Dr Ashesh Bhumkar, Bhumkar ENT Hospital, Thane, Maharashtra, India.

SUGGESTED READING

1. Czachor A, Diaz JD, Cho SH, Lockey RF. The Use of Flexible Rhinolaryngoscopy for Allergy-Immunology Practice. J Allergy Clin Immunol Pract. 2023;11(1):149-157.e1.

CHAPTER 10

How to Maintain an Asthma Diary?

Akshay Holla, Soundarya M

INTRODUCTION

Asthma is a common respiratory disease among children in India, with its incidence increasing each year, due to rapid urbanization and worsening air pollution. When compared to the developed nations, both the mortality and morbidity rates are higher in India, highlighting the urgent need for a comprehensive approach toward asthma management. Effective patient follow-up is an equally important step after appropriate medical treatment. An asthma diary serves as a simple and cost-effective tool for tracking symptoms and medication usage in children with asthma. They serve as an easy-to-understand visual cue for patients, which helps in treatment adherence. To the treating doctor, they help in keeping track of the patient's triggers and symptoms, so that preventive and therapeutic measures can be taken up appropriately.

An asthma diary can be crafted depending on the individual's requirements for the diary.

For example:

- To document daytime symptoms of asthma, asthma daytime symptom diary (ADSD) can be used, and to document nighttime symptoms, asthma nighttime symptom diary (ANSD) can be used. This data can be used to start appropriate treatment as per standard guidelines.
- To indicate the change in symptoms with respect to new treatment, that is, to assess the response to new treatment.
- To document daily peak expiratory flow rate, which can help predict acute exacerbation/acute asthma attacks.
- Diary should also include a column for the common triggers that a patient feels were responsible for exacerbations, identification of which helps them to seek early preventive measures.

ADVANTAGES OF AN ASTHMA DIARY TO PATIENTS

Maintenance of a daily record by patients ensures adherence to their medications. Gaps in such records can identify reasons for noncompliance/skipped days in the treatment. By regularly documenting potential triggers in their diary, patients can work with their doctors to develop strategies to avoid them, such as allergens, which have been proven to be the cause. They also help patients understand acute asthma exacerbations. Early recognition of symptoms such as shortness of breath, chest tightness, or worsening cough, or a change in frequency of symptoms/reducing in peak expiratory flow (PEF) value seen from past records of the diary can lead to early visits to healthcare facilities and avoid unnecessary admissions and healthcare-related expenditure.

ADVANTAGES OF AN ASTHMA DIARY TO THE PHYSICIAN

For doctors, these records help monitor treatment response compliance with medication, thereby optimizing medical management. Decisions on step-up or step-down treatment plans become easier based on documented evidence of asthma symptoms rather than relying on recall of symptoms over the last month. The treating physician can keep track of the cumulative steroid exposure over a year, this can help identify potential complications and comorbidities expected and help patients take appropriate measures. Based on the severity of symptoms and frequency of reliever medications needed, and PEF records, they can help doctors decide on early referrals to specialists or severe asthma clinics. Furthermore, the prospective data obtained from a pool of children is a valuable source of data, for clinical trials and developing biomarkers that are predictive of asthma exacerbations, asthma control, and asthma-related quality of life.

LIMITATIONS OF THE DIARY

Although keeping a regular diary has many benefits, it can have a few drawbacks. Daily exposure to the visual representation of their symptoms, medications used, and the frequent hospital visits may be difficult to maintain as the parents of asthmatics are already burdened with health care expenditure and time lost in hospital visits, and the children may not have accurate symptom representation. If the child is young, the responsibility for maintaining the record falls on the parents, which can be difficult for working parents.

The asthma diary **(Table 10.1)** is read with guidelines from the Global Initiative for Asthma (GINA) 2024.

- *Well-controlled asthma:*
    - Not more than twice per week, daytime symptoms
    - No nighttime symptoms
    - No restriction in school or play/activity
    - No daily use of salbutamol/reliever (occasional use <1/week)
    - Normal peak expiratory flow rate (PEFR)
- *Partly controlled asthma:*
    - One to two of these symptoms are present.
    - Use of salbutamol/reliever >1/week
- *Uncontrolled asthma:*
    - All of the above
    - Use of salbutamol/reliever daily

TABLE 10.1: Asthma diary.

Day/date	Daytime symptoms	Nighttime symptoms	Need for salbutamol/day	School attendance	Play and activity	PEFR	Any fever

(PEFR: peak expiratory flow rate)

Flowchart 10.1: Pediatric asthma diary maintained by child.

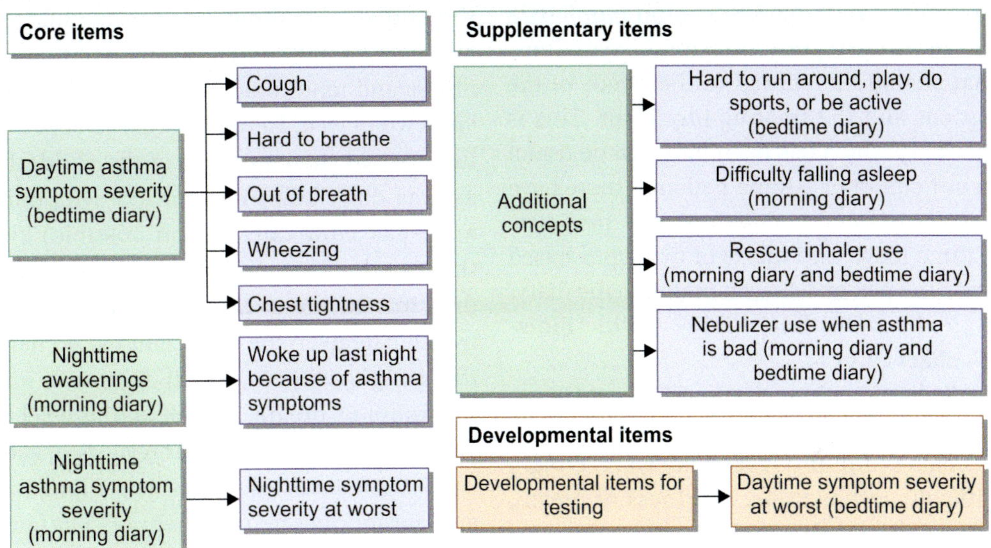

Flowchart 10.2: Pediatric asthma diary maintained by caregiver.

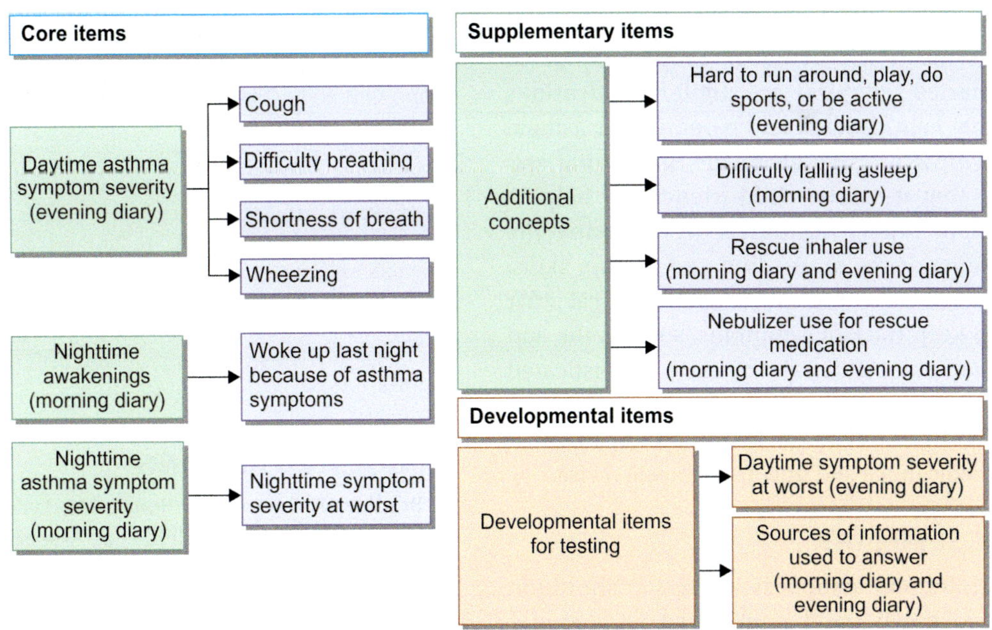

By regularly charting the child's symptoms, the actual control of asthma can be deciphered. Many physicians rely more on this diary than the parent's description, as at times the parent could exaggerate or downplay the child's symptoms.

There is no universally standardized asthma diary format. Organizations such as

GINA, the European Respiratory Society, and the American Lung Association emphasize the need for regular tracking of symptoms that should be tailored to the needs of the patient and the treating physician. This is our diary which has been found to be useful in our cohort of asthma patients. There have been attempts at developing a pediatric asthma diary, and this is of two types based upon the person who can maintain the diary:

1. Pediatric asthma diary—Child **(Flowchart 10.1)**
2. Pediatric asthma diary—Observer **(Flowchart 10.2)**.

The symptoms assessed were cough, difficulty in breathing, shortness of breath, wheezing, and chest tightness. The domains impacting the quality of life that were assessed were physical activity, school performance, sleep, social functioning, and emotional wellbeing.

Electronic pediatric asthma symptom diaries (ePASDs) are digital applications that help children and parents track asthma symptoms. The advantage of a digital app is that it can be child-friendly by helping them report accurately by reducing the dependence on reading and writing skills. ePASDs can be as simple as a digital calendar to keep track of symptoms, such as the app made by IAP Kerala, or more sophisticated apps such as FindAir and Omron, that even send reminders for taking daily controller medications and upcoming hospital visits.

SUMMARY

Childhood asthma is a chronic condition and needs good monitoring and regular checking of inhaler and medication compliance along with technique revisions. Single OPD visits cannot help understand the status of asthma control as children tend to visit more often during intermittent illness and tend to delay/miss health check visits when well. Hence in order to correctly understand the condition of the child, the asthma diary helps plot the key symptoms and Peak Flow rates (when possible) and thus guides the clinician in appropriate drug management. The diary is maintained by the caregiver/the older child and charts the cough, wheeze, chest tightness and shortness of breath as well as the level of activity of the child. Regular reviews of such carefully maintained diaries help a long way and appropriate management of childhood asthma and achieve good control.

KEY POINTS

- Asthma diary is a carefully maintained diary by the caregiver/older child regarding the asthma symptoms and activity of the child as advised by GINA.
- It helps in monitoring asthma control and in helping taper down or scale up asthma medications as well as gives a guide regarding reinforcing of inhaler technique and compliance.
- Maintenance of the diary must be taught to all caregivers and children and must be brought on all OP or ER visits for appropriate asthma control

SUGGESTED READING

1. Bradley H, Trennery C, Jones AM, Lydon A, White F, Williams-Hall R, et al. Assessing asthma symptoms in children: qualitative research supporting the development of the Pediatric Asthma Diary-Child (PAD-C) and Pediatric Asthma Diary-Observer (PAD-O). J Patient Rep Outcomes. 2023;7(1):104.

CHAPTER 11

Asthma Diary: A Mobile App for Asthma Symptom Assessment

Peter P Vazhayil

INTRODUCTION

Living with asthma can often feel like balancing a lot at once—symptoms, inhalers, action plans, and hospital visits. Tracking symptoms regularly and following an asthma action plan are vital steps in improving patient outcomes. With the advancements in mobile health (mHealth) technologies, innovative solutions are now available to empower patients. One such solution is this handy app, acting as your personal asthma sidekick to help you log symptoms, stick to your action plan, and generate detailed symptom reports with ease, all from the comfort of your phone.

Link: https://play.google.com/store/apps/details?id=com.asthma.diary

WHAT DOES THE APP DO?

When you open the app, the first thing you see is a colorful *calendar view*. It is like your personal health diary. Click on a date and log your symptoms **(Figs. 11.1 and 11.2)**.

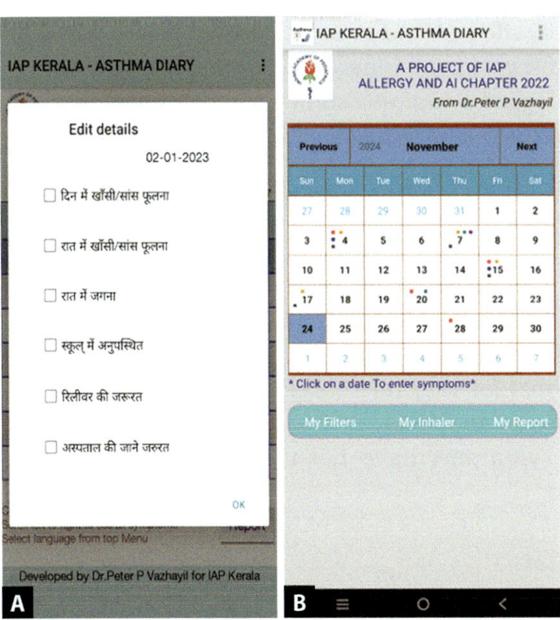

Figs. 11.1A and B: App screenshots. (A) Log symptoms; (B) Calendar view.

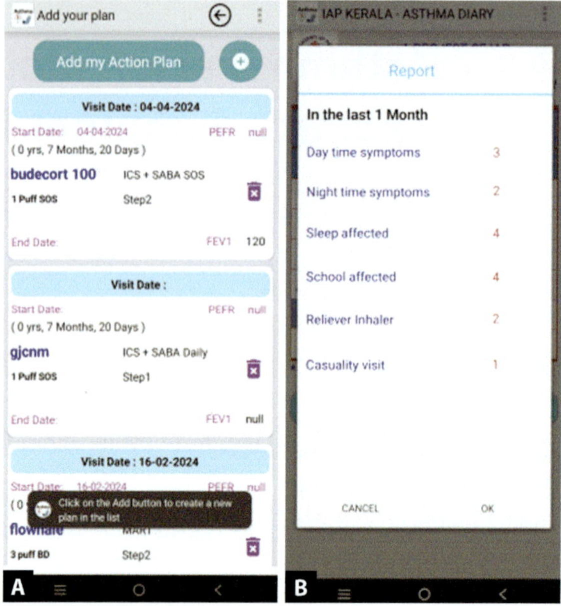

Figs. 11.2A and B: App screenshots. (A) Action plan; (B) Report generation.

Log Symptoms

When you click on a date, a pop-up window opens with the symptoms such as daytime symptoms, nighttime symptoms, use of a reliever inhaler, activity affected, and casualty visit. Tick the boxes for your symptoms, and you are done. Your logged symptoms show up as colorful dots on the calendar, making it super easy to spot patterns at a glance.

Report Generation

The app allows you to generate detailed reports spanning the past 4 weeks to an entire year. These reports are also presented in a clear, Excel-style format for easy reference. This means your doctor can quickly review how your asthma symptoms have been progressing over time.

Asthma Action Plan

You can document action plans, including details of inhalers (e.g., medication names, dose, start dates, and end dates) and other diagnostic details.

Track and Filter Symptoms

Want to know how often you have been using your inhaler or how many cough-free days you have had? Use the filter option to focus on specific symptoms.

Multilanguage Support

You can log your symptoms in three languages: English, Hindi, or Malayalam.

UTILITY FOR PATIENTS AND PHYSICIANS

You can always know what is going on with your asthma. Tracking your symptoms can help you spot triggers, stay on top of your action plan, and feel more in control.

This will help you consult your doctor with a detailed report instead of trying to remember when you last had a bad night.

COOL FEATURES

Simple logging: No complicated menus—just click, tick, and done.

Color-coded calendar: Those tiny colorful dots on the calendar make symptom tracking surprisingly easy!

Symptom logging: A simple and intuitive interface to log symptoms for any selected date.

Language selection: A pop-up menu for language selection.

Privacy first: All your data stays on your phone—no sneaky sharing with anyone.

POTENTIAL IMPACT

The asthma diary app is not just a tool—it is a health companion. It simplifies life for people with asthma, making it easy to stay on top of symptoms and treatment plans.

FUTURE DIRECTIONS

To expand its utility, future versions of the app will include:

- Medication reminders to enhance adherence
- Educational modules to improve patient knowledge of asthma management.

SCREENSHOTS

Figures 11.1 and 11.2 are the screenshots of asthma diary app.

SUMMARY

The Asthma Diary app is a mobile tool designed to help children with asthma, to track their symptoms and generate reports for physicians. It provides a simple, user-friendly calendar interface where symptoms can be logged. The app supports multilingual use (English, Hindi, Malayalam), ensures privacy by storing data only on the device, and allows the physicians to better assess the level of control of asthma.

KEY POINTS

- *Symptom logging:* Patients can record daytime/nighttime symptoms, reliever use, activity limitation, and hospital visits with a simple, intuitive interface.
- *Calendar and reports:* A color-coded calendar and Excel-style reports (covering 4 weeks to 1 year) help track trends and share progress with physicians.
- *Asthma action plan:* Users can document medications, dosages, and treatment timelines for better adherence.
- *Filtering and tracking:* The app allows filtering by specific symptoms (e.g., inhaler use, cough-free days) for personalized monitoring.
- *Patient–physician utility:* Empowers patients to spot triggers and provides doctors with objective, detailed symptom reports.
- *Cool features and future add-ons:* Multilanguage support (English, Hindi, Malayalam), privacy-first design, with upcoming features like medication reminders and educational modules.

SUGGESTED READING

1. Digital Health Technology in Asthma: A Comprehensive Scoping Review. J Allergy Clin Immunol Pract. 2021;9(6):2377-98.
2. Chan AHY, Drummond D, Ramakrishnan S, van Boven JFM, Gibson PG, Thomas D. Digitally mapping the asthma journey—from diagnosis to remission. EClinicalMedicine. 2025;83:103204.
3. Use of a digital tool to support and optimise high-risk asthma patients NHS UK;2022.

12 CHAPTER

Peak Expiratory Flow Rate

Hima Mathews P

INTRODUCTION

It is defined as "the highest flow achieved from a maximal forced expiratory maneuver started without hesitation from a position of maximal lung inflation" (Miller et al. 2005).

The maximum flow rate generated during a forceful exhalation, beginning from the level of maximal lung inflation, i.e., full inspiration, is called peak expiratory flow rate (PEFR). Peak flow meter is a portable handheld simple flow gauge device with defined standards of reproducibility and accuracy. PEFR measurement is a cost-effective outpatient procedure to identify airway obstruction, to predict impending asthma exacerbation, and also an indicator of the severity of disease. Spirometry can also measure the peak flow rate. PEFR reflects the caliber of the large or proximal airways, with a diameter >2 mm, and it is conventionally measured in liters per minute. As distal airways have no cartilaginous support, they are likely to be affected by mucus plugging and collapse, and asthma being a disease of both small and large airways, PEFR may not always be a good tool.

PEAK EXPIRATORY FLOW RATE AND SPIROMETRY

Forced expiratory volume in 1 second (FEV1) is the amount of air forcibly exhaled during the forced maneuver and recorded as part of spirometry. PEFR and FEV1, are both used to quantify the degree of obstruction, and the correlation between PEFR and FEV1 is controversial. PEFR is widely available and easy to perform. In those with significant air trapping (residual volume/total lung capacity >30%) PEFR may not accurately detect the severity of airway obstruction. PEFR assesses obstruction predominantly in larger airways, and spirometry can be abnormal even with normal PEFR.

FACTORS AFFECTING THE PEAK EXPIRATORY FLOW RATE

- *Anthropometry:* Standing height is the single best predictor in children, also having almost a linear relationship with weight, body surface area, and chest expansibility.
- *Age and sex:* PEFR decreases with age from 30 to 40 years onward after an increase in the pediatric and adolescent age group. The association is linear in females and curvilinear in males.
- *Ethnicity:* Predicted normal values vary according to population.
- *Environmental factors:* Particulate air pollution and environmental smoke cause a decline in PEFR in children.
- *Respiratory tracts and chest wall abnormalities:* Thoracic cage deformity and respiratory tract infection can affect the PEFR adversely.

- *Malnutrition:* As the growth of the large airways is affected by acute and chronic malnutrition, it can also cause a reduction in PEFR.
- *Diurnal variation:* Diurnal variation of 20% or more in PEFR is a good indicator of asthma.

PEAK EXPIRATORY FLOW RATE AND THE CIRCADIAN RHYTHM

There is a normal circadian rhythm for PEFR in the absence of external stimuli, with a daylight maximum and night-time minimum, with a difference in the circadian bronchomotor tone between normal and asthmatic individuals. Minimum PEFR occurs at about *04:00 hours*, which is when plasma histamine is at its maximum and plasma cyclic adenosine monophosphate (cAMP) and epinephrine are at their minimum. Plasma cortisol achieves its minimum around midnight. It has been found that validation of the morning dip by PEFR was a good indicator of the severity of asthma in various studies.

Peak Flow Meter

Figure 12.1 shows the parts of peak flow meter.

HOW TO PERFORM PEAK EXPIRATORY FLOW RATE

Peak flow rate requires patient cooperation and with appropriate training it can be performed in children over 5 years. Small children and those who lack coordination or have difficulty in understanding the instructions, may not be able to perform PEFR **(Figs. 12.2A to D and Box 12.1)**.

ERRORS IN PERFORMING PEAK EXPIRATORY FLOW RATE

- Failure to achieve maximum inspiration
- Delay in blowing into the meter after maximal inhalation
- Teeth or tongue obstructing the mouth-piece
- Cough during exhalation
- Mouthpiece leaks

ROLE OF PEAK FLOW METER IN PRACTICE

- To diagnose asthma
- To predict the impending exacerbation in asthma
- To identify the triggers
- As a follow-up tool in asthma
- To diagnose occupational asthma

INTERPRETATION OF PEAK EXPIRATORY FLOW RATE

Even though a PEFR >80% of the reference value can be considered as normal, there is a wide variation in the normal reference range. PEFR should be ideally interpreted in

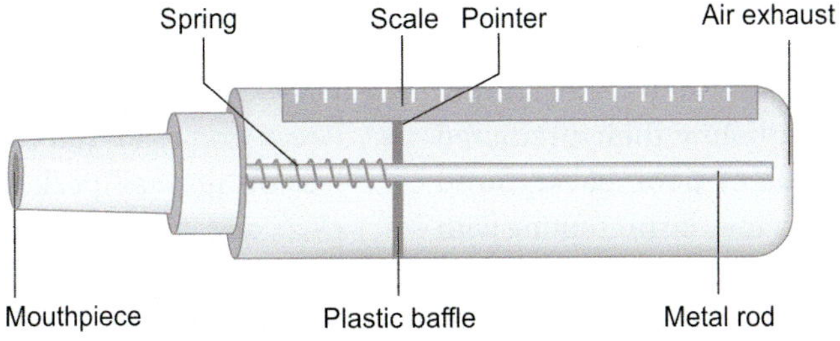

Fig. 12.1: Parts of peak flow meter.

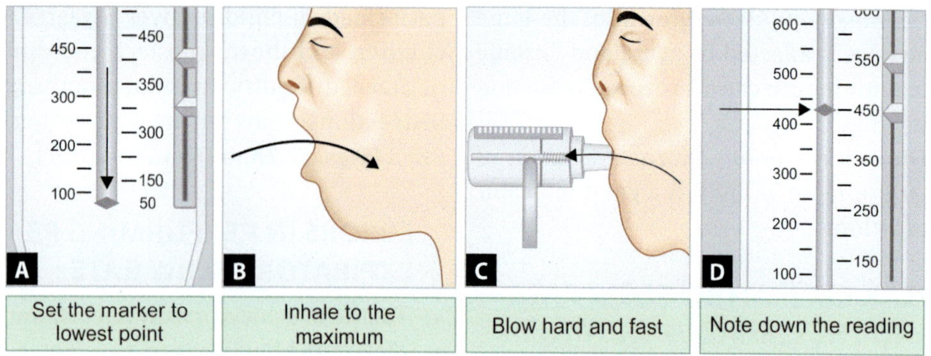

Figs. 12.2A to D: Peak expiratory flow rate (PEFR) testing technique.

BOX 12.1: Steps in performing peak expiratory flow rate (PEFR).

1. Standing or sitting straight is preferred, and the same posture should be maintained while repeating the PEFR daily
2. Slide the marker down and set it at the bottom of the scale
3. Fit the mouthpiece correctly
4. Take a deep breath in and hold
5. Place the mouthpiece in the mouth with the tight seal of lips around it
6. Blow out as hard and fast as possible
7. Remove the device and note the number
8. Repeat the same steps two more times, resetting the marker to zero each time, with proper relaxation between the attempts, and peak flow is the highest of these three readings

BOX 12.2: Steps in finding the personal best peak expiratory flow (PEF).

The "personal best" peak flow is the highest number you can perform over a 2-week period when asthma is under good control.

1. Perform peak flow testing twice a day for 2 weeks following the correct steps.
2. It has to be done at the same time in the morning and in the early evening using the same device.
3. It should be preferably done before taking any inhalers.
   To calculate the patient's PEF as a percentage of the reference value or best ever reading:

$$\frac{\text{PEF recording}}{\text{Reference value or patient's best}} \times 100$$

the pediatric age group in comparison with a patient's best reading **(Box 12.2)**. Personal best reading should ideally be recorded over a period of 2 weeks and should be revised regularly as the child grows. Nomograms or calculators can be used to give a "predicted" value if the personal best value is not known. If it is significantly below their predicted value, this may reflect poor background control, and the child may be presenting with very significant airway obstruction even with a small fall from their personal best. Similarly, a child who has previously been able to perform PEFR but is unable to do so in the emergency department (ED) points toward a more severe exacerbation.

Regular use of peak flow will help you to recognize early decreases in airflow, and the asthma action plan should be prepared using peak flow readings in different zones:

- *Green zone:* 80–100% of your personal best or "normal" peak flow rate signals all clear, and it is no-problem zone.
- *Yellow zone:* 50–80% of your personal best and signals caution and warrants the need for quick reliever medications.

- *Red zone:* <50% of your personal best and signals a medical alert and need referral to the emergency room (ER).

For example, if your personal best *peak expiratory flow (PEF) is 200 L/min,* the zones will be:

- *Green zone:* 160–200 L/min (80–100%)
- *Yellow zone:* 100–160 L/min (50–80%)
- *Red zone: <100 L/min (<50%)*

SIGNIFICANCE OF PEAK EXPIRATORY FLOW RATE

When reliable spirometry cannot be performed in a child, PEFR can aid in documenting airway obstruction. It is highly recommended to document airway obstruction and to confirm the asthma diagnosis before starting treatment.

Criteria that would suggest variable expiratory flow limitation include:

- *Bronchodilator responsiveness (BDR):* Increase in baseline PEF ≥15% (4 × 100 µg salbutamol and retesting after 15 minutes or anticholinergics 4 × 40 µg ipratropium bromide and retesting after 30 minutes).
- *Increase in lung function after 4 weeks of treatment:* Increase in baseline PEF ≥15%
- *Positive bronchial challenge test:* Fall in PEF >15% predicted after a standardized exercise challenge
- *Excessive variation in lung function between the visits:* Variation in PEF ≥15% between visits
- *Diurnal variation of PEFR indicates sensitivity of airways:* Excessive variability in twice daily PEFR monitoring over 2 weeks with average daily diurnal PEF variability >13%.

(Variability is calculated from twice daily readings as the daily amplitude percent mean, i.e., highest reading of the day-lowest reading/mean of both values × 100, then the average of each day's value is calculated over 1–2 weeks).

To calculate diurnal variability in serial PEF measurements:

$$\frac{\text{Highest PEF reading-lowest PEF reading}}{\text{Highest PEF reading}} \times 100$$

Recordings above 70% of personal best are an indicator of reducing the drug dosage, and below 70% is an indicator of starting or increasing the dose. Average PEFR continues to increase and diurnal PEFR variability decreases for about 3 months after the initiation of treatment. Excessive variation in PEFR recordings (20–30%) suggests suboptimal asthma control and increases the risk of exacerbations. If there is a change of >15% after use of bronchodilator, in a child on treatment for asthma, indicates suboptimal control. If there is a diurnal variability of >20%, for at least 3 days in a week can be considered an indicator of poor asthma control.

Low PEFR can help in identifying triggers causing worsening of asthma symptoms (especially when the exposure to allergens outside the home). Long-term home monitoring of PEFR can be suggested for poorly controlled asthma and those having a low perception of worsening of asthma symptoms. Accuracy of interpretation increases by plotting PEFR on a standardized chart. Children who perceive airflow limitation poorly can have a significant decline in lung function without any worsening of symptoms, progression to near-fatal asthma, and regular PEF monitoring at home should be considered for such patients. A written asthma action plan specifying short-term treatment changes, including PEFR values based on their personal best, along with symptoms, helps the parents to identify and take the necessary steps to prevent ER visits.

SUMMARY

PEFR is a simple, objective test that measures the maximum rate of airflow from the lungs during a forceful exhalation. PEFR values reflect the degree of airway obstruction, which is a hallmark of asthma. PEFR can predict the control and impending worsening of asthma. The patient's "personal best" PEFR should be measured and the readings should be interpreted according to that value. PEFR should be a part of asthma action plan and it can also be used in diagnosing asthma if spirometry is not available.

KEY POINTS

- Peak expiratory flow rate is a good test to document variable expiratory airflow limitation if spirometry is unavailable or not able to be performed.
- It is a good tool to be included in the asthma action plan, to assess the severity of the asthma episode, and to monitor response to therapy.
- In cases of severe airway obstruction and air trapping, the PEFR may underestimate the degree of obstruction, especially in the smaller airways.
- PEFR should not be considered as a replacement for spirometry, and the value cannot be compared with FEV1.

SUGGESTED READING

1. Ahmed M, Gavhane J, Goel S. Age-specific peak expiratory flow nomogram in children. Indian J Pediatr. 2017;84(9):678-82.
2. Davis SD, Eber E, Koumbourlis AC (Eds). Diagnostic Tests in Pediatric Pulmonology: Applications and Interpretation. New York: Springer; 2014.
3. Dobra R, Equi A. How to use peak expiratory flow rate. Arch Dis Child Educ Pract Ed. 2017;102(6):296-300.
4. Global Initiative for Asthma (GINA). Global Strategy for Asthma Management and Prevention, 2024 Update.
5. Lebowitz MD. The use of peak expiratory flow rate measurements in respiratory disease. Pediatr Pulmonol. 1991;11(3):166-74.
6. Long J. Peak Expiratory Flow Rate: Monograph. University of Glasgow.
7. Miller MR, Hankinson J, Brusasco V, Burgos F, Casaburi R, Coates A, et al. ATS/ERS Task Force: standardisation of spirometry. Eur Respir J. 2005;26(2):319-38.
8. Mridha MAA, Amin MR, Kabir ARML. Peak expiratory flow rate (PEFR): a simple ventilatory lung function test. J Shaheed Suhrawardy Med Coll. 2011;3(2):44-7.
9. Proceedings of the 16th International Congress of Pediatric Pulmonology; 2017 Jun 22-25; Lisbon, Portugal. Pediatr Pulmonol. 2017;52(Suppl 46):S1-S181.
10. Ruffin R. Peak expiratory flow (PEF) monitoring. Thorax. 2004;59(11):913-4.
11. Srisingh K, Phuaksaman C. The reference values of peak expiratory flow rate in Thailand children. J Thorac Dis. 2021;13(1):31-8.
12. Taussig LM, Landau LI (Eds). Pediatric Respiratory Medicine, 2nd edition. Philadelphia: Mosby Elsevier; 2008.
13. Wilmott RW, Deterding RR, Li A, Ratjen F, Sly PD, Zar HJ, et al. (Eds). Kendig's Disorders of the Respiratory Tract in Children, 9th edition. Philadelphia: Elsevier; 2019.

13

CHAPTER

Spirometry

Hima Mathews P

INTRODUCTION

Spirometry is a simple test, which measures lung volume changes during the forced breathing maneuvers with graphical display along with the numerical values. It gives an estimation of lung function, and it is a good tool for the diagnosis of airway obstruction and follow-up for asthma and chronic obstructive pulmonary disease (COPD).

Lung volume is divided, according to normal physiological function. Each subdivision is called a volume, whereas any combination of two or more volumes is called a capacity **(Fig. 13.1)**.

LUNG VOLUMES

- *Tidal volume:* It is the volume of air inhaled or exhaled during each respiratory cycle.
- *Expiratory reserve volume (ERV):* It is the volume of air that can be exhaled forcibly after exhalation of normal tidal volume.
- *Inspiratory reserve volume (IRV):* The volume of air, which could be forcibly inhaled above the normal tidal volume. IRV is attained during deep breathing.
- *Residual volume (RV):* It is the volume of air remaining in the lungs after a maximal exhalation.

LUNG CAPACITY

- *Inspiratory capacity (IC):* Inspiratory capacity is the sum of inspiratory reserve volume and tidal volume. IC = IRV + TV. The maximum volume of air that can be inhaled is known as inspiratory capacity.
- *Total lung capacity (TLC):* TLC is calculated by summation of the four

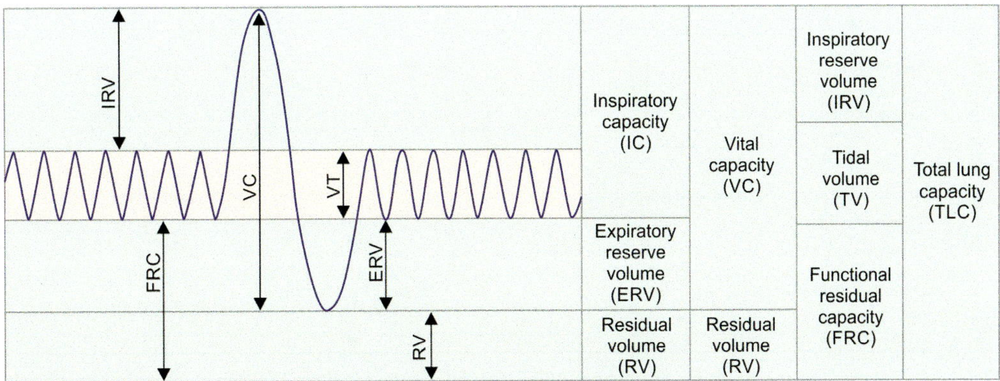

Fig. 13.1: Lung volume and capacities.

primary lung volumes (TV + IRV + ERV + RV). The maximum volume of air, which could be accommodated in the lungs after maximum inspiration, is called TLC.

- *Vital capacity (VC):* It is the total amount of air exhaled after maximal inhalation. It is calculated by summing tidal volume, inspiratory reserve volume, and expiratory reserve volume. VC = TV + IRV + ERV.
- *Functional residual capacity (FRC):* It is the amount of air remaining in the lungs at the end of a normal exhalation. It is calculated by adding together residual and expiratory reserve volumes. FRC = RV + ERV.

SPIROMETRIC MEASURES (FIG. 13.2)

- *Forced vital capacity (FVC):* Following a maximal inspiration the volume of air in liters, which can be forcefully and maximally exhaled, is known as FVC.
- *Forced expiratory volume in 1 second (FEV_1):* Volume of air exhaled in 1 second of FVC is known as FEV_1, i.e., volume of air in liters that can be forcefully and maximally exhaled in 1 second after a maximal inspiration.
- *FEV_1/FVC ratio:* This ratio is used to differentiate an obstructive from a restrictive pattern. The ratio will be decreased in obstructive disorders, because the decrease in FEV_1 is higher compared to FVC. In restrictive disorders, the drop in FEV_1 is less marked than drop in FVC, and the ratio is either normal or increased. The ratio is higher in children up to 0.9 and 0.7 in adults. The ratio decreases with age due to decrease in elastic recoil of the lungs.
- *Forced expiratory flow at 25% and 75% of the pulmonary volume (FEF 25–75%):* It is the mean FEF during the middle half of the FVC and measures average flow rates on the FVC segment and includes flow from medium-to-small airways. FEF 25–75% is supposed to be the most sensitive indicator of airflow in peripheral airways where primary airflow

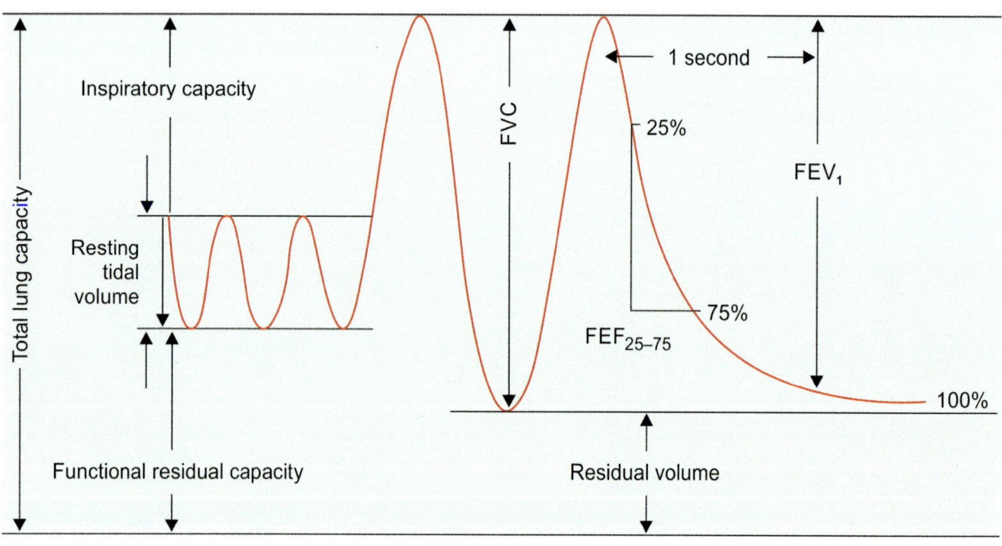

Fig. 13.2: Parameters measured in spirometry. (FEF: forced expiratory flow; FEV_1: forced expiratory volume in 1 second; FVC: forced vital capacity)

obstruction originates, and it is reduced in early bronchial impairment, which is associated with small airway disease.

- *Peak expiratory flow (PEF):* The maximum flow of air soon after the start of forceful exhalation.

STEPS IN PERFORMING SPIROMETRY

Steps in performing spirometry are shown in **Box 13.1**.

Checklist to Avoid before Spirometry Test

Checklist to avoid before spirometry test is mentioned in **Box 13.2 and Table 13.1**.

PEDIATRIC SPIROMETRY INDICATIONS

Pediatric spirometry indications are shown in **Box 13.3**.

Common clinical scenarios requiring spirometry in children include:

- Persistent wheezing
- Diagnosis and prognostication of asthma
- Chronic cough
- Cystic fibrosis
- Assessing the control of asthma and disease activity of cystic fibrosis in children
- Assessing the pediatric lung function, in transfusion-dependent thalassemia major and sickle-cell anemia, connective tissue disorders, and chest wall deformities
- Preoperative spirometry is found to be helpful in assessing the postoperative lung status of the pediatric population.

BOX 13.1: Steps in performing spirometry.

1. Make sure quality control and standards for equipment performance
2. Prepare the child
3. Get a detailed history and analyze the indication
4. Check for contraindications (any recent illness or medications)
5. Enter patient demographics accurately (age, gender, height, weight, and race)
6. Explain how to perform the test, instruct, and demonstrate
7. Perform maneuver and repeat for a minimum of three maneuvers
8. Check for acceptability, usability, and repeatability
9. Check for bronchodilator responsiveness
10. Interpret the graph and values

BOX 13.2: Checklist before performing spirometry.

- Check the medication list
- Avoid alcohol consumption within 4 hours and other intoxicants within 8 hours before testing (as it can affect coordination, comprehension, and physical ability)
- Avoid smoking within 1 hour as it may cause bronchoconstriction
- Wearing restrictive clothing as it may prevent proper chest expansion
- Performing vigorous exercise within 1 hour to avoid exercise-induced bronchospasm)
- Eating large meal within 2 hours

TABLE 13.1: Drug withholding time prior to spirometry.

Bronchodilator medication	***Withholding time***
SABA (e.g., albuterol or salbutamol)	4–6 hours
SAMA (e.g., ipratropium bromide)	12 hours
LABA (e.g., formoterol or salmeterol)	24 hours
Ultra-LABA (e.g., indacaterol, vilanterol, or olodaterol)	36 hours
LAMA (e.g., tiotropium, umeclidinium, aclidinium, or glycopyrronium)	36–48 hours

(LABA: long-acting beta-agonist; LAMA: long-acting muscarinic antagonist; SABA: short-acting beta-2 agonist; SAMA: short-acting muscarinic antagonist)

- Effective tool for assessing the lung health of school-going children

Contraindications

Although there is no absolute contraindication for spirometry, the following conditions are considered relative contraindications:

- *Cardiovascular:* Recent myocardial infarction or pulmonary embolism, uncontrolled systemic or pulmonary hypertension, significant arrythmias, and cough syncope
- *Raised intracranial or intraocular pressure:* Cerebral aneurysms, recent concussion injury, recent eye surgery (1 week) or recent brain surgery (4 weeks)
- *Raised thoracic and abdominal pressure:* Hemoptysis of unknown origin, pneumothorax, recent thoracic or abdominal surgeries
- Sinus/middle ear infection or recent surgery, transmissible respiratory infections
- Acute illness such as fever, nausea, or vomiting, which may affect the performance

BOX 13.3: Indications in performing spirometry in children.

- To establish whether pulmonary mechanics are normal in a child with symptoms
- To define the nature and severity of any pulmonary dysfunction (obstructive vs. restrictive defect).
- To define the site of airway obstruction-central vs. peripheral or intrathoracic vs. extrathoracic
- To follow the course of pulmonary disease or assess the effect of therapy
- To establish the presence or absence of airway reactivity
- To assess the risks of diagnostic or therapeutic procedures
- To monitor the adverse effects of chemotherapy or radiation therapy
- To predict prognosis or assess disability
- To assess the effect of disease on lung growth

Any of the above can be considered as a relative contraindication, and spirometry could be performed after complete recovery.

PATIENT POSITIONING

- *Sit upright:* Standing position and sitting up straight without leaning forward with no restrictions is the ideal posture.
- Feet should be flat on floor with legs uncrossed to avoid the use of abdominal muscles
- Avoid tight-fitting clothing as they can give falsely lower volumes, i.e., restrictive pictures on spirometry
- A chair with arm support is preferred as the forceful exhalation may cause fainting and light headedness.

Different Techniques in Performing Forced Breathing Maneuver

Different techniques in performing forced breathing maneuver are shown in **Box 13.4**.

There is no consensus about the benefits of using a nasal clip in open-circuit spirometry. It can depend on the experience of the technician, and can be decided on individual basis to obtain the best results.

BOX 13.4: Techniques in performing spirometry.

- Before performing the forced expiration, normal tidal breaths can be taken initially followed by a deep breath taken in through the mouthpiece, without pausing for >2 seconds, followed by a quick, full inspiration, i.e., blast air out as hard and fast as possible and for as long as possible, measuring expiratory and inspiratory flow *(closed-circuit method)*
- Alternatively, a deep breath can be taken in then the mouthpiece placed tightly around the mouth before a full expiration is performed, measuring expiratory flow *only (open-circuit method)*
- Or child can be asked to completely empty their lungs then take in a quick full inspiration, followed by a full expiration

Performing Spirometry in Children

- Explain the procedure to the child in a simple way and allow the child to have one or two practice trials in a relaxed fashion
- Re-emphasize by exaggerated demonstration rather than words on how to do it correctly with a positive reinforcement technique
- With good training prior to the spirometry encouraging the child to prolong blowing the air, toward the end of the maneuver, children as young as 5 years of age are often able to perform acceptable spirometry
- Different interactive programs such as games and animated incentives in software designed to encourage rapid and prolonged expiration help in pediatric spirometry.
- The study should be brief, lasting no >15 minutes and if the patient cries during the study, there should be no further attempt, and the test should be done later only.

ACCEPTABILITY AND USABILITY CRITERIA (NEW AMERICAN THORACIC SOCIETY GUIDELINES)

Table 13.2 depicts the acceptability and usability criteria [new American Thoracic Society (ATS) guidelines].

Repeatability Criteria

Repeatability criteria is shown in **Box 13.5**.

Back-extrapolated Volume (Fig. 13.3 and Box 13.6)

Back-extrapolation method can determine the beginning of forced expiration **(Box 13.6)**. A large back-extrapolated volume (BEV) will usually result in an erroneously high FEV_1. There should be <0.025 L change in volume for at least 1 s, which is the most reliable indicator of complete expiration.

End of Forced Expiration

Children as well as those with restrictive lung disease cannot expire long enough to achieve a plateau due to high elastic recoil and in that scenario, the measure of whether end of forced expiration (EOFE) has been reached is for the patient to repeatedly achieve the same FVC.

- The two best values should meet the repeatability criteria, and if the criteria are not met more attempts are required.
- As performing forced exhalations is extremely tiring, a maximum of eight maneuvers kept as an upper limit and beyond that point its unlikely to obtain better values.
- There should be ≥30 seconds between forced maneuvers to avoid bronchoconstriction.

FACTORS AFFECTING SPIROMETRY VALUES

- *Age:* After an increase with age up to ~25 years, spirometry values decline with advancing age.
- *Sex:* Lung function remains same in both sex in the prepubescent period. As growth of the thorax is more in males, after puberty lung volumes are more in males.
- *Height:* Lung volume increases with height.
- *Weight:* Till the point of obesity lung function increases and after that lung function has an opposite effect.
- *Ethnicity*
- *Smoking:* It causes rapid decline in the lung function compared with nonsmokers.

NORMAL PATTERN

In a normal spirometry, FVC, FEV_1, and FEV_1/FVC values will be the predicted range. Spirometry values in the normal range

TABLE 13.2: Acceptability and usability criteria (new ATS guidelines).

	Required for acceptability		***Required for usability***	
Acceptability and usability criterion	***FEV_1***	***FVC***	***FEV_1***	***FVC***
Must have BEV ≤ 5% of FVC or 0.100 L, whichever is greater	Yes	Yes	Yes	Yes
Must have no evidence of a faulty zero-flow setting	Yes	Yes	Yes	Yes
Must have no cough in the 1 second of expiration	Yes	No	Yes	No
Must have no glottic closure in the 1 second of expiration	Yes	Yes	Yes	Yes
Must have no glottic closure after 1 second of expiration	No	Yes	No	No
Must achieve one of these three EOFE indicators: 1. Expiratory plateau (≤0.025 L in the last 1 second of expiration) 2. Expiratory time ≥15 seconds 3. FVC is within the repeatability tolerance of or is greater than the largest prior observed FVC	No	Yes	No	No
Must have no evidence of obstructed mouthpiece or spirometer	Yes	Yes	No	No
Must have no evidence of a leak	Yes	Yes	No	No
If the maximal inspiration after EOFE is greater than FVC, then FIVC-FVC must be ≤0.100 L or 5% of FVC, whichever is greater	Yes	Yes	No	No

(ATS: American Thoracic Society; BEV: back-extrapolated volume; EOFE: end of forced expiration; FIVC: forced inspiratory vital capacity; FEV_1: forced expiratory volume in 1 second; FVC: forced vital capacity)

Source: Stanojevic S, Kaminsky DA, Miller MR, Thompson B, Aliverti A, Barjaktarevic I, et al. ERS/ATS technical standard on interpretive strategies for routine lung function tests. Eur Respir J. 2022;60(1):2101499.

BOX 13.5: Repeatability criteria for spirometry.

Repeatability criteria (applied to acceptable FVC and FEV_1, values)

- *Age 6 years:* The difference between the two largest FVC values must be ≤0.150 L, and the difference between the two largest FEV_1, values must be 0.150 L
- *Age 6 years:* The difference between the two largest FVC values must be 0.100 L or 10% of the highest value, whichever is greater, and the difference between the two largest FEV_1, values must be ≤0.100 L or 10% of the highest value, whichever is greater

(FEV_1: forced expiratory volume in 1 second; FVC: forced vital capacity)

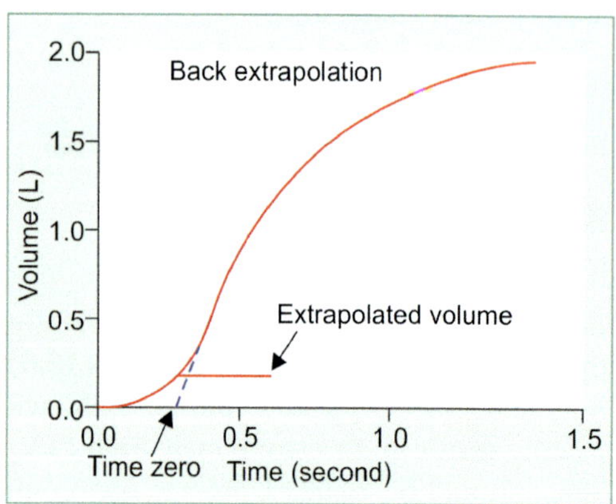

Fig. 13.3: Graphical representation of back-extrapolated volume.

cannot completely rule out lung disease, especially if the pretest probability of disease is elevated and if the recorded values are near the lower limit of normal (LLN). In asthmatics, spirometry can be normal during asymptomatic period.

Flow-volume Loop

Flow-volume loop is shown in **Figures 13.4 and 13.5**.

Slow start, glottic closure, submaximal effort, and tongue occlusion are examples of unacceptable spirometry **(Figs. 13.6 and 13.7)**.

BOX 13.6: Definition of back-extrapolated volume.

The back-extrapolated volume (BEV) is the volume of gas that has already been expired from maximal lung volume to time 0 and is included in the FEV_1 and FVC measurements. To ensure that the FEV_1 comes from a maximal effort, the BEV must be 5% of the FVC or 0.100 L, whichever is greater.

(FEV_1: forced expiratory volume in 1 second; FVC: forced vital capacity)

Volume-time Curve

Volume-time curve is shown in **Figure 13.8**.

INTERPRETING SPIROMETRY

Results should be compared against reference values or predicted values. Even though there are so many reference charts available, which are derived from data from population surveys derived using different reference equation. The Global Lung Function Initiative (GLI) reference equations, provides a single suite of pulmonary function test (PFT) equations

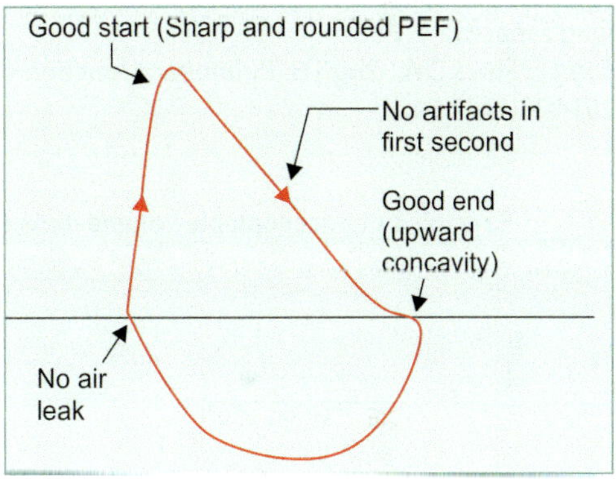

Fig. 13.4: Ideal flow-volume loop. (PEF: peak expiratory flow)

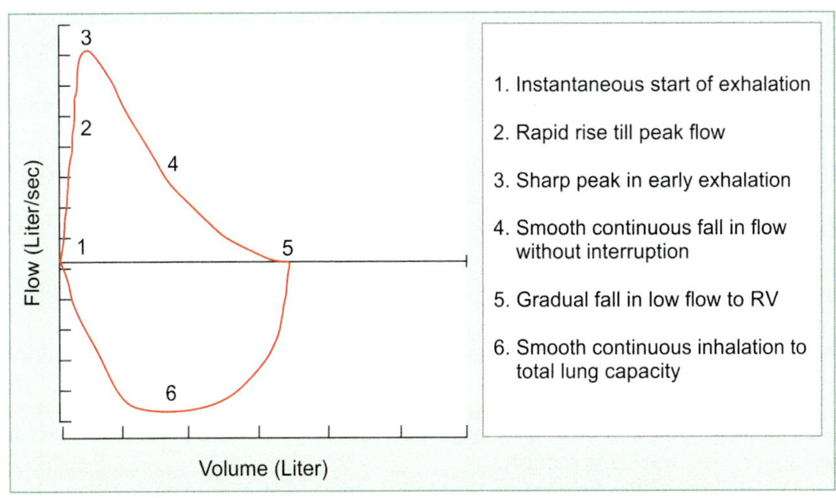

Fig. 13.5: Explanation of an ideal flow-volume loop. (RV: residual volume)

Acceptable efforts
Flow
Volume
Submaximal effort
Not at TLC
Cough
Start not rapid
Steps prematurely or glottic closure
Submaximal inspiration
Tongue occlusion

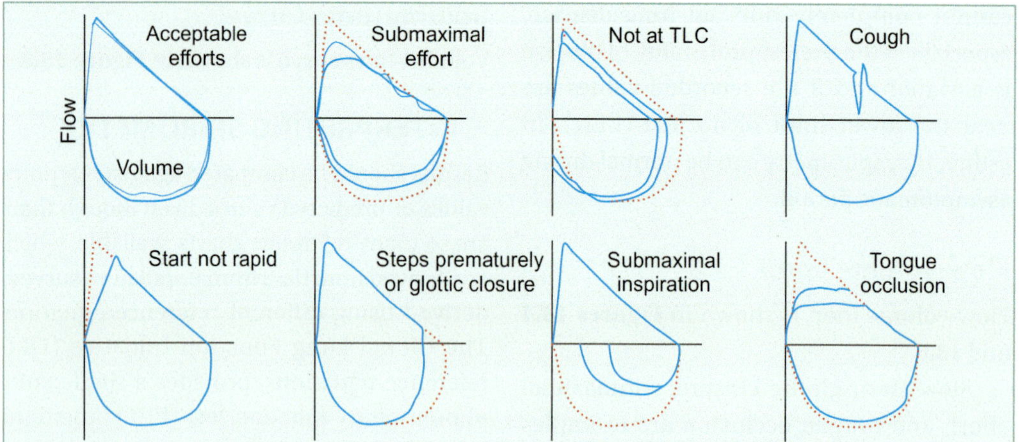

Fig. 13.6: Comparison between acceptable and unacceptable flow volume loops in spirometry. (TLC: total lung capacity)
Source: Sewa DW, Ong TH. Pulmonary function test: Spirometry. Proceedings of Singapore Healthcare. 2014;23(1):57-64.

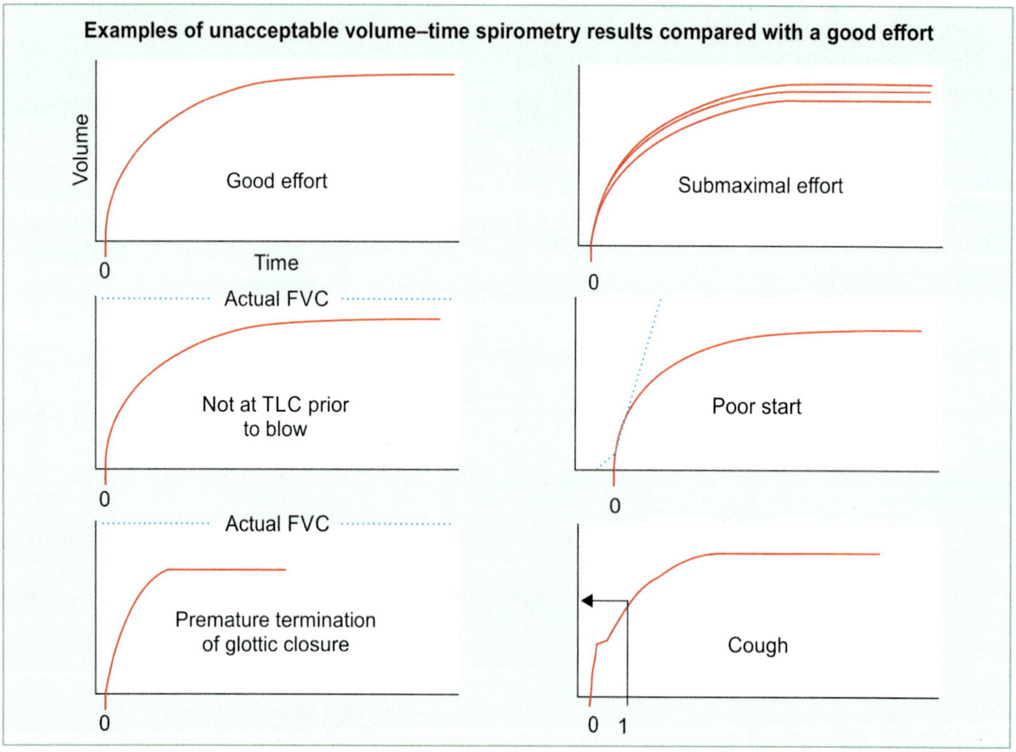

Examples of unacceptable volume–time spirometry results compared with a good effort
Volume
Good effort
0
Time
Submaximal effort
0
Actual FVC
Not at TLC prior to blow
0
Poor start
0
Actual FVC
Premature termination of glottic closure
0
Cough
0 1

Fig. 13.7: Comparison between acceptable and unacceptable volume-time curve in spirometry. (FVC: forced vital capacity; TLC: total lung capacity)
Source: Pierce R, Johns DP (1995). Spirometry: The Measurement and Interpretation of Ventilatory Function in Clinical Practice. University of Tasmania. Book. https://hdl.handle.net/102.100.100/539748

for spirometry. The 5th and 95th percentile limits (–1.645 and +1.645, *z*-scores) of the healthy population can be used to identify individuals with unusually low or high results, respectively. Ideally limits of normal ought to be based on an individual's predisease measure, or baseline. As there are no standards available to take that into consideration, careful medical history of an individual is necessary when interpreting lung function results when using the limits of normal. The concept of LLN provides an indication of whether the observed result can be expected in otherwise healthy individuals of similar age, sex, and height, and may not necessarily indicate a pathophysiological abnormality or a clinically meaningful threshold to diagnose disease. A spirometry value in the expected range for a particular subject cannot exclude the presence of a disease process. For example, a drop from 90th to 10th percentile is a very significant change but still leaves lung function within normal limits. The widely used absolute cut-offs of 80% of predicted for FEV_1 and the 0.70 cut-off for the FEV_1/FVC ratio have to be strongly discouraged as per the new ATS guidelines.

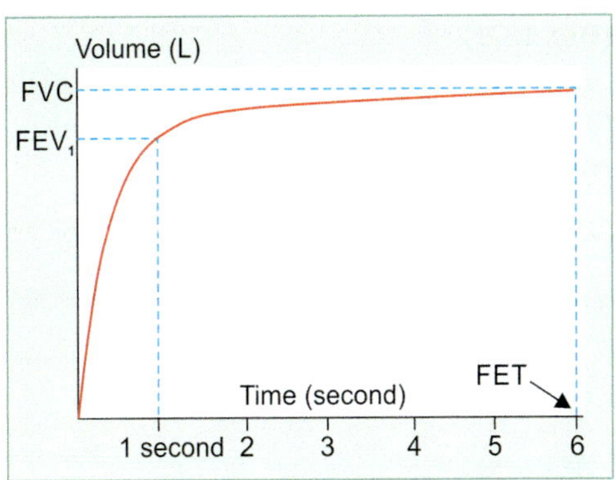

Fig. 13.8: Normal volume-time curve. (FEV_1: forced expiratory volume in 1 second; FET: forced expiratory time; FVC: forced vital capacity)

Bronchodilator Responsiveness Testing

A baseline spirometry has to be performed meeting acceptability and repeatability criteria. After that, a bronchodilator is given preferably using a spacer, which is either a short-acting β-agonist (SABA) (4 × 100 μg salbutamol and retesting after 15 minutes) or anticholinergics (4 × 40 μg ipratropium bromide and retesting after 30 minutes). Changes in FEV_1 and FVC following the bronchodilator should be expressed as the percent change relative to the individual's predicted value. "A change >10% of the predicted value in FEV_1 or FVC indicates a positive response" **(Box 13.7)**.

CLASSIFICATION OF LUNG FUNCTION IMPAIRMENT

The following classification using *z*-score values should be used to grade the lung function impairment, according to the new guidelines **(Box 13.8)**.

BOX 13.7: Equation to determine BDR.

Determination of a bronchodilator response

$$\text{Bronchodilator response} = \frac{[\text{Postbronchodilator value (1)} - \text{Prebronchodilator value (1)}]}{\text{Predicted value (1)}} \times 100$$

A change of >10% is considered a significant BDR response.
Predicted value should be determined using the appropriate GLI spirometry equation.

(BDR: bronchodilator response; GLI: Global Lung Function Initiative)

Source: Stanojevic S, Kaminsky DA, Miller MR, Thompson B, Aliverti A, Barjaktarevic I, et al. ERS/ATS technical standard on interpretive strategies for routine lung function tests. Eur Respir J. 2022;60(1):2101499.

Both the European Respiratory Society (ERS) and the ATS have endorsed the LLN as 1.645 standard deviation (SD) below the mean value applying the 5th percentile LLN **(Fig. 13.9)**.

Identifying Abnormal Ventilatory Patterns

- Is the shape of the flow-volume curve normal?
- Is FEV_1/FVC ratio normal? FEV_1/FVC ratio <LLN identifies expiratory airflow obstruction. Use $FEV_1\%$ predicted to assess severity.
- Is FVC normal? FVC <LLN identifies potential restriction.

BOX 13.8: Lung impairment classification using scores.

- *z*-score >–1.645 (normal)
- *z*-score between –1.645 and –2.5 (mild)
- *z*-score between –2.5 and –4 (moderate)
- *z*-score <–4.1 (severe)

OBSTRUCTIVE AIRWAY DEFECT

An obstructive airway defect is characterized by FEV_1/FVC ratio <LLN. If there is no airway obstruction, major part of FVC will be exhaled in 1 second of the forced exhalation. In obstructive pattern, FEV_1 will show a lower peak flow and a scooped/concave expiratory loop **(Fig. 13.10)**. Airway narrowing can occur either by a physical obstruction or by dynamic collapse of the airway. Airflow resistance, at large lung volumes, is determined by proximal airways and distal airway determine airflow resistance at small lung volumes and determine measurements toward the end of maximal exhalation. As lung emptying is affected by airway obstruction there will be air trapping and hyperinflation, which can reduce the FVC **(Box 13.9)**.

Bronchodilator responsiveness (BDR) is the characteristic feature of asthma **(Figs. 13.11 and 13.12)**.

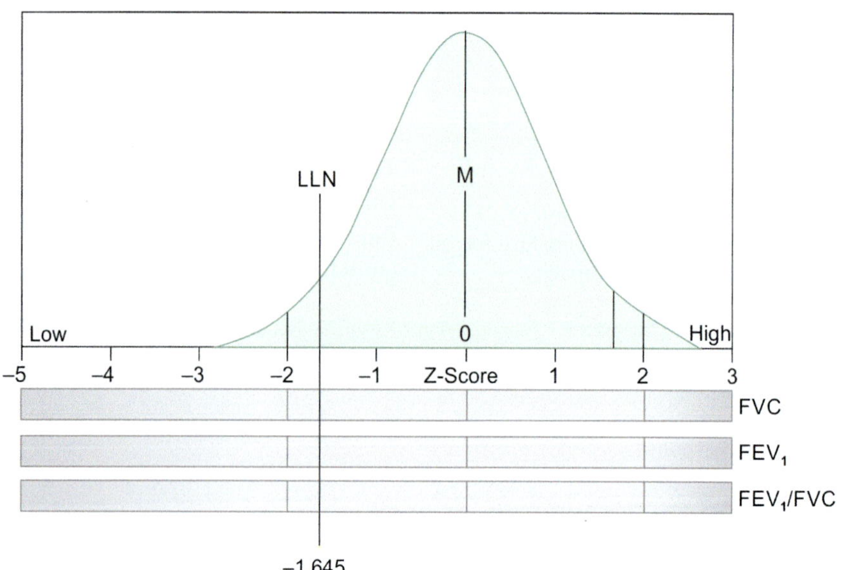

Fig. 13.9: Interpretation of spirometric parameters, according to the lower limit of normal (LLN) (FEV_1: forced expiratory volume in 1 second; FVC: forced vital capacity)

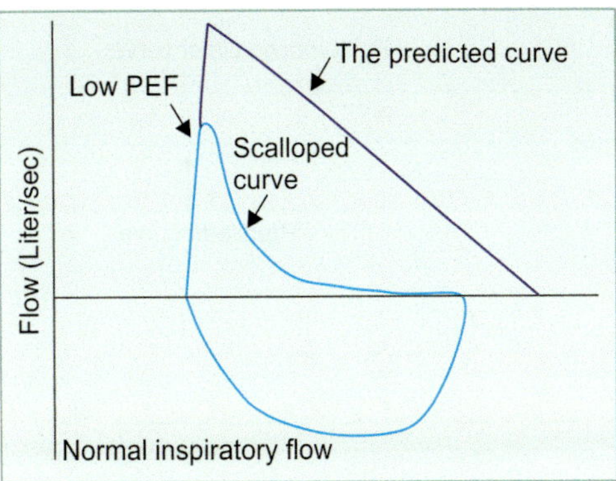

Fig. 13.10: Flow-volume loop in obstructive airway defect. (PEF: peak expiratory flow)

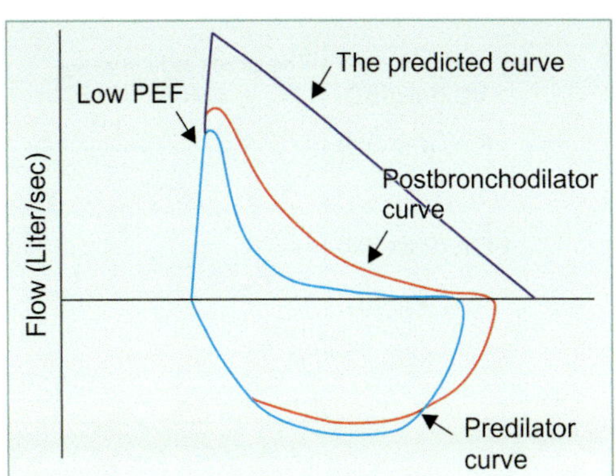

Fig. 13.11: Postbronchodilator effect in flow-volume loop in obstructive airway defect.

BOX 13.9: Abnormalities in obstructive airway defects.

- *Obstructive airway defects:*
  - ↓ FEV_1
  - ↓ or normal FVC
  - ↓ FEFs and MMEF (FEF_{25}, FEF_{50}, FEF_{75}, and FEF_{25-75})
  - ↓ PEF
  - ↑ FET
- Possible significant bronchodilator response
- The height of the curve (PEF) is less than predicted. The descending limb is concave (scooped), with the concavity being more pronounced with more severe obstruction. The slope of the descending limb, which represents MMEF and FEFs is reduced due to airflow limitation at low lung volumes

(FEF: forced expiratory flow; FET: forced expiratory time; FEV_1: forced expiratory volume in 1 second; FVC: forced vital capacity; MMEF: maximal mid-expiratory flow; PEF: peak expiratory flow)

Small Airway Dysfunction

Identification of small airway obstruction remains still as a challenge, especially when FEV_1 and the FEV_1/FVC ratios are normal. Attempts to quantify small airway defect, using $FEF_{25-75\%}$ (mid-range flow measurements), also have insufficient evidence due to high variability and poor reproducibility. Spirometry is not a good tool to diagnose small airway obstruction.

Restrictive Airway Defect (Box 13.10)

In restrictive airway defect, FVC and FEV_1 will be below the LLN. Even though spirometry can suggest restrictive lung disease, it should be confirmed by measuring lung volumes and total lung capacity below the LLN (5th percentile). In spirometry FVC is reduced, FEV_1/FVC is normal or increased, and the flow-volume curve shows a convex pattern due to high elastic recoil **(Fig. 13.13)**. In a "simple restrictive" pattern FVC, FEV_1, and TLC are typically reduced almost in the same proportion.

If the reduction in FVC is out of proportion to the reduction in TLC, indicating a disproportionately elevated RV, in "complex restriction" there is a disproportionate decline in FVC values compared to TLC, and usually occur with conditions that impair lung emptying like chest wall or neuromuscular disease or any unidentified obstruction with gas trapping **(Fig. 13.14)**. A "mixed" disorder is characterized by obstructive airway pattern associated with a low FEV_1 ratio.

APPROACH TO INTERPRETATION OF SPIROMETRY

Approach to interpretation of spirometry is depicted in **Flowchart 13.1**.

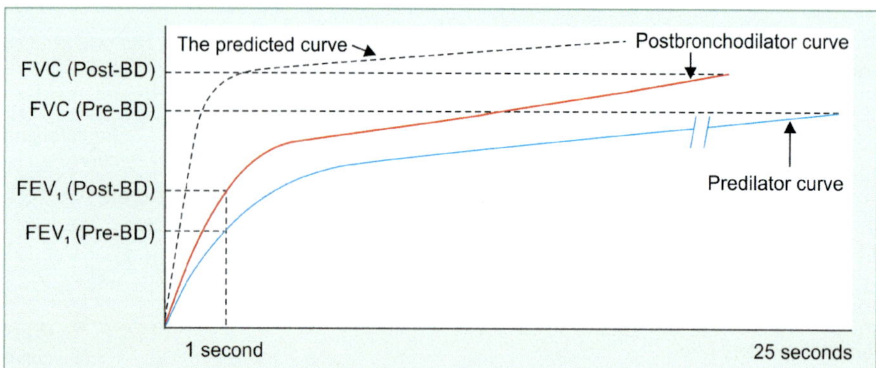

Fig. 13.12: Postbronchodilator effect in volume time curve in obstructive airway defect. (BD: bronchodilator; FEV_1: forced expiratory volume in 1 second; FVC: forced vital capacity)
Source: Altalag A, Road J, Wilcox P, Aboulhosn K (Eds). In: Pulmonary Function Tests in Clinical Practice, 2nd edition. New York: Springer International Publishing AG; 2019.

BOX 13.10: Abnormalities in restrictive airway defect.

- *Restrictive disorders:*
  - ↓ FVC and normal
  - ↑ FEV_1/FVC ratio
  - ↓ FEV_1 (proportional to FVC), but it can be normal
  - ↓ MMEF
- *PEF:* Normal, increased or decreased
- Descending limb of FV curve will be steep

(FEV_1: forced expiratory volume in 1 second; FV: flow volume; FVC: forced vital capacity; MMEF: maximal mid-expiratory flow; PEF: peak expiratory flow)

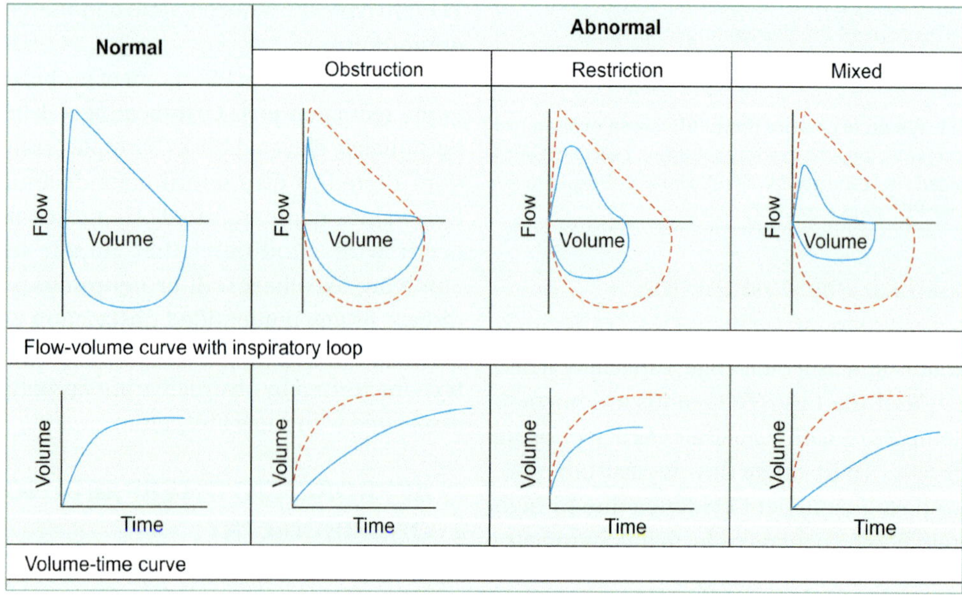

Fig. 13.13: Summary of abnormal spirometry curves.

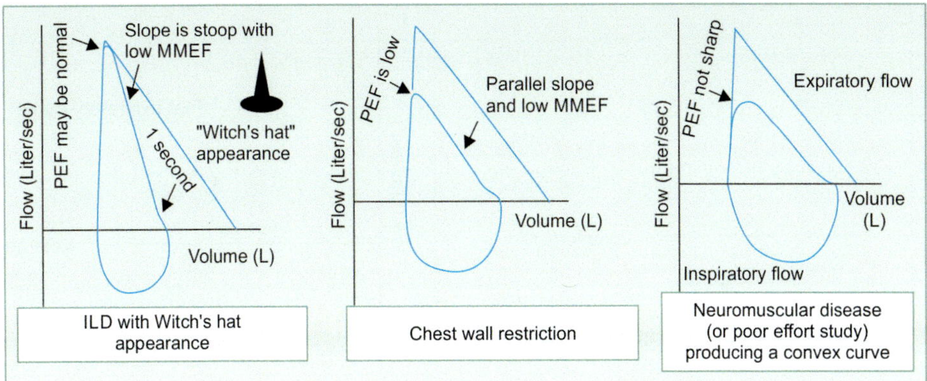

Fig. 13.14: Restrictive airway defects in different diseases. (FEV1: forced expiratory volume in 1 second; FVC: forced vital capacity; ILD: interstitial lung disease; MMEF: maximal mid-expiratory flow; PEF: peak expiratory flow)

Source: Altalag A, Road J, Wilcox P, Aboulhosn K (Eds). In: Pulmonary Function Tests in Clinical Practice, 2nd edition. New York: Springer International Publishing AG; 2019.

Flowchart 13.1: Algorithm to interpret spirometry.

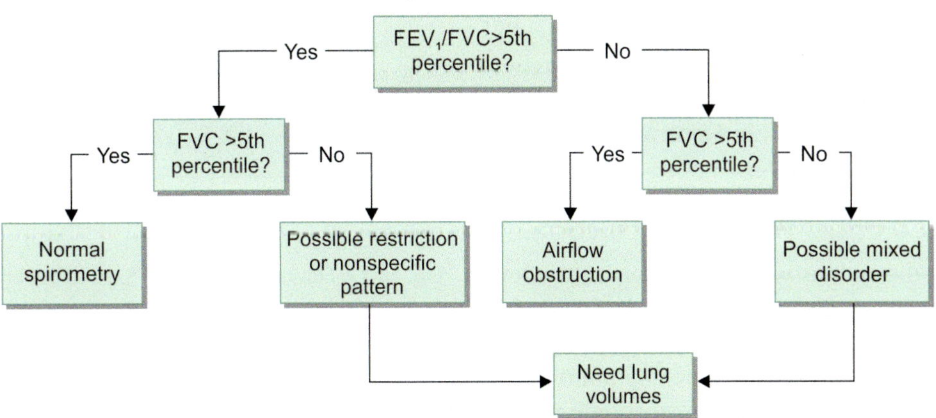

(FEV_1: forced expiratory volume in 1 second; FVC: forced vital capacity)

Source: Stanojevic S, Kaminsky DA, Miller MR, Thompson B, Aliverti A, Barjaktarevic I, et al. ERS/ATS technical standard on interpretive strategies for routine lung function tests. Eur Respir J. 2022;60(1):2101499.

Spirometry in Upper Airway Obstruction

Variable Extrathoracic Obstruction

In variable extrathoracic obstruction, which is dynamic or mobile, during inspiration due to the negative airway pressure, obstruction takes place during inspiration hence resulting in reduction of inspiratory flow and flattening of inspiratory limb of the flow volume **(Fig. 13.15)**. Examples include tumors of hypopharynx or upper trachea, paralysis of vocal cord, subglottic stenosis, and external compression of upper trachea.

Variable Intrathoracic Obstruction

In variable intrathoracic obstruction, as major intrathoracic airways such as trachea

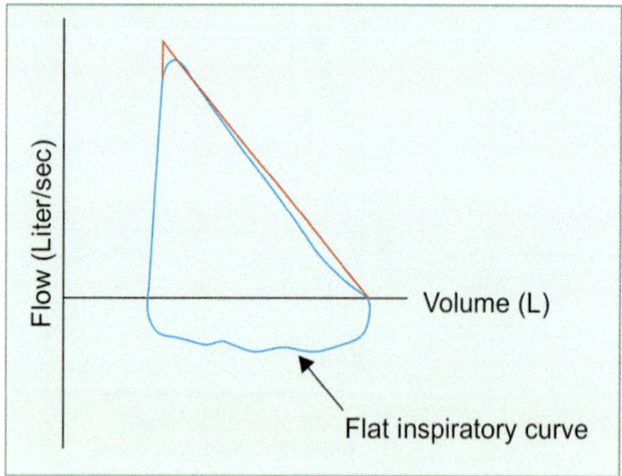

Fig. 13.15: Flow volume loop in variable extrathoracic obstruction.

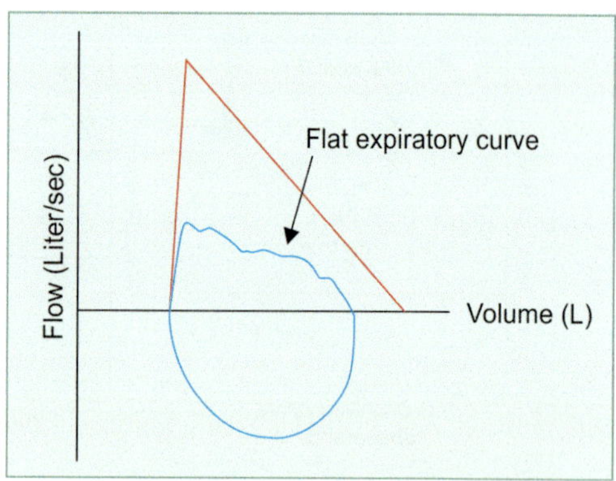

Fig. 13.16: Flow volume loop in variable intrathoracic obstruction.

(intrathoracic part) and main bronchi are compressed during expiration, due to the raised intrathoracic pressure. In flow volume loop, expiratory limb will be deformed form at the beginning including the PEF **(Fig. 13.16)**. Examples include tracheomalacia, tumors of the lower trachea, mobile tracheal strictures, and external compression of lower trachea.

Fixed Upper Airway Obstruction

Fixed upper airway obstruction at any level will cause flattening of both inspiratory and expiratory limbs of flow volume loop **(Fig. 13.17)**. Examples include nondynamic tumors and fibrotic strictures of upper airways.

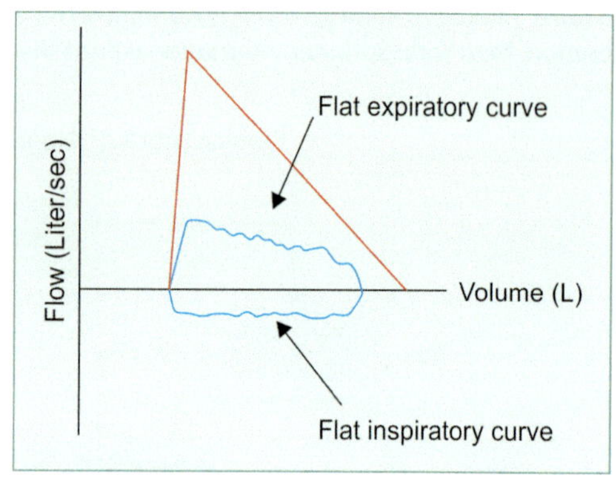

Fig. 13.17: Flow volume loop in fixed upper airway obstruction.

GLOBAL INITIATIVE FOR ASTHMA GUIDELINES 2024 ON ASTHMA DIAGNOSIS IN CHILDREN USING SPIROMETRY

Documentation of variable expiratory flow limitation include any of the criteria given here.

- *Bronchodilator responsiveness:* Increase in baseline FEV_1 ≥12% (10–15 minutes after 200–400 μg of salbutamol/albuterol or equivalent)
- *Increase in lung function after 4 weeks of treatment:* Increase in baseline FEV_1 ≥12%
- *Positive bronchial challenge test:* Fall in FEV_1 >12% predicted after a standardized exercise challenge
- *Excessive variation in lung function between the visits:* Variation in FEV_1 ≥12% between the visits

SUMMARY

Spirometry is a standard, noninvasive pulmonary function test that measures the volume and flow rate of air during forced breathing maneuvers. It is a foundational and gold standard tool for assessing lung function.

Spirometry is clinically useful for confirming diagnoses especially in obstructive airway diseases, monitoring disease progression, treatment effectiveness, and assessing risk for surgery. Spirometry is not suitable for definitive diagnosis for restrictive conditions without further tests. The reliability of the test is highly dependent on patient effort and proper technique. Interpretation should be done considering the clinical scenario.

KEY POINTS

- Spirometry should be interpreted only based on the history and clinical examination.
- Spirometry is an important tool in diagnosing obstructive airway defect in children and should be performed based on clear indication only.
- A well-trained technician with the help of modified spirometry equipment with a positive reinforcement technic can attain a good spirometry result in children above 5 years.
- As per the new ATS guidelines, it should be interpreted in comparison with the LLN values and use of absolute numbers are discouraged.

SUGGESTED READING

1. Aconf. (2017). Pediatric Pulmonology: 16th International Congress of Pediatric Pulmonology (CIPP 2017). Lisbon Portugal, June 22-25, 2017. [online] Available from www.aconf.org/conf_103395.html. [Last accessed April, 2025].
2. Altalag A, Road J, Wilcox P, Aboulhosn K (Eds). In: Pulmonary Function Tests in Clinical Practice, 2nd edition. New York: Springer International Publishing AG; 2019.
3. Beydon N, Davis SD, Lombardi E, Allen JL, Arets HGM, Aurora P, et al. An official American Thoracic Society/European Respiratory Society statement: pulmonary function testing in preschool children. Am J Respir Crit Care Med. 2007;175(12):1304-45.
4. Centers for Disease Control and Prevention. (2011). National Health and Nutrition Examination Survey (NHANES): respiratory health spirometry procedures manual. [online] Available from https://stacks.cdc.gov/view/cdc/26507. [Last accessed April, 2025].
5. Chhabra SK, Kumar R, Mittal V. Prediction equations for spirometry for children from Northern India. Indian Pediatr. 2016;53:781-5.
6. Davis SD, Eber E, Koumbourlis AC (Eds). In: Diagnostic Tests in Pediatric Pulmonology: Applications and Interpretation, 1st edition. New York: Humana Press; 2015.
7. Dombkowski KJ, Hassan F, Wasilevich EA, Clark SJ. Spirometry use among pediatric primary care physicians. Pediatrics. 2010;126(4):682-7.
8. Galant SP, Nickerson B. Lung function measurement in the assessment of childhood asthma: recent important developments. Curr Opin Allergy Clin Immunol. 2010;10(2):149-54.
9. Global Initiative for Asthma (GINA). (2022). 2022 GINA report, global strategy for asthma management and prevention. [online] Available from https://ginasthma.org/gina-reports/. [Last accessed April, 2025].
10. Graham BL, Steenbruggen I, Miller MR, Barjaktarevic I, Cooper BG, Hall GL, et al. Standardization of spirometry 2019 update. An official American Thoracic Society and European Respiratory Society technical statement. Am J Respir Crit Care Med. 2019;200(8):e70-88.
11. Haynes JM. Basic spirometry testing and interpretation for the primary care provider. Can J Respir Ther. 2018;54(4):92-8.
12. Hill S, Winter R. (2013). A Guide to Performing Quality Assured Diagnostic Spirometry. [online] Available from www.brit-thoracic.org.uk/media/70454/spirometry_e-guide_2013.pdf. [Last accessed April, 2025].
13. Jat KR. Spirometry in children. Prim Care Respir J. 2013;22(2):221-9.
14. Kaslovsky R, Sadof M. Spirometry for the primary care pediatrician. Pediatr Rev. 2014;35(11):465-71.
15. Miller MR, Hankinson J, Brusasco V, Burgos F, Casaburi R, Coates A, et al. Standardisation of spirometry. Eur Respir J. 2005;26(2):319-38.

16. National Asthma Council Australia. The Spirometry Handbook for primary care. Melbourne: National Asthma Council Australia; 2023.
17. O'Connor T, Manning P. (2005). Spirometry: Performance and Interpretation - A Guide for General Practitioners. [online] Available from https://irishthoracicsociety.com/wp-content/uploads/2017/05/SpirometryGuidelinespdf.pdf. [Last accessed April, 2025].
18. Pellegrino R, Viegi G, Brusasco V, Crapo RO, Burgos F, Casaburi R, et al. Interpretative strategies for lung function tests. Eur Respir J. 2005;26(5):948-68.
19. Queensland Health. (2013). Spirometry (Paediatric) Respiratory Science: Document Number QH-GDL-393. [online] Available from https://metronorth.health.qld.gov.au/refer-your-patient/spirometry-training-program. [Last accessed April, 2025].
20. Stanojevic S, Kaminsky DA, Miller MR, Thompson B, Aliverti A, Barjaktarevic I, et al. ERS/ATS technical standard on interpretive strategies for routine lung function tests. Eur Respir J. 2022;60(1):2101499.
21. Taussig LM, Landau LI. Pediatric Respiratory Medicine, 2nd edition. Missouri: Mosby; 2008.
22. Wilmott RW, Bush A, Deterding RR, Ratjen F, Sly P, Zar H, Li A. Kendig's Disorders of the Respiratory Tract in Children, 9th edition. Amsterdam: Elsevier; 2019.

CHAPTER 14

Fractional Exhaled Nitric Oxide

Shebna A Khader

INTRODUCTION

Fractional exhaled nitric oxide (FeNO) is a simple, reproducible, quantitative, and noninvasive test to measure nitric oxide (NO)—a marker of inflammation in the exhaled air.

NITRIC OXIDE

The presence of NO in exhaled air was first described in 1991 by Gustafsson. In 1992, NO was voted "Molecule of the year". Scientists from Karolinska Institute reported significance of FeNO in asthmatics in the year 1993.

Nitric oxide, the smallest signaling molecule, is produced in our body by nitric oxide synthase (NOS). NOS is mainly of three types **(Fig. 14.1)**:

1. *nNOS (neuronal NOS):* Expressed in the central and peripheral nervous systems
2. Actions—central control of BP, learning, memory, gut peristalsis *iNOS (inducible NOS)*:
   - By airway epithelial cells, eosinophils
   - Marker of inflammation
   - Assessed by FeNO
3. *eNOS (endothelial NOS):* Vasodilator

Inducible Nitric Oxide Synthase

Nitric oxide by iNOS is produced by airway epithelial cells and eosinophils. It is usually not expressed in cells, but induced by

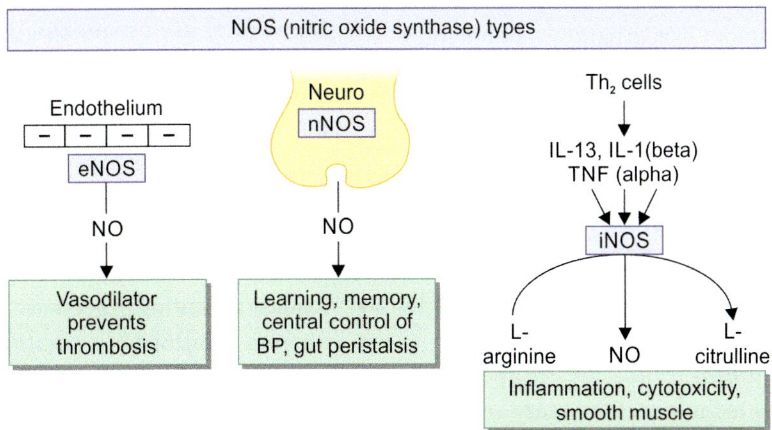

Fig. 14.1: Nitric oxide synthase (NOS) types and functions. (eNOS: endothelial NOS; IL: interleukin; iNOS: inducible nitric oxide synthase; nNOS: neuronal NOS; Th2 cells: T helper type 2 cells; TNF: tumor necrosis factor)

bacteria and cytokines. NO by iNOS is a marker of eosinophilic airway inflammation. Measuring the fraction of this gas during a steady state exhalation is called FeNO, and it correlates with airways inflammation in type 2 asthma.

ASTHMA-ENDOTYPES AND NITRIC OXIDE

Asthma is a chronic inflammatory heterogeneous disease with specific mechanistic pathways (Endotypes) and clinical presentations (phenotypes). Endotypes and phenotypes can be explained based on patterns of symptoms, biomarkers, and response to treatment.

In pediatric onset asthma, the major endotype (80%) is type 2 (T2) asthma with elevated type 2 biomarkers, blood or sputum eosinophils, increased FeNO, causing less exacerbations and a very good response to corticosteroids. In T2 high asthma, IL-13 upregulates iNOS, leading to increased NO production. The amount of exhaled NO is proportionate with sputum eosinophils and peak flow variation. Non-type 2 asthma is less frequent, refractory to corticosteroids, causing frequent exacerbations, and is more common in preschool age children. FeNO levels do not correlate with this type of inflammation.

FRACTIONAL EXHALED NITRIC OXIDE MEASUREMENT

Nitric oxide is analyzed quantitatively by different methods:

- *Chemiluminescence technique:* Gold standard technique. Stationary analyzers, complex method.
- *Electrochemical technique:* By newer handheld devices, widely used portable.

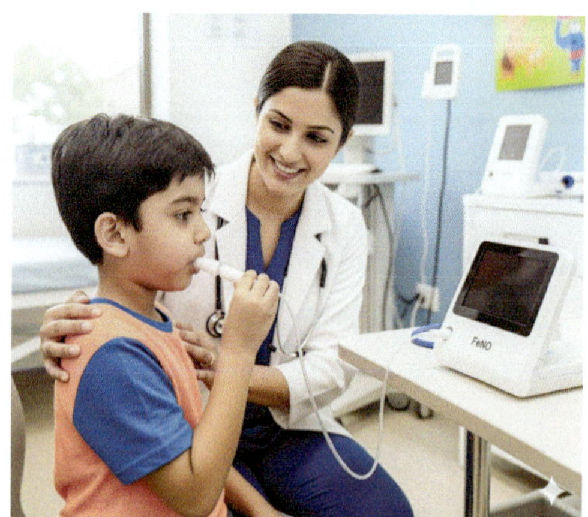

Fig. 14.2: Fractional exhaled nitric oxide (FeNO) device.

In newer electrochemical sensors, patients should exhale for at least 10 seconds at a pressure ensuring a flow rate of 50 +/– 5 mL/s. An expiratory flow of 50 mL/s is recommended to increase the involvement of the lower respiratory tract **(Fig. 14.2)**.

Preparation for Procedure

- Refrain from eating and drinking for at least 1 hour before the test.
- Avoid the use of nitrate-rich foods such as beetroot, spinach, lettuce, 3 hours before the procedure.
- No alcohol use or smoking 1 day before the test.
- Rule out upper and lower respiratory viral infections.
- No vigorous exercise within 1 hour before procedure.

Procedure

- Explain regarding procedure
- Sit in a comfortable position or stand upright.
- Insert mouthpiece and inhale through mouth to reach total lung capacity.
- Exhale immediately at a constant flow rate of 50 mL/sec.

- The indicator on the machine shows the rate at which flow is to be maintained.
- FeNO levels are shown on screen and interpreted.

Note:

- *Avoid nose clip:* As nasal NO accumulates, it can leak into the nasopharynx, affecting the value.
- FeNO value is flow rate dependent change in flow rate affects NO transfer from wall to lumen.

Reference Value for Fractional Exhaled Nitric Oxide

The American Thoracic Society (ATS) and the European Respiratory Society (ERS) have recommended cut-off values for FeNO to aid in asthma diagnosis and treatment **(Table 14.1)**.

TABLE 14.1: Cut-off values for fractional exhaled nitric oxide (FeNO) to aid in asthma diagnosis and treatment.

FeNO (ppb)	*Adult*	*Children (<12 years)*
Low	<25	<20
Intermediate	25–50	20–35
High	>50	>35

(ppb: parts per billion)

Factors Affecting Fractional Exhaled Nitric Oxide

There are multiple factors which can affect FeNO including hereditary, dietary factors, infections, comorbidities, drugs, etc. which has to be considered before interpreting the results. Factors influencing FeNO are shown in **Table 14.2**.

Clinical Applications of Fractional Exhaled Nitric Oxide in Asthma

- *Diagnosis:* High FeNO levels are considered as supporting evidence for diagnosis while low values do not necessarily exclude diagnosis. Values are most reliable in patients not started on inhaled corticosteroids (ICS); confounding factors that increase or reduce NO have to be noted. GINA highlights factor the limitation of confounding factors, as it can be elevated in eosinophilic bronchitis, atopy, allergic rhinitis, eczema, and can be normal in T2 low asthma. GINA recommends FeNO ≥20 ppb cutoff for type 2 inflammation in severe asthma along with blood eosinophil (≥300 cells/μL) and sputum eosinophil (≥3%) count **(Flowchart 14.1)**.
- *To predict response to treatment:* High FeNO predicts a better clinical response

TABLE 14.2: Factors affecting fractional exhaled nitric oxide.

Factors increasing FeNO	*Factors reducing FeNO*
• Atopy • Eczema • Nitrate-containing food, e.g., beetroot, spinach • Viral infections, e.g., Rhinovirus • Chronic rhinosinusitis • Nasal polyposis • Air pollution • HIV infection • Patient characteristics, e.g., male sex, increasing age, increased height	• Inhaled corticosteroids use • Cigarette smoking—cumulative • Alcohol ingestion • Spirometry done before FeNO test • Drugs, leukotriene receptor antagonist, prostaglandin • Exercise before the test

Flowchart 14.1: For supporting diagnosis of asthma with fractional exhaled nitric oxide (FeNO).

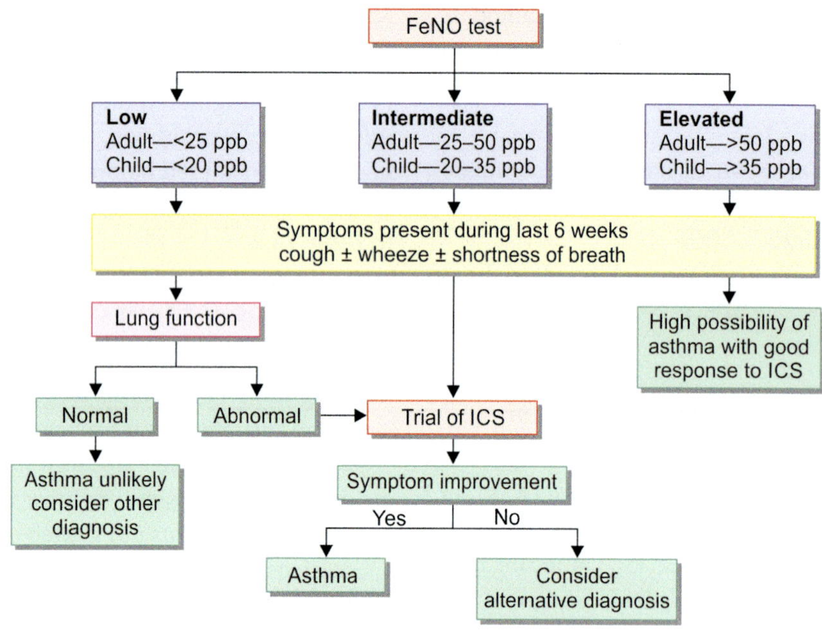

(ICS: inhaled corticosteroids; ppb: parts per billion)

Flowchart 14.2: For monitoring treatment and compliance using FeNO. (FeNO: fractional exhaled nitric oxide; ICS: inhaled corticosteroids)

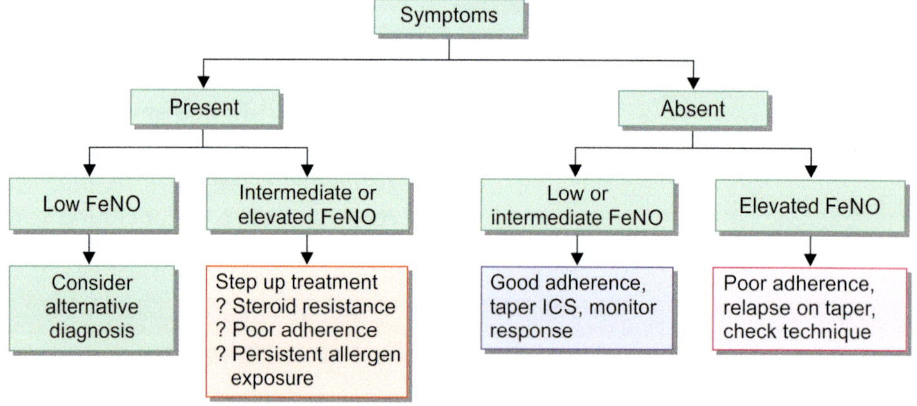

to corticosteroid, both in improvement of lung function. It also helps guide in stepping down the treatment.

- *To predict exacerbations:* High NO along with high blood eosinophil count, has prognostic value in predicting patients prone to frequent exacerbations.
- *As a test for treatment adherence:* Nonadherence to treatment with ICS is a common cause of poor asthma control. In patients who show a visible response of reduction in FeNO on taking ICS under direct supervision FeNO can be used to monitor adherence **(Flowchart 14.2)**.

TABLE 14.3: Comparison of treatment responses to biologics in terms of concentration and efficacy.

Omalizumab	>19.5 ppb	43% response
Dupilumab	>25 ppb	47% response
Mepolizumab	>41 ppb	26% response
Benralizumab	>40 ppb	14% response

- *To predict response to biologics:* Elevated NO has been shown to predict response to biologics. This ability has a cost-saving benefit to plan on treatment. Response to mepolizumab was better predicted by NO along with eosinophilia **(Table 14.3)**.

Fractional Exhaled Nitric Oxide in Other Illnesses

- *Nonasthmatic eosinophilic bronchitis (NAEB):* FeNO levels are significantly elevated as inflammatory cells infiltrate the bronchial mucosa. The FeNO level can predict the possible favorable response to ICS.
- *Chronic obstructive pulmonary disease (COPD):* There will be only a slight increase in FeNO, but factors such as smoking, ICS use can affect the levels. ↑ FeNO has an association with increased risk of COPD exacerbation and correlates well with steroid responsiveness for exacerbation.
- *Alpha 1 antitrypsin deficiency:* Alpha 1 antitrypsin deficiency has low FeNO when compared to COPD and healthy individuals. FeNO helps in monitoring disease progression to COPD, where FeNO will be elevated.
- *Interstitial lung disease:* FeNO is significantly elevated in interstitial lung disease (ILD) secondary to connective tissue disease, unlike in idiopathic ILD. Hence, it can be used as a screening tool to know the pathology of ILD.
- *Cystic fibrosis:* Nasal NO is altered in cystic fibrosis, primary ciliary dyskinesia, and allergic rhinitis. Nasal NO is extremely low in primary ciliary dyskinesia (PCD). Low levels of NO in cystic fibrosis are related to the absence of NOS2 expression. Nasal NO can be used as a screening test for primary ciliary dyskinesia.

SUMMARY

- Fractional exhaled nitric oxide is an easy-to-measure, quantitative, noninvasive test to assess eosinophilic airway inflammation.
- FeNO test supports asthma diagnosis, especially in differentiating the phenotypes—type 2 asthma phenotype.
- FeNO helps clinicians to plan the management of asthma, check compliance, and predict response to treatment.
- FeNO utility in the diagnosis and management of other inflammatory airway diseases and allergic disorders is promising and is widely studied.

SUGGESTED READING

1. Dweik RA, Boggs PB, Erzurum SC, Irvin CG, Leigh MW, Lundberg JO, et al. An official ATS clinical practice guideline: interpretation of exhaled nitric oxide levels (FeNO) for clinical applications. Am J Respir Crit Care Med. 2011;184(5):602-15.
2. Hoggins R, Velpula M, Woodward S, Tighe MP. How to use the fractional exhaled nitric oxide test. Arch Dis Child Educ Pract. 2021;107(2).
3. Ragnoli B, Radaeli A, Pochetti P, Kette S, Morjaria J, Malerba M. Fractional nitric oxide measurement in exhaled air (FeNO): perspectives in the management of respiratory diseases. Ther Adv Chronic Dis. 2023;14: 20406223231190480.
4. Sen P, Khatri SB, Tejwani V. Measuring exhaled nitric oxide when diagnosing and managing asthma. Cleve Clin J Med. 2023;90(6):363-70.

CHAPTER 15

Impulse Oscillometry

Neeraj Gupta

INTRODUCTION

Asthma is one of the most common non-infectious diseases worldwide, significantly affecting both quality and quantity of life. It's appropriate and timely management is warranted to reduce both symptoms and medication scores in the indigents. Lung function testing plays a vital role in the diagnosis, monitoring, and management of respiratory diseases including asthma. Although spirometry has traditionally been the gold standard technique for monitoring pulmonary functions, it has notable limitations, especially among certain patient populations such as children, the elderly, and those with significant respiratory impairments particularly in the small airway diseases. Patients who are unable to perform the vigorous breathing maneuvers required by spirometry, due to limited neuromuscular capacity or following cardiothoracic or abdominal or spine surgery, require an alternative reliable method for monitoring the lung function. Children with limited attention spans, cognitive impairments like autism, or various genetic-neurometabolic syndromes further increase the demand for alternative assessment tools. Forced oscillation technique (FOT) is gaining wider recognition as a simpler and more reliable method that assesses respiratory mechanics by introducing small pressure oscillations during the normal breathing. This technique provides detailed insights into the mechanical properties of the respiratory system with minimal effort from the patient, presenting potential benefits over traditional spirometry.

PRINCIPLE OF OSCILLOMETRY

Oscillometry operates on the concept that the respiratory system can be modeled as a combination of resistive, elastic, and inertial elements. When pressure oscillations are introduced to the respiratory system, the corresponding flow response is measured. These oscillations, generated by either a loudspeaker or an oscillating piston, are applied to the respiratory flow produced during normal breathing that is why it is termed as the FOT. Built-in pressure and flow transducers measure these parameters at different frequencies after filtering the signals. The machine then analyses the relationship between pressure and flow to determine respiratory impedance (Zrs), which includes both resistance (Rrs) and reactance (Xrs), using Ohm's law (Resistance = Pressure/Flow) **(Fig. 15.1)**.

Loudspeaker generated impulses (green arrow) travel through airways along with tidal breathing (blue arrow) in the tracheobronchial tree. During expiration, signals are transmitted backward (red arrow) and are captured by transducers, after signal filtering using fast Fourier's equation to dampen the effects of respiratory flow, in

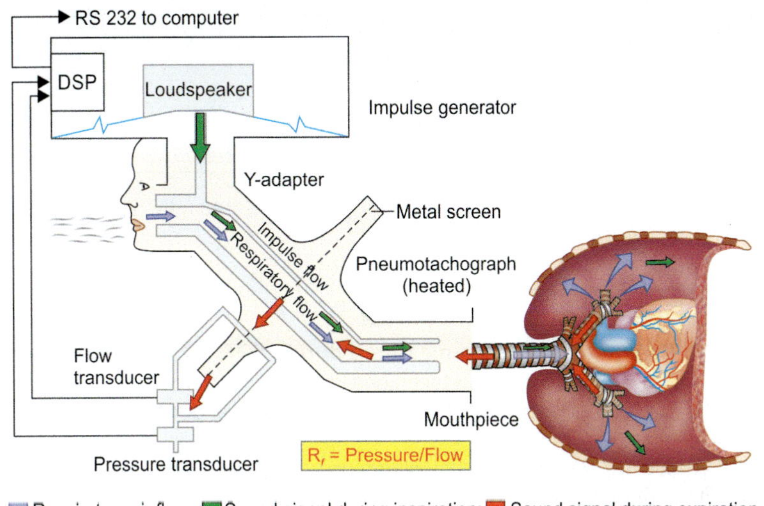

Fig. 15.1: Schematic diagram depicting superimposition of sound impulses over airflow during FOT. (DSP: digital signal processing; FOT: forced oscillation technique)
Source: Gupta N, Sachdev A, Gupta D, Gupta S. Oscillometry—The future of estimating pulmonary functions. Karnataka Pediatr J. 2020;35(2):79-87.

order to directly measure flow and pressures on individual frequencies. Later, resistance is calculated by the machine using Ohm's law and directly displayed on the screen.

Mathematical Modeling

The respiratory system is typically represented by simple linear equations that define the pressure-flow relationships. This model generally includes parameters such as airway resistance (R), tissue compliance (C), and inertance (I), allowing for a detailed examination of both airway and tissue mechanics.

Parameters Measured (Figs. 15.2A and B)

- *Resistance (Rrs):* It reflects the resistive properties of the airways. It is a measure of opposite force encountered during airflow in the airways.
- *Reactance (Xrs):* It represents the combined effects of airway and tissue elasticity/capacitance (of smaller airways) and inertance (of mid-size airways). It mainly depicts the recoiling ability of peripheral airways. It is typically measured at 5 Hz and shown as negative values from the baseline because the force occurs in the opposite direction and reflective of peripheral airway properties.
- *Impedance (Zrs):* It is a complex value representing combined effect of both Rrs and Xrs, often displayed as a function of frequency.
- *Resonant frequency (Fres):* The frequency at which the (negative) capacitive and (positive) inertial components of Xrs cancel each other out, meeting at the zero line (baseline). Capacitive forces represent small airways whereas mid-size airways are represented by inertial forces.
- *Reactance area (Ax):* It is also known as Goldman's triangle or area of reactance. This is the area below the baseline (in the negative direction) up to X_5 (reactance

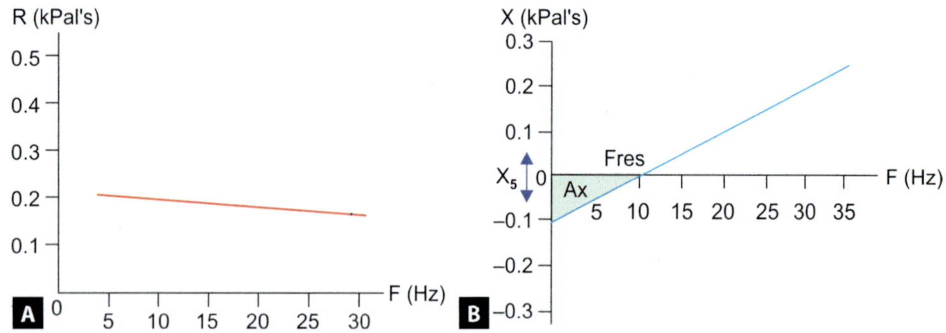

Figs. 15.2A and B: Common parameters measured during FOT. [Ax: reactance area (green zone); F: frequency in hertz; FOT: forced oscillation technique; Fres: resonant frequency; Hz: hertz; R: resistance in kilopascal per liter per second (red line); X: reactance in kilopascal per liter per second (blue line); X_5: reactance at 5 Hz]

Source: Gupta N, Sachdev A, Gupta D, Gupta S. Oscillometry—The future of estimating pulmonary functions. Karnataka Pediatr J. 2020;35(2):79-87.

at 5 Hz), which extends until Fres on the *x*-axis in the right side.

TYPES OF FORCED OSCILLATION TECHNIQUE AND WAVEFORMS (FIGS. 15.3A TO C)

In clinical practice, frequencies ranging from 3 to 41 Hz are typically used. FOT can be categorized based on the frequencies of oscillations employed:

1. *Mono/single/sinusoidal frequency* **(Figs. 15.3A and 15.4A)**: It uses single frequencies (5 Hz for adults and 7/8 Hz for children) to demonstrate airflow characteristics at a specific moment. This method is time-consuming because different frequencies can only be tested sequentially, and it is recommended only in special cases with significantly high-airway resistance.
2. *Impulse oscillometry (IOS)* **(Fig. 15.3B)**: It utilizes multiple impulses of a fundamental frequency (5 Hz) simultaneously, creating a square wave pattern due to overlapping sine waves **(Fig. 15.4B)**. IOS reduces test duration but can alter the characteristics of the 5 Hz frequency due to impulse overlap at regular intervals. Resistance (Rrs) measured with recurrent impulses is slightly (nonsignificantly) higher than pseudorandom noise (PRN) due to impedance distortion.
3. *Pseudorandom noise* **(Fig. 15.3C)**: It uses prime number frequencies (5, 11, and 19 Hz) to save time without compromising data integrity. A nonspecific waveform pattern is observed **(Fig. 15.4C)**, hence called as pseudorandom pattern. When available, PRN is considered a superior modality to IOS.

Machines and Devices

There are various devices available for FOT across the globe, each offering different features and applications **(Table 15.1)**. These devices typically include advanced software for data acquisition, signal processing, and interpretation, with features such as real-time data display, automated quality control, and patient-specific analysis.

Analysis of Waveforms

Since frequency is inversely related to wavelength, lower frequency impulses (5 Hz)

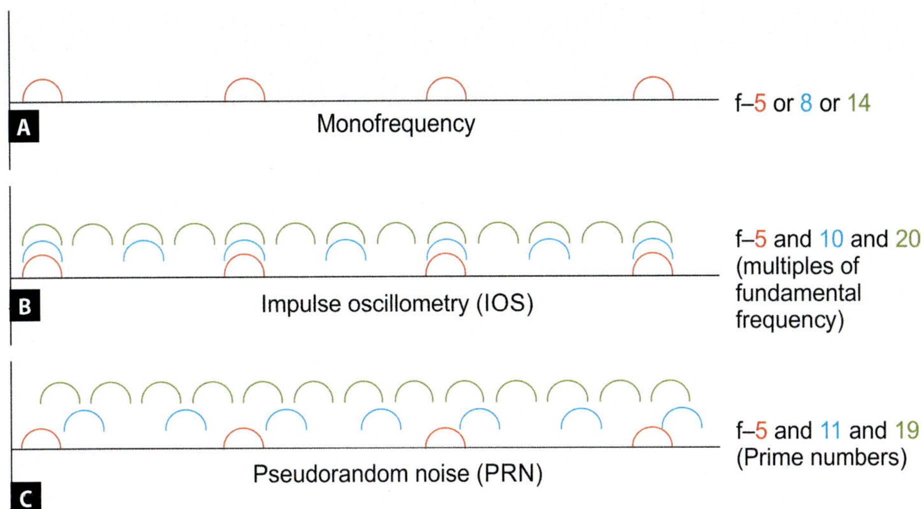

Figs. 15.3A to C: Types of FOT. (A) Individual frequency sound waves are generated at a time; (B) Multiples of fundamental frequency (5 Hz) are transmitted simultaneously with overriding of impulses; (C) Frequencies of prime numbers are transmitted simultaneously without any overlap. (f: frequency in Hz; FOT: forced oscillation technique; IOS: impulse oscillometry; PRN: pseudorandom noise)

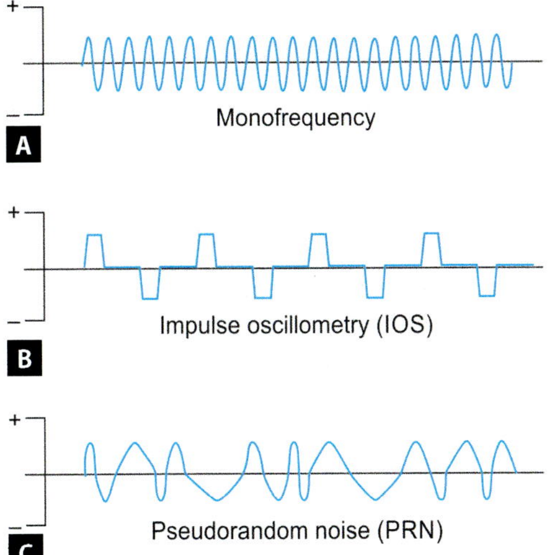

Figs. 15.4A to C: Types of waveforms in different FOTs. (A) Typical sinusoidal waves are generated in monofrequency FOT; (B) Square wave pattern is produced due to aggregation of overlapping sinusoidal waves; (C) Pseudorandom pattern is produced due to nonoverlapping multiple sinusoidal waves in random order generated over prime number frequencies. (FOT: forced oscillation technique; IOS: impulse oscillometry; PRN: pseudorandom noise)

travel deeper into the airways than higher frequencies (19/20 Hz) **(Fig. 15.5)**. Consequently, low-frequency oscillations (e.g., 5 Hz) reflect the entire airways, while high-frequency oscillations (e.g., 19 or 20 Hz) are more sensitive to large or central airway functions **(Fig. 15.5, Table 15.2)**. In healthy adults, the contribution of smaller airway resistance is negligible, making it frequency-independent. However, in young children and during conditions such as asthma-induced peripheral obstruction, this resistance becomes frequency-dependent. The frequency-dependence of resistance and reactance can provide valuable insights into different lung regions and the nature of airway obstruction. The coefficient of variation (CoV) in R_5 values within consecutive efforts should not exceed 10% in adults or 15% in children. A mean of three acceptable efforts (within a range of CoV) out of maximum eight attempts are considered for deriving oscillometry values. Postbronchodilator

TABLE 15.1: Types and frequency contents of available FOT machines.

Device	*Frequencies (Hz)*	*Signal types*	*Recording time*
Wave tube	5, 11, 13, 17, 19, 23, 29, 31, 37	Pseudorandom, relative primes	16 seconds
TremoFlo C-100	5, 11, 13, 17, 19, 23, 29, 31, 37	Pseudorandom, relative primes	16 seconds
MasterScreen IOS*	5, 10, 15, 20, 25, 35	Recurrent impulses	30 seconds
MostGraph-O_2 imp	5, 10, 15, 20, 25, 30, 35	Recurrent impulses	60 seconds
MostGraph-O_2 prn	5, 10, 15, 20, 25, 30, 35	Pseudorandom	60 seconds
Quark-i2m	4, 6, 8, ..., 32, 34, 36	Pseudorandom	8 seconds
Resmon Pro*	5, 11, 13, 17, 19, 23, 29, 31, 37	Pseudorandom, relative primes	30 seconds
Resmon Pro 3f*	5, 11, 19	Pseudorandom, relative primes	5 breaths
PulmoScan*	4–32	Pseudorandom	10 breaths
Antlia Pro*	5, 10, 14, 20 5, 11, 19	Monofrequency Multifrequency	24 seconds

*Available in Indian market for clinical use.
(FOT: forced oscillation technique; IOS: impulse oscillometry)

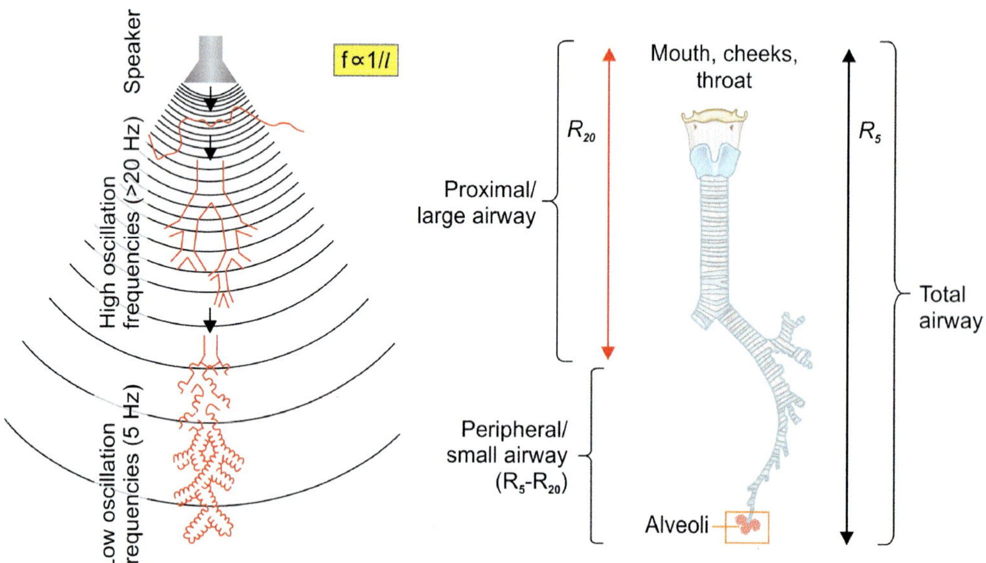

Fig. 15.5: Different frequencies travelling to varying length of airways. (*f*: frequency; *l*: length; R_{20}: resistance at 20 Hz; R_5: resistance at 5 Hz reflective of total airway; R_{20}: resistance at 20 Hz reflective of proximal or large airway; $R_5 - R_{20}$: reflective of peripheral or small airway resistance)

Source: Gupta N, Sachdev A, Gupta D, Gupta S. Oscillometry—The future of estimating pulmonary functions. Karnataka Pediatr J. 2020;35(2):79-87.

TABLE 15.2: Interpretation of FOT parameters.

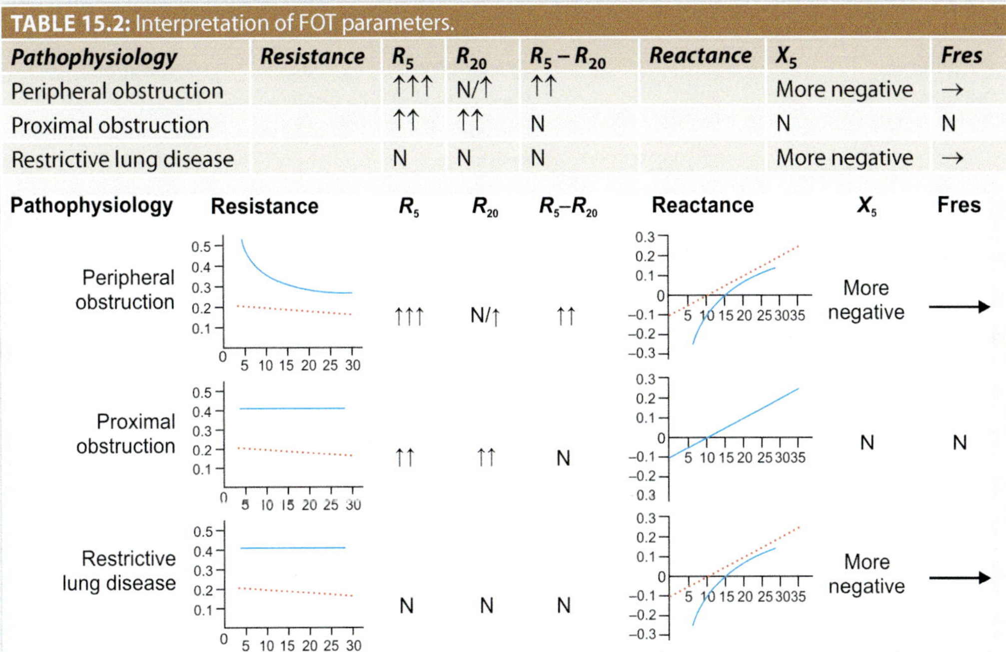

Pathophysiology	*Resistance*	R_5	R_{20}	$R_5 - R_{20}$	*Reactance*	X_5	*Fres*
Peripheral obstruction		↑↑↑	N/↑	↑↑		More negative	→
Proximal obstruction		↑↑	↑↑	N		N	N
Restrictive lung disease		N	N	N		More negative	→

(Blue solid line: baseline; Red dotted line: postbronchodilator; FOT: forced oscillation technique; N: normal; R_5: resistance at 5 Hz; R_{20}: resistance at 20 Hz; X_5: reactance at 5 Hz; Fres: resonant frequency; ↑: increase; →: rightward shift)

Source: Gupta N, Sachdev A, Gupta D, Gupta S. Oscillometry—The future of estimating pulmonary functions. Karnataka Pediatr J. 2020;35(2):79-87.

reversibility is considered significant if there is a reduction in R_5, X_5, or Ax by at least 40%, 50%, or 80%, respectively. However, recent studies suggest lower cut-off values for significant reversibility.

COMPARISON AGAINST SPIROMETRY

Table 15.3 outlines the key differences between the two techniques for measuring pulmonary functions: spirometry and oscillometry. As a noninvasive and relatively passive technique, FOT is suitable for children, the elderly, and those with severe respiratory conditions, both at diagnosis and during follow-up. Unlike traditional spirometry, FOT generates minimal aerosols, making it safer during pandemics **(Fig. 15.6)**. Additionally, FOT has better sensitivity for detecting restrictive diseases compared to spirometry. However, interpreting the complex data generated by FOT requires expertise. There is an urgent need to disseminate knowledge about FOT's utility and to develop region-specific nomograms. Until then, changes in baseline parameters, either after bronchodilator use or during subsequent follow-ups, can guide clinicians in adjusting treatment plans.

APPLICATIONS OF FORCED OSCILLATION TECHNIQUE

Current Applications

- *Pulmonary conditions (***Flowchart 15.1** *suggests a working algorithm to be used in office practice for oscillometry):*

TABLE 15.3: Comparison of spirometry and oscillometry.

Parameters	***Spirometry***	***Oscillometry***
Principle	Flow rates and lung volumes are considered reflective of airway resistance	Depicts airway resistance at various levels
Parameters measured	FVC, FEV_1, FEF_{25-75}, PEFR	Z, R, X, Fres, Ax
Type of breath required	Forced maneuver	Tidal breath
Level of patient cooperation needed	High	Minimal
Can be performed in children	>7 years	>2 years
In patients with neuromuscular weakness, intellectual disability, or postcardiothoracic surgery	Procedure cannot be done	Can be done
Sensitivity for detection of peripheral airway dysfunction (obstructive and/or restrictive)	Low	High
Within breath respiratory parameter analysis	Not possible	Possible
Aerosol generation **(Fig. 15.6)**	High	Very low
Standardization of method	Yes	Yet to be done
Reference values	Available for different ethnicities	Need more studies

(Ax: reactance area; FEF_{25-75}: forced expiratory flow at 25–75% of FVC; FEV_1: forced expiratory volume in 1 s; FVC: forced vital capacity; PEFR: peak expiratory flow rate; R: resistance; X: reactance; Fres: resonant frequency; Z: impedance)

Source: Gupta N, Sachdev A, Gupta D, Gupta S. Oscillometry—The future of estimating pulmonary functions. Karnataka Pediatr J. 2020;35(2):79-87.

- *Asthma:* FOT's ability to detect small airway obstruction early is a distinct advantage over spirometry. Reversibility after bronchodilator inhalation is a hallmark of the disease.
- *Chronic obstructive pulmonary disease (COPD):* FOT significantly affects reactance at 5 Hz (X_5) in COPD, compared to asthma where resistance at 5 Hz (R_5) is more impacted. FOT has also been used to monitor the therapeutic efficacy of high-flow nasal cannula therapy in COPD patients.
- *Pulmonary fibrosis:* In restrictive lung diseases, end-inspiratory reactance (Xi) is more affected than end-expiratory reactance (Xe).
- *Congenital lung malformation:* FOT can be used in children with hypoplastic lungs to assess respiratory function.

▪ *Extrapulmonary conditions:*
- *Obstructive sleep apnea (OSA):* FOT can assess functional impairment due to airway narrowing during adenoid hypertrophy and help titrate noninvasive ventilation support by demonstrating effects on airway resistance in real time.
- *Obesity hypoventilation syndrome:* FOT is useful for showing the clinical impact of obesity on lung mechanics. Intrabreath oscillometry can detect tidal expiratory flow limitation and assist in titrating continuous positive airway pressure (CPAP) therapy.
- *Neuromuscular weakness:* FOT is feasible for patients with poor neuromuscular reserves, such as those with spinal muscular atrophy.
- *Extratracheal compression:* Nonreversible central airway obstruction can

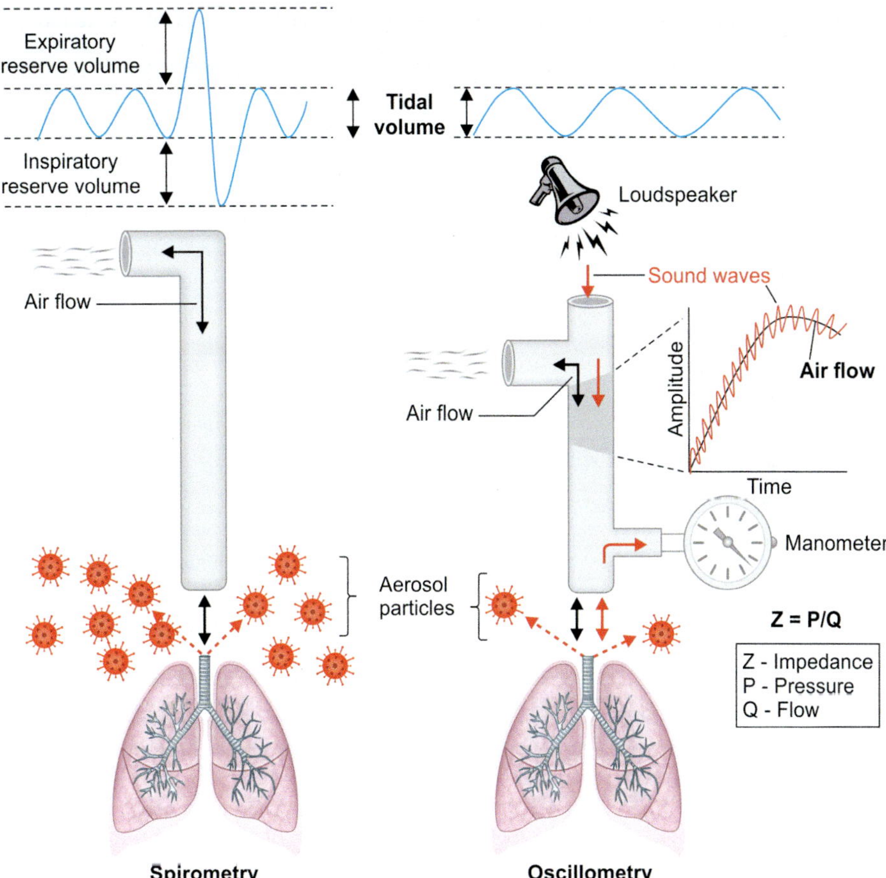

Fig. 15.6: Aerosol generation in spirometry versus oscillometry. Aerosol particle generation is much lesser in oscillometry compared to spirometry.
Source: Gupta N, Sachdev A, Gupta D. Oscillometry-A reasonable option to monitor lung functions in the era of COVID-19 pandemic. Pediatr Pulmonol. 2021;56(1):14-5.

serve as an early indicator of extratracheal fixed obstruction.

- *Systemic conditions:*
  - *Parkinson's disease:* FOT can measure airway tonicity as a marker of cholinergic activity and monitor therapeutic efficacy.
  - *Spinal cord injuries:* FOT can assess functional and structural impairments of the pulmonary system.
  - *Nephrotic syndrome:* In children with nephrotic syndrome, FOT can monitor respiratory function before and after diuretic therapy, demonstrating the presence of pulmonary edema due to extravascular fluid leakage.
  - *Metabolic syndrome:* FOT can be used to monitor pulmonary function in patients with metabolic syndrome.

Future Applications

Forced oscillation technique has potential for future applications in various areas:

- *Allergic rhinitis (AR):* Nasal oscillometry can measure nasal resistance before and

Flowchart 15.1: Algorithmic approach for oscillometry procedure and interpretation.

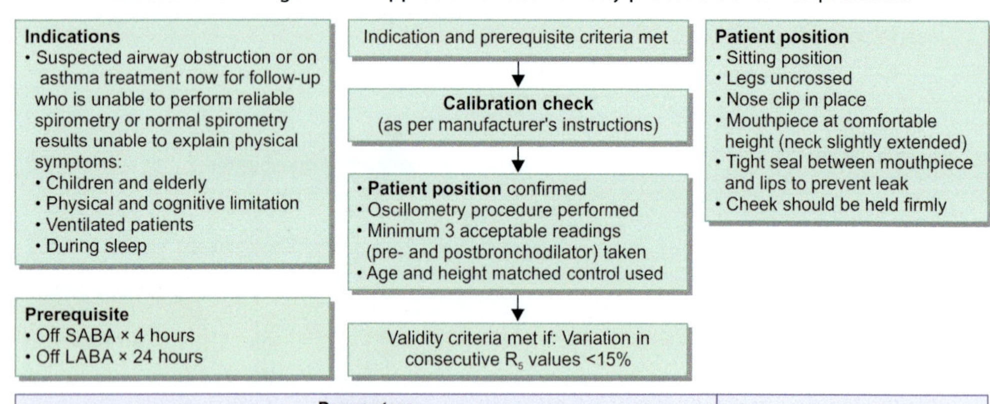

Parameters (as compared to age and height matched controls for respective ethnicity)						Interpretation
R_5	$R_{19/20}$	R_5–$R_{19/20}$	X_5	Ax	Fres	
↑	N	↑	↑	↑	→	Small airway obstruction
↑	↑	N	N	N	N	Proximal airway obstruction
↑↑	↑	↑	↑	↑	→	Combined airway obstruction
N	N	N	↑	↑	→	Restrictive pathology

*Reduction in R_5 (40%), X_5 (50%), Ax (80%) and Fres (leftward shift) from baseline suggests postbronchodilator reversibility

(Ax: reactance area; Fres: resonant frequency; LABA: long-acting beta agonist; N: normal; R: resistance; SABA: short-acting beta agonist; X: reactance; ↑: increase; →: rightward shift)

Source:

- Gupta N, Sachdev A, Gupta D, Gupta S. Oscillometry—The future of estimating pulmonary functions. Karnataka Pediatr J. 2020;35(2):79-87.
- King GG, Bates J, Berger KI, Caverley P, de Melo PL, Dellacà RL, et al. Technical standards for respiratory oscillometry. Eur Respir J. 2020;55(2):1900753.

after drug administration and during immunotherapy in patients with AR and chronic rhinosinusitis (CRS).

- *Bronchiolitis and asthma:* Early diagnosis of bronchiolitis obliterans and early intervention in children with bronchopulmonary dysplasia may be possible with FOT.
- *Cystic fibrosis:* Oscillometry can be used to assess peripheral airway involvement and track lung function decline.
- *Immunodeficiencies:* It may detect lung dysfunction early in patients with chronic lung disease due to primary or acquired immunodeficiency.

LIMITATIONS

- *Technique sensitivity:* Oscillometry requires the subject to remain quiet and calm during testing.
- *Data interpretation:* The complex nature of oscillometry data demands specialized knowledge.
- *Lack of standardization:* Limited reference ranges exist for FOT, making standardization challenging across different populations and regions.
- *Artefacts and noise:* Artefacts caused by irregular breathing or other involuntary movements can affect data accuracy.

- *Limited clinical adoption:* Despite its potential, FOT is not yet widely adopted in clinical practice due to a lack of awareness and understanding of its applications.

SUMMARY

Oscillometry has emerged as a promising technique for evaluating lung function, particularly inpatient populations where spirometry is not feasible. While FOT offers unique advantages and shows potential across various applications, it is not without limitations. The need for further research, education, and standardization remains critical to unlocking its full potential in clinical practice. Future efforts should focus on optimizing the technique, improving interpretation accuracy, and expanding its use to a broader range of conditions.

KEY POINTS

- *Principle of oscillometry:* Oscillometry, specifically the FOT, is a noninvasive method for assessing respiratory mechanics by introducing small pressure oscillations during normal breathing. It measures parameters such as resistance (Rrs) and reactance (Xrs) to evaluate the mechanical properties of the respiratory system, providing a more detailed and less effort-intensive alternative to traditional spirometry.
- *Types of FOT and waveforms:* This chapter describes three main types of FOT based on oscillation frequencies—mono/single/sinusoidal frequency, IOS, and PRN. Each type has specific applications and advantages, with PRN considered superior due to its ability to save time without compromising data integrity.
- *Comparison with spirometry:* Oscillometry offers several advantages over spirometry, including minimal patient cooperation and effort, suitability for younger children and patients with limited neuromuscular capacity, and better sensitivity in detecting peripheral airway dysfunction. Additionally, FOT generates minimal aerosols, making it safer for use during pandemics.
- *Current and potential applications:* FOT is currently used to diagnose and monitor a variety of pulmonary conditions (e.g., asthma, COPD, and pulmonary fibrosis) and extrapulmonary conditions (e.g., obesity hypoventilation syndrome and neuromuscular weakness). Future applications may include the diagnosis and management of allergic rhinitis, bronchiolitis, cystic fibrosis, and immunodeficiencies.
- *Limitations of FOT:* Despite its benefits, oscillometry faces several challenges, including the need for calm and quiet conditions during testing, the complexity of data interpretation, limited standardization across different populations, and artifacts caused by irregular breathing or movements. The limited clinical adoption of FOT is primarily due to a lack of awareness and understanding of its potential applications.

SUGGESTED READING

1. Global Initiative for Asthma (GINA). (2024). 2024 GINA Main Report: Global Strategy for Asthma Management and Prevention. [online] Available from https://ginasthma.org/2024-report/. [Last accessed April, 2025].
2. Gupta N, Kumar D. Functional evaluation of a child with hypoplastic lung using oscillometry. Lung India. 2024;41(1):73-4.
3. Gupta N, Sachdev A, Gupta D, Gupta S. Oscillometry - The future of estimating pulmonary functions. Karnataka Pediatr J. 2021;35(2):79-87.
4. Gupta N, Sachdev A, Gupta D. Oscillometry-a reasonable option to monitor lung functions in the era of COVID-19 pandemic. Pediatr Pulmonol. 2021;56(1):14-15.
5. Kaminsky DA, Simpson SJ, Berger KI, Caverley P, de Melo PL, Dandurand R, et al. Clinical significance and applications of oscillometry. Eur Respir Rev. 2022;31(163):210208.
6. King GG, Bates J, Berger KI, Caverley P, de Melo PL, Dellacà RL, et al. Technical standards for respiratory oscillometry. Eur Respir J. 2020;55(2):1900753..

16 CHAPTER

Questionnaires in Pediatric Asthma

Shebna A Khader

INTRODUCTION

In children, asthma is the most common chronic disease. Regular monitoring has to be done to tailor the treatment. Questionnaires are easy-to-use tools widely used in monitoring asthma control. It can also be used to measure the extent to which quality of life is affected and as a screening tool.

TYPES OF QUESTIONNAIRES

Questionnaires are mainly used for asthma to assess symptom control. These can be broadly classified as discussed here.

Simple Screening Tools

These questionnaires are used in primary care to quickly identify those who need detailed assessment.

For example, Global initiative for asthma (GINA) symptom control tool, 30-second asthma test.

Categorical Questionnaires

These questionnaires can measure categorical variables by assigning responses to specific groups.

For example, asthma APGAR tool, GINA symptom control tool, and PCT 3-questions asthma tool.

Numerical Questionnaires

These provide scores and cut off points to assess asthma control, and result is expressed as a number. This is simpler both for the physician and for the patient. It also gives a quick observation of change in control over time.

For example: ACT—Asthma Control Test, C-ACT—Childhood Asthma Control Test, and ACQ—Asthma Control Questionnaire.

QUESTIONNAIRES FOR ASSESSING ASTHMA CONTROL

The achievement and maintenance of asthma control are considered as main goal of asthma treatment. Asthma control is assessed by symptom control and the future risk of adverse outcomes. Directed questioning is important based on the presence of symptoms, limitations of daily activities, and use of rescue medications. Recent symptom control can be assessed over 1–4 weeks using questionnaires. In order to reduce recall error, patients are advised to maintain a symptom diary.

Symptom Diary

This should be an important communication tool to share with healthcare provider. It helps patients and doctors to identify triggers, understand symptoms, assess the effectiveness of treatment, and tailor treatment accordingly.

GINA advises recording the following data in the asthma diary.

- Asthma symptom (cough/wheezing breathlessness/chest tightness):
  - Daytime symptoms
  - Nighttime symptoms
- Activity limitation due to asthma
- Controller and reliever medication use

Peak Expiratory Flow Diary

Global Initiative for Asthma also advises a PEF (peak expiratory flow) diary. It has to be recorded every day morning and evening—highest of three peak flows (if not able to do daily, at least 2 weeks prior to hospital visit is recommended).

Symptom diary helps the clinician to carry out questionnaires more faster and to tailor the treatment without recall errors during consultation.

COMMON QUESTIONNAIRES FOR ASTHMA CONTROL

Global Initiative for Asthma Symptom Control Tool (Fig. 16.1)

- This is a simple and reliable short questionnaire for use in primary care.
- Age group—children 6 years and above, adults
- Recall period—4 weeks (can ask patient about whole period since last review)
- *Questions included*:
  - Daytime asthma symptoms more than twice/week?
  - Any night walking due to asthma?
  - Short-acting beta-agonist (SABA) reliever > twice/week?
  - Any activity limitation due to asthma?
- *Assessment*: Each question are given Yes/No options and is categorized as:
  - Well controlled—none of these
  - Partly controlled—1-2 of these
  - Uncontrolled—3-4 of these
- *Advantages:*
  - Easy and quick assessment
  - GINA also includes future risk factor assessment (discussed later)
  - Can be done for ages 6 years and above
- *Disadvantages*:
  - It is a categorical and not numerical questionnaire—hence, quick observation of changes on review is difficult.
  - Cannot be used <6 years of age.

Asthma Control Test

Asthma Control Test (ACT) is one of the best-known and most widely used questionnaires for clinical assessment of asthma control.

- Age group—12 years of age and above
- Recall period—4 weeks
- Self-administered questionnaire
- Questions included—5 questions:
  1. How much of your time did asthma keep you from getting work done at school or at home?
  2. How often does shortness of breath?
  3. How often do night symptoms?

Asthma symptom control		Level of asthma symptom control		
In the past 4 weeks, has the patient had:		Well controlled	Partly controlled	Uncontrolled
• Daytime asthma symptoms more than twice/week?	Yes■ No■	None of these	1–2 of these	3–4 of these
• Any night waking due to asthma?	Yes■ No■			
• SABA reliever for symptoms more than twice/week?	Yes■ No■			
• Any activity limitation due to asthma?	Yes■ No■			

Fig. 16.1: GINA asthma symptom control. (GINA: Global Initiative for Asthma; SABA: short-acting beta-agonist)

4. How often rescue inhaler?
5. How would you rate your asthma control?

- *Assessment:* To each answer, a point value from 1 to 25 is assigned:
  - Maximum—25 points (total control)
  - 20–24 points (partial control)
  - 19 and below (insufficient control)
- *Clinical correlation:*
  - Good correlation of scoring with clinical assessment, but poor correlation with forced expiratory volume in 1 second (FeV1) (as spirometry cannot be used as a single tool for control)
  - A score difference of three from the previous visit means it is time to make changes in treatment.
- *Disadvantages:*
  - Cannot be used for <12 years of age. Hence, a special version of ACT, the childhood asthma control test, was developed for 4–11 years of age.
  - Does not include lung function or risk assessment.

Childhood Asthma Control Test (C-ACT)

This is a version of ACT especially designed for 4–11 years of age **(Fig. 16.2)**.

- Age group—4–11 years
- Recall period—4 weeks
- To be answered by the child and the parent
- Questions included:

Seven questions—first four are answered by child. The next three are answered by parents:

1. How is your asthma?
2. Does it affect play or exercise?
3. Do you cough?
4. Is your sleep disturbed?
5. Daytime symptoms
6. Wheeze during the day
7. Night symptoms

- *Assessment:* Answers contain the graphic elements to help the child provide the right answer. Similar to ACT, points 19 or less—uncontrolled asthma.
- *Advantage:* It gives child's perspective on disease control.

Asthma Control Questionnaire

Asthma Control Questionnaire (ACQ) is a questionnaire with strong measurement properties. It was developed in 1999 by Elizabeth Juniper of McMaster University, Canada.

- Age group—6 years and above
- Recall period—1 week
- >10 years—self administered
- 6–10 years—with the help of a trained interviewer FeV1—by clinician
- *Questions included:* The original test (ACQ-7) has seven questions:
  1. Nocturnal awakenings due to asthma
  2. Limitation of daily activity
  3. Severity of morning symptom
  4. Shortness of breath
  5. Wheezing
  6. Use of short-acting beta-2 agonist
  7. FeV1
- *Assessment:* Each answer is given values from 0 to 6. The final result is the mean value of the results:
  - <0.75—well controlled asthma
  - >1.5—poorly controlled asthma
  - A change of 0.5 points from the previous value should be considered significant.
- *Clinical correlation:* ACQ correlates well with asthma severity. It is negatively associated with quality of life, FeV1, high ACQ scores are associated with recent use of oral corticosteroids, hospitalization, and exacerbations.
- *Disadvantages:* Measurement of FeV1 for scoring ACQ-7 requires access

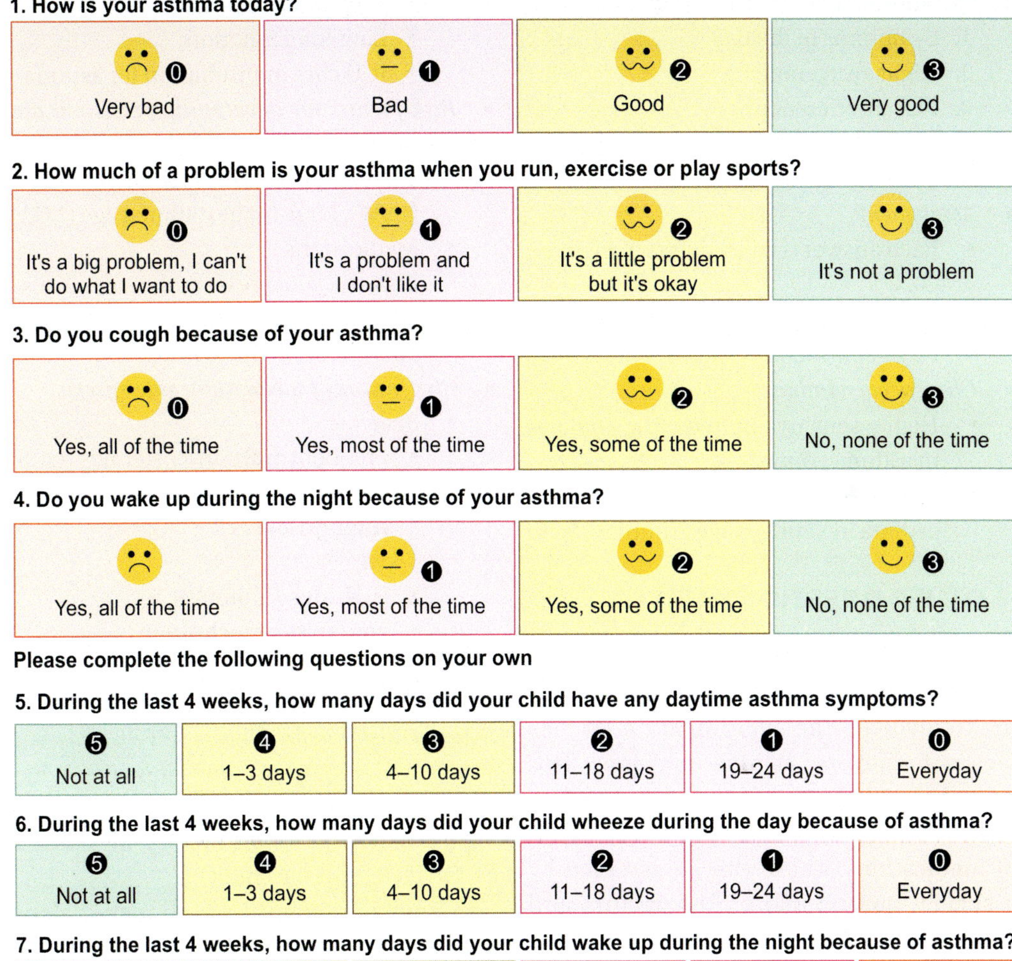

1. How is your asthma today?

0	1	2	3
Very bad	Bad	Good	Very good

2. How much of a problem is your asthma when you run, exercise or play sports?

0	1	2	3
It's a big problem, I can't do what I want to do	It's a problem and I don't like it	It's a little problem but it's okay	It's not a problem

3. Do you cough because of your asthma?

0	1	2	3
Yes, all of the time	Yes, most of the time	Yes, some of the time	No, none of the time

4. Do you wake up during the night because of your asthma?

	1	2	3
Yes, all of the time	Yes, most of the time	Yes, some of the time	No, none of the time

Please complete the following questions on your own

5. During the last 4 weeks, how many days did your child have any daytime asthma symptoms?

5	4	3	2	1	0
Not at all	1–3 days	4–10 days	11–18 days	19–24 days	Everyday

6. During the last 4 weeks, how many days did your child wheeze during the day because of asthma?

5	4	3	2	1	0
Not at all	1–3 days	4–10 days	11–18 days	19–24 days	Everyday

7. During the last 4 weeks, how many days did your child wake up during the night because of asthma?

5	4	3	2	1	0
Not at all	1–3 days	4–10 days	11–18 days	19–24 days	Everyday

Fig. 16.2: Childhood asthma control test.

to spirometry, prolongs the time, and requires the patient to withhold bronchodilator before the visit.

- *Versions:* Three new versions were developed (Symptoms only, symptoms + bronchodilator use, symptoms + FeV1). All these versions are well validated, but complete ACQ (ACQ-7) has the strongest measurement properties.

Test for Respiratory and Asthma Control in Kids

Test for Respiratory and Asthma Control in Kids (TRACK) is a special questionnaire specifically designed for kids under 5 years of age, and it corresponds well with the guidelines.

- Age—<5 years
- Recall period—4 weeks
- To be filled by a caregiver

- Questionnaire included five questions:
  1. Symptoms in the day
  2. Night awakening
  3. Play interference
  4. Use of a reliever
  5. Use of oral corticosteroids
- *Assessment:*
  - Each answer is given points 0, 5, 10, 15, 20.
  - Total score <80—not controlled
  - >80—controlled
- *Clinical correlation:*
  - Highly sensitive in detecting changes in asthma control
  - Can be used as a screening tool for asthma in younger age groups

OTHER QUESTIONNAIRES

Questionnaires to Assess Risk Factors

According to GINA, asthma control assessment involves the identification of risk factors for adverse asthma outcomes. This includes risk factors for exacerbations, persistent airflow limitation, and side effects of medications. These can be assessed by a special questionnaire. Risk factors and comorbidities that are modifiable are called treatable traits, and assessment helps in implementing measures to improve asthma outcomes.

- *Risk factors for exacerbations:*
  - Uncontrolled asthma symptoms.
  - Factors, even if less symptoms.
    - SABA over use (>3 × 200 dose canisters)
    - Inadequate inhaled corticosteroids (ICS)
    - Medical conditions—obesity, chronic rhinosinusitis, gastroesophageal reflux disease (GERD), food allergy.
    - Allergen exposure
    - Psychosocial problems
    - Low-long function
    - ICU care or intubation for asthma
- *Risk factors for developing persistent airflow limitation:*
  - History—preterm, low birth weight (LBW), large for gestational age (LGA)
  - Medications
  - Irritant exposure—smoke, chemicals
  - Low FeV1
  - Sputum or blood eosinophilia
- *Risk factors of medication side effects:*
  - *Systemic:*
    - Frequent oral corticosteroids (OCS)
    - Long-term ICS
    - High-dose ICS
  - *Local:*
    - High-dose/potent ICS
    - Poor inhaler technique.

Asthma Predicting Questionnaires

Asthma Risk Factor Scale (ARFS): This is a simple and easy-to-use questionnaire. It has questions in three sections: (1) Environmental exposure, (2) Parental history of asthma, (3) Diet habits of the child.

Cumulative exposure with toxins, along with positive family history and specific diet habits, was associated with asthma. This is a questionnaire that can predict asthma. Another version of ARFS, preschool-ARFS (PS-ARFS) can predict asthma with 1-year follow-up in preschool kids.

Asthma APGAR System

(APGAR is Poor Activities, Persistent triggers, Asthma medications and Response to therapy). This is developed for ages 5 and above. Questions to be answered by both parents and children together. Newer questionnaire is to be validated further, but it is found to be very sensitive to predict asthma severity.

TABLE 16.1: Comparison of commonly used questionnaires.

	Age	*Recall period*	*No. of questions*	*Expertise needed*	*Numerical*
GINA	>6 years	4 weeks	4	No	No
ACT	>12 years	4 weeks	5	No	Yes
C-ACT	4–11 years	4 weeks	5	No	Yes
ACQ-7	>6 years	1 week	7	Yes	Yes
TRACK	0–4 years	4 weeks	5	No	Yes
APGAR	>5 years	2 weeks	6	No	No

(ACQ-7: Asthma Control Questionnaire-7; ACT: Asthma Control Test; C-ACT: Childhood Asthma Control Test; GINA: Global Initiative for Asthma; TRACK: Test for Respiratory and Asthma Control in Kids)

Asthma Quality of Life Questionnaire

This is to assess both the physical and emotional impact of the disease. Asthma Quality of Life Questionnaire (AQLQ) is a self-administered questionnaire with 2-week recall. It assesses four domains—activities limitations, emotional function, environmental stimuli and symptoms in mild-to-moderate asthma.

Other questionnaires are risk factor assessment by GINA, 30-second asthma test, and Royal College of Physicians three Questions Asthma Tool (RSP3Q).

HOW TO SELECT A QUESTIONNAIRE

- An ideal questionnaire for children needs to be:
  - Relatively quick to complete
  - Able to identify children with uncontrolled asthma
  - Easily reproducible with less recall error
  - Can indicate need for changing treatment strategy
- Choice of questionnaire should be primarily based on
  - Age of child
  - Whether expertise is essential
  - Intellectual level of the child
  - Symptoms evaluated
  - Repeatability
  - Availability
  - Validity according to guidelines

As with all questionnaires, the answers depend on factors such as cultural, psychological, and social factors. Overstatement and understatement of symptoms to physicians can also produce differences in responses. Large variations in perception of symptoms are a limiting factor of questionnaires. But still in a busy clinical practice, a simple scoring system with the questionnaire is highly desirable **(Table 16.1)**.

SUMMARY

- Questionnaires are simple tools used in primary care to assess asthma control in a short period of time.
- Numerical questionnaires help in the easy assessment of asthma control and guide in tailoring treatment.
- Maintaining an asthma diary is essential to reduce recall error and also increase the sensitivity of the questionnaire.
- GINA, ACT, C-ACT, ACQ, and TRACK are simple questionnaires, which are well validated, but proper selection of questionnaires is crucial.

KEY POINTS

- Questionnaires are practical and time-efficient tools for assessing asthma control in children across various healthcare settings.
- Numerical questionnaires like ACT, C-ACT, ACQ, and TRACK provide objective scoring that helps clinicians tailor treatment and track progress.
- Maintaining an asthma symptom or peak flow diary enhances the accuracy of questionnaires by reducing recall bias.
- The choice of questionnaires should be guided by age, clinical setting, intellectual level of the child, and ease of administration.
- Widely validated tools include the GINA symptom control tool, ACT, C-ACT, ACQ and TRACK, each suited for different age groups.
- Despite cultural and perceptual variations in reporting, questionnaires remain invaluable in busy clinical practice to monitor control, assess risk, and guide therapy adjustments.

SUGGESTED READING

1. Bohnen AM, Bindels PJE, Elshout G. A systematic review of questionnaires measuring asthma control in children in a primary care population. NPJ Prim Care Respir Med. 2023;33:25.
2. Global Initiative for Asthma (GINA). Global Strategy for Asthma Management and Prevention. 2024 update. Available from: https://ginasthma.org/2024. [Last accessed April, 2025].
3. Juniper EF, Jones G, Ward S, Svensson K. Asthma control questionnaire in children: validation, measurement properties, interpretation. Eur Respir J. 2010;36:1410-6.
4. Przybyszowski M, Bochenek G. The role of questionnaires in the assessment of asthma control. Pneumonol Alergol Pol. 2015; 83:220-8.

CHAPTER

17

Tools in Asthma for Assessing Recent Symptom Control

Charu Chandwani

INTRODUCTION

Asthma is a prevalent chronic condition among children and adolescents, entailing effective management strategies to ensure optimal symptom control. Accurate assessment of asthma control is crucial for tailoring treatment and improving health outcomes.

IMPORTANCE OF ASTHMA CONTROL ASSESSMENT

Asthma control is defined as the degree to which the symptoms of asthma are minimized and the goals of therapy are met. Regular assessment of asthma control is essential for:

- Optimizing treatment
- Preventing exacerbations
- Enhancing quality of life
- Monitoring long-term outcomes

The Global Initiative for Asthma (GINA) guidelines provide various tools to evaluate asthma symptoms and their impact on daily life. This chapter focuses on primary assessment tools:

- The Asthma Control Test (ACT)
- The Asthma Control Questionnaire (ACQ)
- Asthma action plan
- Peak Expiratory Flow Rate Monitoring

This write-up summarizes these tools, framing their usage, reliability, and relevance in clinical practice.

ASTHMA CONTROL TEST

The ACT is a validated, patient-reported outcome measure designed to assess asthma control in individuals aged 12 years and older. It helps both patients and healthcare providers evaluate how well asthma is managed and identify areas needing attention.

Overview

- *Purpose:* The ACT aims to measure asthma symptoms and their impact on daily life, providing a simple way to assess control over the condition.
- *Structure:* The ACT consists of five questions assessed over a period of 4 weeks that cover:
    - Frequency of symptoms (e.g., wheezing, shortness of breath)
    - Nighttime awakenings
    - Impact on daily activities
    - Use of rescue medications
    - Overall self-assessment of asthma control
- *Scoring:* Each question is scored from 1 to 5, with a total possible score ranging from 5 to 25. Score interpretation:
    - *19–25*: Well controlled
    - *16–18*: Not well controlled
    - *<16*: Poorly controlled

Implementation in Clinical Practice

- *Regular assessment:* The ACT should be administered periodically to monitor asthma control and track changes over time.

- *Patient engagement:* Involving patients in completing the ACT fosters awareness and encourages discussions about their condition and treatment options.
- *Guiding treatment decisions:* Results from the ACT can inform treatment adjustments, helping clinicians decide if medications need to be increased, decreased, or changed.
- *Identifying exacerbations:* The test can help identify patients at risk of asthma exacerbations, prompting proactive management strategies.

Benefits of the Asthma Control Test

- *Simplicity and accessibility:* The ACT is straightforward and can be completed quickly, making it easy for both patients and healthcare providers to use.
- *Improved communication:* Provides a common framework for discussing asthma control between patients and clinicians.
- *Empowerment:* Encourages patients to take an active role in managing their asthma, leading to better adherence to treatment plans.
- *Data for research and quality improvement:* Aggregated ACT scores can provide valuable insights for healthcare systems looking to improve asthma management and outcomes.

Regular use of the ACT can lead to better communication between patients and healthcare providers, ultimately enhancing the quality of asthma care.

ASTHMA CONTROL QUESTIONNAIRE

The Asthma Control Questionnaire (ACQ) is a widely used tool that helps assess asthma control, as recommended by the GINA guidelines.

Overview of the Asthma Control Questionnaire

- *Purpose:* The ACQ is designed to evaluate the level of asthma control over a specific period, typically the past week or 2 weeks.
- *Structure:* The questionnaire consists of several items that address key aspects of asthma control, including:
  - Frequency of daytime symptoms
  - Nighttime awakenings due to asthma
  - Use of rescue medications
  - The impact of asthma on daily activities
  - Overall self-assessment of asthma control
- *Scoring system:* The ACQ is scored on a scale from 0 to 6:
  - *0* indicates complete control of asthma
  - *6* reflects very poor control

A score of 1.5 or higher typically suggests that asthma is not well controlled.

Implementation in Clinical Practice

- *Regular use:* GINA guidelines recommend that the ACQ be administered regularly to monitor asthma control over time. This helps in identifying patterns and guiding treatment adjustments.
- *Personalized action plans:* The results of the ACQ can inform individualized asthma action plans, ensuring that management strategies are tailored to the patient's specific needs and control levels.
- *Tracking progress:* By comparing scores over time, clinicians can evaluate the effectiveness of treatment interventions and make necessary adjustments based on the patient's progress.
- *Patient engagement:* Involving patients and their families in the completion of

the ACQ fosters better understanding and engagement in asthma management, promoting adherence to treatment plans.

Conclusion

The ACQ is a crucial component of asthma management as outlined by GINA guidelines. By facilitating regular assessment and promoting personalized care, the ACQ helps improve asthma outcomes and enhances the quality of life for patients. Regular use of the ACQ enables healthcare providers to make informed decisions, ensuring that children with asthma receive optimal care tailored to their needs.

COMPARISON OF ASTHMA CONTROL TEST AND ASTHMA CONTROL QUESTIONNAIRE

Both the ACT and ACQ are valuable tools for assessing asthma control, but they differ in their design and application:

- *Length and complexity:* The ACT is shorter and may be preferred for routine assessments, while the ACQ offers a more detailed evaluation.
- *Age suitability:* The ACT is designed for individuals aged 12 and older, whereas the ACQ can be adapted for younger children.
- *Focus areas:* The ACT emphasizes the patient's overall perception of control, while the ACQ combines symptoms and the use of rescue medications for a more comprehensive assessment.

ASTHMA ACTION PLAN

Key Components

- *Personal information:* Importance of including personal and emergency contact details.
- *Recognizing triggers:* Techniques to identify and avoid specific triggers and keep a symptom diary.
- *Medication management:* Overview of controller versus rescue medications and the importance of adherence to prescribed medication schedules.

Monitoring your Asthma

Symptom Tracking

- How to log daily symptoms and peak flow readings
- Tools and apps available for tracking

Understanding Peak Flow Measurements

- Explanation of peak flow meters and how to use them
- Importance of knowing personal best peak flow readings

Response Plan (Fig. 17.1)

Green Zone (Well Controlled)

Description of symptoms in this zone and actions to maintain control.

Yellow Zone (Caution)

- Signs indicating the need for intervention.
- Steps to take and when to consult a healthcare provider.

Red Zone (Emergency)

- Identifying severe symptoms and immediate actions required
- Importance of having a clear emergency plan

Emergency Contacts and Resources

- Listing emergency services and nearest healthcare facilities
- Importance of having an updated contact list for asthma specialists

ASTHMA ACTION PLAN

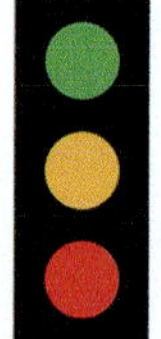

Asthma and Allergy Foundation of America
aafa.org

Name:	Date:
Doctor:	Medical Record #:
Doctor's Phone #: Day	Night/Weekend
Emergency Contact:	
Doctor's Signature:	

The colors of a traffic light will help you use your asthma medicines.

GREEN means Go Zone! Use preventive medicine.

YELLOW means Caution Zone! Add quick-relief medicine.

RED means Danger Zone! Get help from a doctor.

Personal Best Peak Flow: ____________

GO

Use these daily controller medicines:

You have *all* of these:
- Breathing is good
- No cough or wheeze
- Sleep through the night
- Can work & play

Peak flow: from ______ to ______

MEDICINE	HOW MUCH	HOW OFTEN/WHEN
For asthma with exercise, take:		

CAUTION

Continue with green zone medicine and add:

You have *any* of these:
- First signs of a cold
- Exposure to known trigger
- Cough
- Mild wheeze
- Tight chest
- Coughing at night

Peak flow: from ______ to ______

MEDICINE	HOW MUCH	HOW OFTEN/ WHEN
CALL YOUR ASTHMA CARE PROVIDER.		

DANGER

Take these medicines and call your doctor now.

Your asthma is getting worse fast:
- Medicine is not helping
- Breathing is hard & fast
- Nose opens wide
- Trouble speaking
- Ribs show (in children)

Peak flow: reading below ______

MEDICINE	HOW MUCH	HOW OFTEN/WHEN

GET HELP FROM A DOCTOR NOW! Your doctor will want to see you right away. It's important! If you cannot contact your doctor, go directly to the emergency room. DO NOT WAIT.
Make an appointment with your asthma care provider within two days of an ER visit or hospitalization.

Fig. 17.1: Asthma and Allergy Foundation of America.

Education and Communication

- Discussing asthma with family, friends, and caregivers
- Importance of education in managing asthma effectively

Review and Adaptation

- Guidance on how often to review and update the action plan
- Encouraging proactive communication with healthcare providers

PEAK EXPIRATORY FLOW MONITORING

What is a Peak Flow Meter?

A peak flow meter **(Fig. 17.2)** is a portable device that measures the maximum speed of expiration, known as peak expiratory flow (PEF). It provides valuable information about how well air is moving out of the lungs.

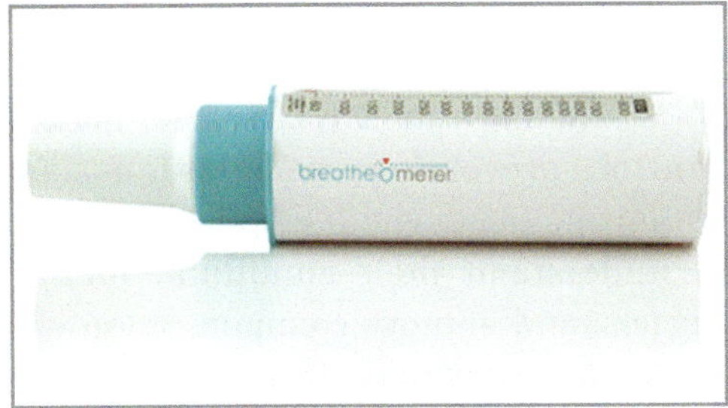

Fig. 17.2: A peak flow meter.

Importance of Peak Expiratory Flow in Pediatric Asthma Management

- *Monitoring lung function:* Regular use of a peak flow meter helps track a child's lung function over time, identifying patterns or changes that may indicate worsening asthma.
- *Early detection of exacerbations:* Decreased peak flow readings can signal an impending asthma attack, allowing for timely intervention and adjustments in treatment.
- *Personalized asthma action plans:* PEF readings can be integrated into asthma action plans, guiding families on when to take specific actions based on the child's condition.

How to Use a Peak Flow Meter?

- *Preparation:* Ensure the device is clean and in good working condition. Explain the process to the child to help them understand.
- *Technique* **(Fig. 17.3):**
  - *Stand up:* The child should stand up straight to allow for optimal lung expansion.
  - *Take a deep breath*: Inhale as deeply as possible.
  - *Seal lips:* Place the mouthpiece in the mouth, sealing lips tightly around it.

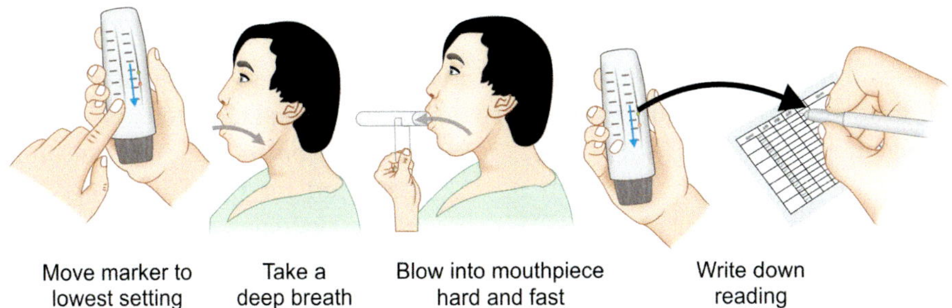

Fig. 17.3: How to use a peak flow meter.

TABLE 17.1: Peak expiratory flow rate (PEFR) readings.

Date	Time	PEFR (L/min)	Notes/Comments
[Date]	[Time]	[PEFR Value]	[Symptoms, medications, environmental factors]
[Date]	[Time]	[PEFR Value]	[Symptoms, medications, environmental factors]
[Date]	[Time]	[PEFR Value]	[Symptoms, medications, environmental factors]

  - *Exhale hard and fast:* Blow out as hard and fast as possible into the meter.
  - *Record the reading:* Note the peak flow reading, which is the highest number displayed.
- *Repeat:* Typically, three readings should be taken, and the highest value should be recorded.
- Documenting **(Table 17.1)**

When to Use the Peak Flow Meter?

- *Daily monitoring:* Recommended to use the meter at the same time each day, preferably in the morning before taking medication.
- *Before and after exercise:* To check how exercise affects lung function.
- *During symptoms:* If the child is experiencing symptoms or feels their asthma is worsening.

Interpreting Peak Flow Readings

- *Green zone:* 80–100% of the child's personal best—indicates good control.
- *Yellow zone:* 50–79% of the personal best—suggests caution and possible need for medication adjustment.
- *Red zone:* <50% of the personal best—requires immediate action, possibly including use of a rescue inhaler or seeking medical help.

Benefits of Using a Peak Flow Meter

- *Empowerment:* Helps children and caregivers take an active role in managing asthma.
- *Data for healthcare providers:* Provides objective data to inform treatment decisions.
- *Improved control:* Regular monitoring can lead to better overall asthma management and reduced hospitalizations.

Conclusion

A peak flow meter is a valuable tool in managing pediatric asthma, offering insights into lung function and helping to prevent exacerbations. By incorporating it into daily routines and asthma action plans, families can enhance their asthma management and improve their child's quality of life. Regular use and proper education on technique are key to maximizing its effectiveness.

Monitoring asthma is crucial for tracking control, preventing exacerbations, and optimizing treatment. It empowers patients to understand their condition, identify triggers, and improve communication with healthcare providers. Ultimately, regular monitoring enhances quality of life by reducing symptoms and allowing for more freedom in daily activities.

SUMMARY

Asthma control tools are vital for effective management and include:

- *Asthma control test:* This questionnaire, designed for individuals aged 12 and older, evaluates asthma symptoms and their effects on daily life. It scores from 5 to 25, aiding in assessing control and guiding treatment decisions.

- *Asthma Control Questionnaire (ACQ):* The ACQ assesses asthma control over a specific timeframe, usually 1–2 weeks. It examines symptom frequency, medication use, and overall management on a scale from 0 to 6, helping to tailor patient care.
- *Peak expiratory flow rate (PEFR) monitoring:* Using a peak flow meter, this method tracks lung function over time. Regular monitoring allows for the early detection of changes, indicating potential asthma exacerbations and informing action plans.
- *Asthma action plan:* This personalized strategy details medication management, recognition of triggers, and a response plan based on symptom severity (green, yellow, red zones). It empowers patients to take proactive steps in managing their asthma.

Collectively, these tools enhance regular assessment, foster communication between patients and healthcare providers, and support individualized asthma management for improved health outcomes.

KEY POINTS

- Asthma control assessment is essential for optimizing treatment, preventing exacerbations, and improving quality of life in children and adolescents.
- *Asthma Control Test (ACT):* A quick, patient-reported tool for ≥12 years; scores 5–25 and helps categorize asthma as well, not well, or poorly controlled.
- *Asthma Control Questionnaire (ACQ):* GINA-recommended; assesses control over 1–2 weeks; score ≥1.5 indicates poor control.
- *Asthma Action Plan:* Personalized, zone-based plan (green, yellow, red) guiding daily management, trigger avoidance, and emergency response.
- *Peak Expiratory Flow Rate (PEFR) monitoring:* Objective lung function tool; helps detect worsening asthma early and supports action plans.
- Combined use of these tools enhances communication between patients and providers, supports individualized care, and improves asthma outcomes.

SUGGESTED READING

1. American Lung Association. (2024). Asthma action plan. [online] Available from https://www.lung.org/asthma/action-plan. [Last accessed April, 2025].
2. Global Initiative for Asthma (GINA). (2024). Global strategy for asthma management and prevention.[online] Available from https://ginasthma.org. [Last accessed April, 2025]
3. National Heart, Lung, and Blood Institute. Asthma. (2024). [online] Available from https://www.nhlbi.nih.gov/health-topics/asthma. [Last accessed April, 2025].

CHAPTER 18

Modified Asthma Predictive Index—How to Use in Practice?

Krishna Mohan R, Francis Kurian

INTRODUCTION

Asthma is one of the most common chronic diseases of childhood. Up to 50% of children wheeze at least once during the preschool years. Although many of these children go on to develop asthma, our ability to predict school-age asthma based on early life characteristics is currently limited. Early identification of persons at risk of disease can be used to identify children who require closer monitoring and may be ideal candidates for prevention strategies or interventions, including allergen immunotherapy. Therefore, accurate prediction of asthma development is highly desirable for clinicians, families, and researchers.

BACKGROUND

The Asthma Predictive Index (API) is simple, inexpensive, and noninvasive and has been well validated. Clinicians can use a positive API score to identify at-risk children and educate parents on the importance of asthma maintenance therapy and treatment of flares. Like any test, the API must be interpreted and acted on appropriately. The use of the API in conjunction with newer antiallergen therapy holds promise for preventing the development and progression of asthma.

The Modified Asthma Predictive Index (mAPI) is an assessment tool that predicts future atopic asthma in pediatric patients with recurrent wheezing. It is applicable for young children with four or more episodes of wheezing per year.

CRITERIA FOR MODIFIED ASTHMA PREDICTIVE INDEX (TABLE 18.1)

The mAPI includes both major and minor criteria along with a prerequisite of four or more wheezing episodes per year. Compared

TABLE 18.1: Criteria for modified Asthma Predictive Index (mAPI).

Major criteria—1 of the following:	*Minor criteria*—2 of the following:
• Parental history	• Allergic sensitization to food (positive skin prick test or blood test)
• Physician diagnosed atopic dermatitis	• Wheezing unrelated to colds
• Allergic sensitization to aeroallergen (dust mite, cat, dog, mold, grass, trees, and weeds)	• Blood eosinophilia ≥4% of WBC count
Modified Asthma Predictive Index (mAPI) • For children under 3 years of age with ALL of the following: – *Four wheezing exacerbations in the past year,* with one physician-confirmed episode – Plus one major criteria or two minor criteria	

to API, mAPI has excluded allergic rhinitis in the criteria.

PREDICTIVE VALUE

Because children with a positive API are at increased risk of developing asthma, the mAPI, which used more objective criteria than the API, was used as entry criteria for many clinical trials. These studies showed decreased exacerbations, decreased controller medication usage, and increased episode-free days in 2- to 3-year-old children with a positive mAPI treated with inhaled corticosteroids compared with placebo.

Negative predictive values are better than positive predictive values. Hence, it is better at excluding rather than predicting.

CLINICAL APPLICATION

Who Might Use this Tool?

- Pediatricians
- Family physicians
- General practitioners
- Nurse practitioners
- Pharmacists
- Certified respiratory educators

When might they Use this Tool?

When providing care to a pediatric patient with suspected asthma.

Why might they Use this Tool?

- To identify the likelihood of preschool-age children developing asthma.
- To aid clinical decision making in assessing future asthma risk for preschool-age children.

What are Important Considerations when Using this Tool?

This tool provides a score that applies to preschool children as they are too young for reliable spirometry, and IgE levels are affected by age.

LIMITATIONS

While the mAPI is a robust predictive tool, it has its own limitations too. Asthma is a complex disease with many phenotypes, and there are still many gaps in our knowledge. There are overlaps between phenotypes associated with different types of inflammation, such as type 2 (T2), non-T2, and mixed. These factors can affect the predictive accuracy of mAPI. Also, its accuracy may vary based on the prevalence of asthma across different populations and settings.

SUMMARY

Although asthma prediction during early life remains challenging, the mAPI's high predictive ability of school-age asthma after a positive test can have clinical value for identifying children at risk of asthma persisting into school age and beyond. Its use in clinical practice can facilitate timely interventions, potentially improving long-term outcomes for pediatric patients with recurrent wheezing.

KEY POINTS

- The Modified Asthma Predictive Index (mAPI) is a validated tool used to predict the likelihood of school-age asthma in children under 3 years of age who have had four or more wheezing episodes in the past year, including at least one confirmed by a physician.
- mAPI has strong negative predictive value, meaning it is better at ruling out future asthma than confirming it—helping clinicians avoid overdiagnosis and unnecessary treatment.
- Clinical use of mAPI supports early identification of at-risk children, allowing timely interventions such as inhaled corticosteroids or allergen immunotherapy to reduce asthma progression and improve outcomes.

- Limitations of mAPI include variability in predictive accuracy due to asthma's heterogeneous nature and population-specific prevalence, and it may not account for all asthma phenotypes such as non-T2 inflammation.

SUGGESTED READING

1. Castro-Rodriguez JA, Cifuentes L, Martinez FD. Predicting asthma using clinical indexes. Front Pediatr; 2019.
2. Chang TS, Lemanske RF Jr, Guilbert TW, Gern JE, Coen MH, Evans MD, et al. Evaluation of the modified asthma predictive index in high-risk preschool children. J Allergy Clin Immunol Pract. 2013;1(2):152-6.
3. MDApp. Modified asthma predictive index (mAPI) calculator. Retrieved from https://www.mdapp.co/modified-asthma-predictive-index-mapi-calculator-337/ [Last accessed June, 2025].

CHAPTER 19

Aerosol Devices in Asthma

Viveka Santhosh Reddy C, Soundarya M

INTRODUCTION

For over 3,500 years, the primary method of treatment for lung diseases, especially asthma, has been therapeutic aerosol delivery. Traditionally, the inhalation of vapor produced by smoking or heating herbal mixes was the method used to provide medicinal aerosols. The industrial revolution brought with it more advanced methods of nebulizing medicinal liquids or producing therapeutic vapors due to advances in manufacturing capacities. Devices made by a firm or individual who had no connection to the patient replaced the custom-made therapeutic aerosols made by a person directly involved in the patient's care. Post the release of the first metered-dose inhaler (MDI) in 1956, the field of medicinal aerosol delivery saw significant advancements. Dry-powder inhalers (DPIs) did not become widely used in the market until the 1990s, even though the first one was created in the middle of the 19th century. The inhaler business as it exists now was created by a spurt of innovation in inhaler creation following the 1987 ratification of the Montreal Protocol. In the future, smart inhalers should find commercial acceptability because of high-tech solutions that enhance medication delivery and patient compliance. But the demands of rising healthcare costs will offset the need for high-tech inhalers, probably guaranteeing that DPI and MDI therapies will continue to be crucial parts of therapeutic aerosol delivery.

AEROSOL DEPOSITION MECHANISM AND LOCALIZATION

The main dynamics underlying aerosol deposition are **(Figs. 19.1A and B)**:

- *Inertial impaction:* Larger (>3 µm), faster-moving particles experience inertial impaction.
- *Diffusion:* Particles <1 µm experience diffusion and
- *Settling or gravitational sedimentation:* Particle mass and time determine the gravitational settling rate, which is proportional to the mass and size of the particles.

The larger particles, measuring between 10 and 15 µm, primarily deposit in the upper airways. Particles, measuring between 5 and 10 µm, reach the major bronchi while the smaller particles, measuring between 1 and 5 µm, enter the lower airways, including peripheries.

SELECTION CRITERIA OF AEROSOL DELIVERY DEVICES

There are four areas into which the criteria for choosing an aerosol generator can be divided:

1. Elements linked to the patient—age, cognitive and physical abilities as well as preference according to end user's comfort.

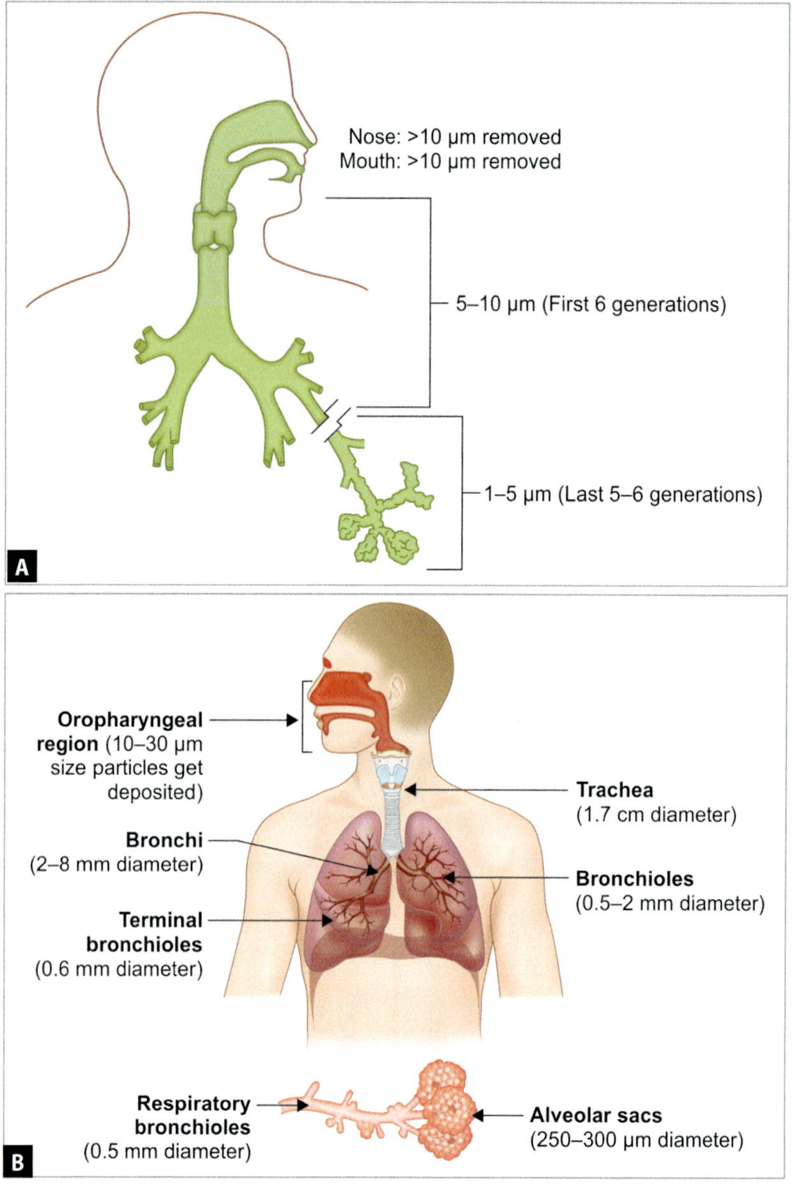

Figs. 19.1A and B: Particle size and localization of deposition in the airway tract.

2. Drug-related—availability in various forms and presence of combination medications.
3. Device related—convenience, durability, and cost of aerosol generator.
4. Environment and clinical considerations.

TYPES OF AEROSOL DELIVERY DEVICES

The three most popular types of aerosol generators used for inhaled medication delivery are as follows:

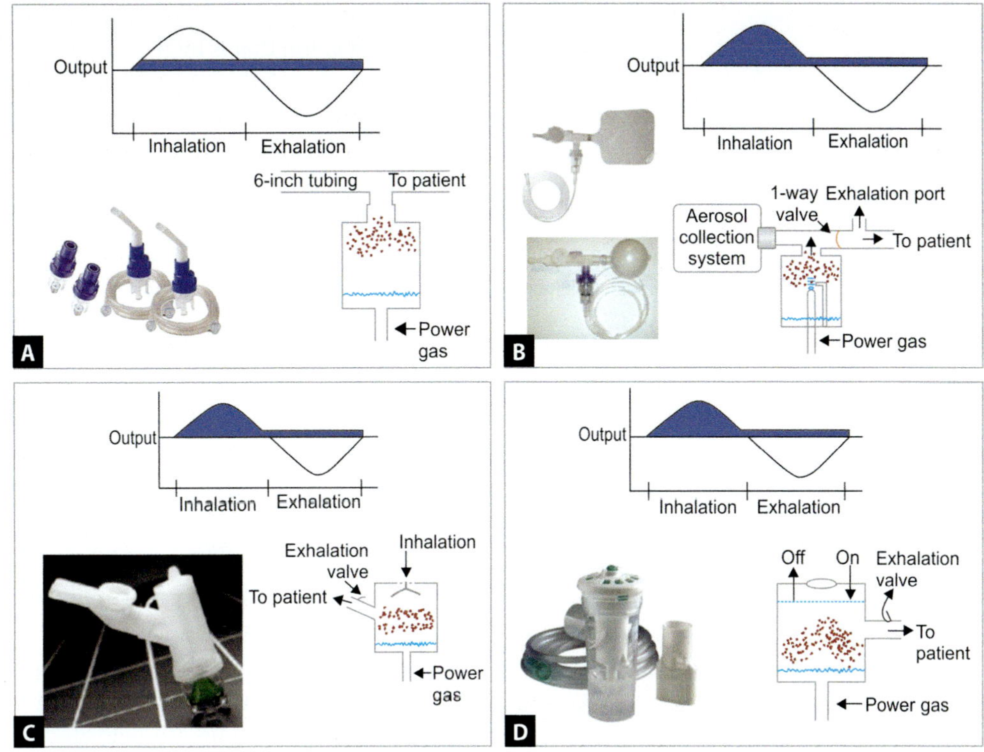

Figs. 19.2A to D: Pneumatic jet nebulizer types—various designs with shaded area indicating the aerosol output: (A) With a reservoir tube; (B) With a collection bag; (C) Breath-enhanced; (D) Breath-actuated.

1. *The small-volume nebulizer (SVN):* Powered by compressed air, oxygen, a compressor, or an electrical device, the SVN is an aerosol generator that turns liquid medication solutions or suspensions into aerosol.
   - Jet, ultrasonic, and mesh nebulizers are different types of SVNs available **(Figs. 19.2A to D)**.
   - In the setting of critical care or acute management, SVNs have been the cornerstone.
   - When it comes to patients who are unable to utilize different inhalers that need active participation and hand-eye coordination, such as infants, young kids, and the elderly, they are often chosen as the device of choice.
   - Advantages include no special technique of breathing required, minimal patient cooperation or coordination, hence useful in very young/old, distressed or debilitated patients, ability to aerosolize drug mixtures and solutions, and possibility of dose/concentration modification.
   - Disadvantages include large, cumbersome equipment requiring a power source, assembly, cleaning, and possible contamination, variable duration of treatment, exposure of the drug to caregivers/clinicians, as well as irritation to the eyes when used with a face mask.
2. *Pressurized metered-dose inhaler (pMDI):* A combination of compact, portable,

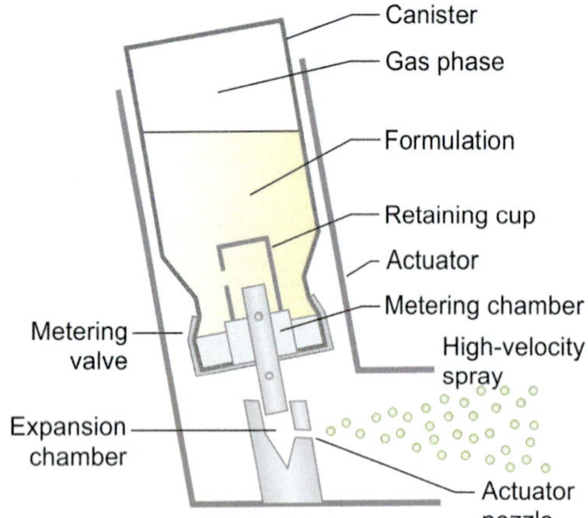

Fig. 19.3: Pressurized metered-dose inhaler (pMDI) components.

self-contained medication devices, deliver several doses based on a metered value. Holding chambers and spacers are frequently utilized as supplementary devices with pMDIs due to the substantial medication loss in the oropharynx and the hand-held coordination difficulties associated with these devices **(Fig. 19.3)**.

- Conventional pMDIs and soft-mist inhalers are the main types of pMDIs.
- The basic parts of the pMDI are the canister, propellants, medication formulary, metering valve, and actuator, irrespective of the manufacturer or ingredient that is being used.
- Advantages include that the devices are light, compact, portable, require shorter convenient treatment time, possibility of multiple dosing, no involvement of drug preparation, with reproducibility of emitted doses, and resistant to contamination.
- Disadvantages include activation from the patient's end, the necessity for hand-breath coordination, correct inhalation technique with breath-holding, drug concentrations that are fixed, and, finally, oropharyngeal deposition that is high.

3. *Dry-powder inhaler:* The DPI is an aerosol drug delivery system that usually uses a breath-actuated dosage mechanism to deliver powdered medication.
   - The energy needed to separate the tiny medication particles from the larger carrier particles and scatter the particles as aerosol released from the device is created by the patient's inspiratory effort, which includes both their respiratory flow rate and the volume breathed.
   - Three categories—single-dose, multiple unit-dose, and multiple-dose DPIs can be distinguished from DPIs according to how their dose containers are designed.
   - Advantages include compact, transportable, integrated dosage counter; propellant-free breath-activated, less time needed for administration and preparation.
   - Disadvantages include depending on the inspiratory flow of the patient, less conscious of the dosage administered, very high impaction of the oropharynx, susceptible to moisture from the surrounding air or from breath entering the mouthpiece, limited selection of medications, dissimilar DPIs for different medications, difficult to understand instructions for using different gadgets **(Fig. 19.4)**.

RECOMMENDATIONS FOR DRUG DELIVERY DEVICES IN NEONATAL AND PEDIATRIC POPULATION

Recommendations for drug delivery devices in neonatal and pediatric population are shown in **Table 19.1**.

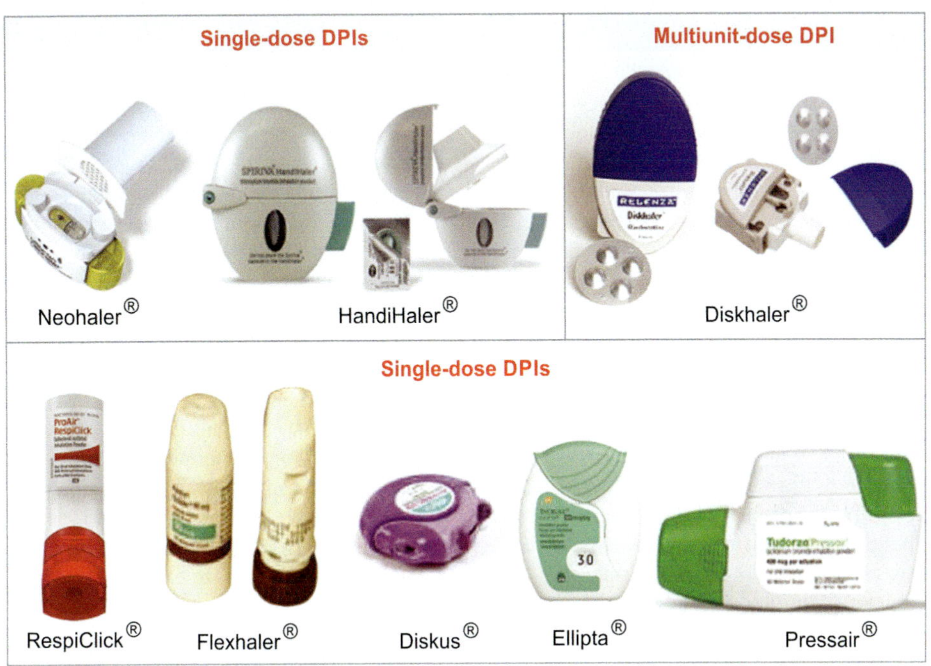

Fig. 19.4: Various types of dry-powder inhalers (DPIs).

TABLE 19.1

S. No.	*Type of aerosol generator*	*Age*
1.	SVN with mask or hood	Infant
2.	SVN with mask	≤3 years
3.	SVN with mouthpiece	≥3 years
4.	pMDI with valved holding chamber/spacer and mask	<4 years
5.	pMDI with valved holding chamber/spacer	≥4 years
6.	Dry-powder inhaler	≥4 years
7.	Metered-dose inhaler	≥5 years
8.	Breath-actuated MDI (e.g., Autohaler)	≥5 years
9.	Breath-actuated nebulizer	≥5 years

(MDI: metered-dose inhaler; pMDI: pressurized metered-dose inhaler; SVN: small-volume nebulizer)

PATIENT EDUCATION

General Instructions and Evaluation

General instructions and evaluation to be followed are mentioned in **Box 19.1**.

Instructions while Using Jet Nebulizers

Instructions while using jet nebulizers are given in **Box 19.2**.

BOX 19.1

- Before instructing others, carefully go over the instructions and practice using a placebo device
- Utilizing a checklist, show patients how to assemble and operate the device correctly
- Give the patient written instructions on how to operate the device and, for patients who are not very literate, a written plan including pictures outlining how often to take the medication based on their symptoms
- While the clinician observes, have the patient practice using the device
- Every time a patient returns, go over how they used the device
- At every follow-up visit, confirm that the patient understands the inhaled drugs (when to use, purpose of the drug, prescribed frequency)
- Whenever inadequate management of airway disease occurs, maintain a high index of suspicion for improper use or nonadherence

BOX 19.2

- Put the mouthpiece (or mask), nebulizer cup, and tubing together
- Place the medication in the cup of the nebulizer
- Maintain an upright posture
- Attach the nebulizer's power supply to it
- Breathe normally, taking intermittent deep breaths, until the nebulization stops or until sputtering starts
- During therapy, keep the nebulizer upright
- After rinsing it with distilled or sterile water, let the nebulizer air dry

Instructions while Using Mesh and Ultrasonic Nebulizers

Instructions while using mesh and ultrasonic nebulizers are listed in **Box 19.3**.

Instructions while Using Pressurized Metered-dose Inhalers Open Mouth Technique

Instructions while using pMDIs open mouth technique are shown in **Box 19.4**.

BOX 19.3

- Assemble the nebulizer correctly, following the manufacturer's instructions
- Transfer the mixture into the prescription drug container. Do not go beyond the manufacturer's suggested volume
- Maintain an upright posture
- Attach the nebulizer's power supply to it
- For these especially crafted mesh and ultrasonic nebulizers, adhere to the manufacturer's recommended breathing method guidelines
- To prevent waste, turn off the unit if it needs to be paused
- As directed by the manufacturer, disassemble and clean when complete
- Avoid touching the mesh when cleaning a mesh nebulizer, as this would spoil the device
- As directed by the manufacturer, clean the nebulizer once or twice a week

BOX 19.4

- Take off the mouthpiece cover, then give the pMDI a good shake
- If the pMDI is brand-new or hasn't been used in a few days, prime it into the air
- Maintain an upright posture either in a sitting or standing position
- Completely exhale
- Two finger widths should separate the pMDI from their lips
- Tilt the pMDI outlet so that it faces the upper rear of the mouth while the patient's mouth is open, and their tongue is flat (tip in contact with the inside of the lower front teeth)
- When the person starts to inhale gently, pMDI is to be activated
- A slow, deep breath through the mouth is to be taken, then held for 10 seconds. As long as they can, if they are unable to hold their breath
- If another dose of medication is to be taken, wait for 1 minute
- Until the dose recommended by the doctor is reached, repeat the above steps
- If the medication used is a corticosteroid, the patient should rinse their mouth after the final dose, spitting out the water rather than ingesting
- Replace the mouthpiece cover post use each time

(pMDI: pressurized metered-dose inhaler)

Instructions while Using Pressurized Metered-dose Inhalers Closed Mouth Technique

Instructions while using pMDIs closed mouth technique are mentioned in **Box 19.5**.

Instructions while Using Breath-actuated Pressurized Metered-dose Inhalers (Autohaler)

Instructions while using breath-actuated pMDIs (Autohaler) are shown in **Box 19.6**.

BOX 19.5

- Take off the mouthpiece cover, then give the pMDI a good shake
- If the pMDI is brand-new or has not been used in a few days, prime it into the air
- Maintain an upright posture either in a sitting or standing position
- Completely exhale
- Make sure the tongue is flat beneath the mouthpiece and does not obstruct the pMDI before placing the device between their teeth
- Lips to be sealed around the mouthpiece
- When the person starts to inhale gently, pMDI is to be activated
- A slow, deep breath through the mouth to be taken, then held for 10 seconds. As long as they can, if they are unable to hold their breath
- If another dose of medication is to be taken, wait for 1 minute
- Until the dose recommended by the doctor is reached, repeat the above steps
- If the medication used is a corticosteroid, the patient should rinse their mouth after the final dose, spitting out the water rather than ingesting
- Replace the mouthpiece cover post use each time

(pMDI: pressurized metered-dose inhaler)

BOX 19.6

- To inspect for foreign items after removal of the mouthpiece cover
- Do not obstruct the air vents and maintain the autohaler upright with the arrow pointing upward
- If the autohaler is brand-new or has not been used in a few days, prime it into the air
- Raise the lever
- To prime the autohaler, push the white test fire slide on the mouthpiece's bottom
- Return the lever to its down position and raise the lever, so that it snaps into place
- Maintain an upright posture either in a sitting or standing position
- Give the autohaler a good three or four shakes
- Exhale normally, keeping the autohaler at a distance
- Make sure the tongue is flat beneath the mouthpiece and does not obstruct the pMDI before placing the device between their teeth
- Lips to be sealed around the mouthpiece
- Using the mouthpiece, inhale deeply and steadily and moderately
- As soon as the autohaler releases the medication, pay attention to the click sound and the sensation of a gentle puff
- Inhale continuously until the lungs are full
- Take the mouthpiece out of your mouth
- Until the dose recommended by the doctor is reached, repeat the above steps
- If the medication used is a corticosteroid, the patient should rinse their mouth after the final dose, spitting out the water rather than ingesting
- Replace the mouthpiece cover post use each time, making sure the lever is down

(pMDI: pressurized metered-dose inhaler)

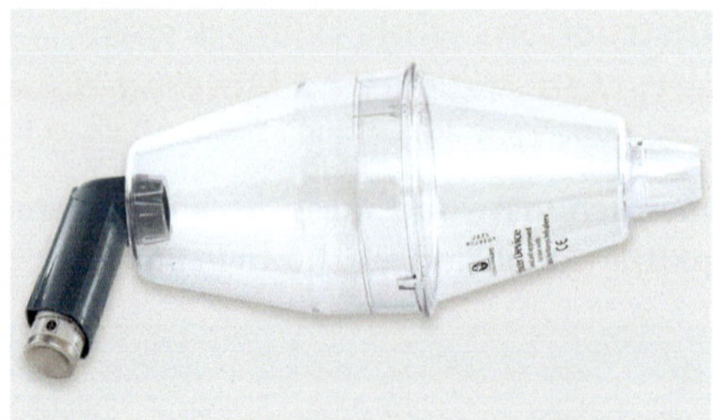

Fig. 19.5: Pressurized metered-dose inhaler (pMDI) with spacer.

Instructions while Using Pressurized Metered-dose Inhalers with Spacer

Instructions while using pMDIs with spacer are shown in **Figure 19.5**.

There is no need to hold one's breath nor any requirement for breath synchronization. The end user needs to take normal breaths for 30 seconds to 1 minute and the remaining steps to follow pre and post.

SUMMARY

Aerosol devices are the mainstay in the treatment of childhood asthma. They deliver the drug to the location of the disease hence mitigating systemic side effects despite prolonged therapy. The primary devices are small-volume nebulizers (SVN), pressurized metered-dose inhalers (pMDIs), and dry-powder inhalers (DPIs) and each has its own specific advantages and limitations. Device selection depends on patient factors, medication formulation, device attributes, and environmental considerations. Correct usage and patient education are crucial for effective treatment and drug delivery.

KEY POINTS

- Aerosol therapy has advanced from traditional breathing of herbal vapors to technologically complex inhalers.
- Device selection considers patient age, ability, comfort, drug availability, device convenience, and environmental factors.
- Three main types:
  1. *SVN:* Suitable for critical care, infants, elderly, or those with difficulty coordinating, but requires maintenance.
  2. *pMDI:* Portable, quick, but need proper hand-breath coordination and technique, often used with spacers.
  3. *DPI:* Breath-activated, compact, but depends on inspiratory effort and sensitive to moisture.
- Detailed instructions and patient education are vital for each device type to ensure effective and safe medication delivery.
- Regular re-evaluation of patient technique and understanding is necessary to ensure ongoing proper use and optimal asthma control.

SUGGESTED READING

1. DiBlasi RM. Clinical controversies in aerosol therapy for infants and children. Respir Care. 2015;60(6):894-914.
2. Gardenhire DS, Burnett D, Strickland S, Myers TR. A Guide to Aerosol Delivery Devices for Respiratory Therapists. 4th edition. American Association for Respiratory Care; 2017.
3. Gardenhire DS. Rau's Respiratory Care Pharmacology. St. Louis: Elsevier; 2016.
4. Newman SP. Principles of metered-dose inhaler design. Respir Care. 2005;50(9): 1177-90.
5. Stein SW, Thiel CG. The history of therapeutic aerosols: a chronological review. J Aerosol Med Pulm Drug Deliv. 2017;30(1):20-41.

CHAPTER 20

Intranasal Steroids in Allergic Rhinitis—Practice Tips

Reyaz A Malik, Asif Ahmed, Asef A Wani

INTRODUCTION

Allergic rhinitis is a common condition affecting almost 40% of children worldwide. These children can present with clinical features such as recurrent sneezing, rhinorrhea, nasal obstruction, and itching in the nose and/or pharynx. Postnasal discharge, cough, and palatal itching may also be present in these patients. The symptoms may be present all the year round or only seasonally. Sometimes the symptoms occur only on exposure to an allergen.

Just like other allergic disorders, the incidence of allergic disorders is increasing. The children with allergic rhinitis may simultaneously be suffering from other allergic disorders such as bronchial asthma, allergic keratoconjunctivitis, etc. It is pertinent to mention that one should be careful to identify other conditions that may mimic allergic rhinitis, viz., sarcoidosis, Sjögren syndrome, systemic lupus erythematosus, deviated nasal septum, and hypertrophied turbinates.

Allergic rhinitis may vary in severity from a mild illness to a severe illness, severely affecting the activities of daily life and leading to school absenteeism and impact on academic performance. Allergic rhinitis can severely impact the quality of life of an affected child and also impact whole of the family of the patient due to need for lifestyle modifications and monetary costs.

The impact of allergic rhinitis can be minimized by early diagnosis and early institution of treatment. The management of allergic rhinitis can be multipronged with options such as allergen avoidance (if it has been identified), specific allergen immunotherapy and drugs.

Drugs commonly used for allergic rhinitis include oral medications—mainly antihistaminics or decongestants, leukotriene antagonists, anticholinergics, chromones and intranasal medications—including steroids, antihistaminics, saline nasal irrigation, and decongestants.

INTRANASAL STEROIDS

Intranasal steroids are very effective and safe for short-term use in allergic rhinitis, especially the moderate to severe disease. Steroids act by blocking the synthesis and release of inflammatory mediators released in response to an allergic stimulus. Hence, they decrease the influx of inflammatory cells into the nasal mucosa. Their effect may start as soon as 6 hours after administration and their peak effects are seen by 14 days of usage. In patients with longstanding untreated illness, these drugs may take more time—days to weeks—to show maximal effect.

Efficacy of Intranasal Steroids

The efficacy of intranasal steroids in allergic rhinitis and their superiority over other drugs in allergic rhinitis has been proven by multiple studies. Various meta-analyses have shown that out of various treatment options available, intranasal corticosteroids are the most effective drugs in moderate to severe allergic rhinitis and are also helpful in improving the associated ocular symptoms. Nasal congestion is better relieved by nasal steroids, where the antihistamines usually do not help.

Various steroids used in allergic rhinitis include:

- Beclomethasone dipropionate
- Budesonide
- Ciclesonide
- Fluticasone furoate
- Fluticasone propionate
- Mometasone furoate
- Flunisolide
- Triamcinolone acetonide

Out of these, ciclesonide, fluticasone furoate, triamcinolone, and mometasone are approved for use in children over the age of 2 years. Beclomethasone and fluticasone propionate are approved for use in children over 4 years of age. Budesonide and Flunisolide are approved for use in children over the age of 6 years. There is no clear-cut evidence to support the superiority of one intranasal corticosteroid over another. The dose for each of these sprays is one puff in each nostril. In case of very severe symptoms, two puffs may be given in each nostril for the initial couple of weeks. As the patient improves, the maintenance dose can be tapered.

Practical Points in Intranasal Steroid Administration

- The efficacy of intranasal steroids will depend on proper deposition of the drug on the nasal mucosa. This will require proper positioning of the head, a clean crust-free nasal mucosa, and proper positioning of the medication delivery device.
- The head needs to be positioned in the midline. If the head is tilted backward, it will lead to medicine going down the throat. It can lead to dryness of throat, stinging/burning/itchy sensation in throat, and more systemic absorption and hence increased systemic side effects. If the head is tilted forward during drug administration, it will lead to lesser medication reaching the desired location at middle turbinate and some medicine may flow down out of the nose.
- If the nasal mucosal crusting is present, these crusts should be removed before administering the drug, so that the drug is deposited directly on the nasal mucosa. This can be achieved by using a saline spray or by rinsing the nose with water before administering the drug.
- If a patient has severe nasal obstruction, there may be a need to initially give a local nasal decongestant before giving an intranasal steroid spray for a few days so that the medicine reaches the desired site.
- The jet of the nasal spray should not be directed at the anterior nasal septum, as this will decrease the incidence of epistaxis. It is desirable to direct the spray tip laterally, away from the septum and directed toward the outer canthus of the ipsilateral eye. It is better to use the contralateral hand for using the spray in each nostril.
- As the drug is sprayed into the nose, the patient is asked to inhale gently through the nose so that the medicine is confined to the nasal cavity and is not lost. Sniffing the medicine is neither required nor recommended. After this same procedure can be repeated in the other nostril.

- We can start with the maximal dose and gradually taper the dose as the patient is optimized.

Safety of Intranasal Steroids

Intranasal steroids are very safe drugs with very few adverse effects. Few local side effects seen with the use of these drugs include itching and burning sensation in the nose, dryness and irritation in the nose and throat, epistaxis and sneezing. Epistaxis is possibly due to the jet of spray directed at the anterior nasal septum, which has a rich vascular supply and it can be decreased by not directing the spray jet at the anterior nasal septum. Very rarely, nasal mucosal atrophy and nasal septal perforation have been reported.

The systemic adverse effects from these drugs are very less due to less systemic absorption and bioavailability. Conclusive data on the effects of these drugs on the hypothalamic-adrenal axis, bone health are not forthcoming with most of the studies showing no adverse effects. However, some studies have shown a reduction in growth velocity in children with long-term use of high dose of these drugs.

SUMMARY

Intranasal corticosteroids are the most effective pharmacological treatment for moderate to severe allergic rhinitis in children. They work by inhibiting inflammatory mediators, providing symptomatic relief including nasal congestion and ocular symptoms. Onset of action may begin within 6 hours, with peak effects by 14 days, though longer duration may be required in chronic cases. Various formulations are approved for different pediatric age groups. Proper administration technique is critical to maximize efficacy and minimize side effects. While generally very safe with minimal systemic absorption, occasional local adverse effects such as dryness, irritation, and epistaxis can occur, often due to incorrect spray direction. Long-term, high-dose use may potentially affect growth velocity in children, although data are inconclusive. Correct positioning, mucosal hygiene, and technique refinement enhance both safety and efficacy.

KEY POINTS

- *Intranasal corticosteroids* are the most effective treatment for moderate to severe allergic rhinitis.
- They act by *suppressing inflammatory mediators*, reducing nasal and ocular symptoms.
- Onset of action occurs within *6 hours*, with *peak effect by 14 days*; longer use may be needed in chronic cases.
- Commonly used steroids include *fluticasone, mometasone, budesonide, and ciclesonide*, among others.
- Proper technique—*head in midline, lateral spray direction, and clear nasal mucosa*—is crucial for effectiveness.
- *Local side effects* like dryness, irritation, and epistaxis are minor and often preventable with correct use.
- *Systemic side effects* are rare due to low bioavailability; however, *growth concerns* exist with prolonged high-dose use.
- Initial higher doses can be used, then *tapered once symptoms are controlled* for maintenance therapy.

SUGGESTED READING

1. Gupta N. Allergy in a Nutshell - A Handbook. 1st edition. New Delhi: Jaypee Brothers Medical Publishers (P) Ltd; 2019.
2. Roberts G, Xatzipsalti M, Borrego LM, Custovic A, Halken S, Hellings PW, et al. Paediatric rhinitis: position paper of the European Academy of Allergy and Clinical Immunology. Allergy. 2013;68(9): 1102-16.
3. Rollema C, van Roon EN, van Boven JFM, Hagedoorn P, Klemmeier T, Kocks JH, et al.

Pharmacology, particle deposition and drug administration techniques of intranasal corticosteroids for treating allergic rhinitis. Clin Exp Allergy. 2022;52(11):1247-63.

4. Sousa-Pinto B, Vieira RJ, Brozek J, Cardoso-Fernandes A, Lourenço-Silva N, Ferreira-da-Silva R, et al. Intranasal antihistamines and corticosteroids in allergic rhinitis: a systematic review and meta-analysis. J Allergy Clin Immunol. 2024;154(2):340-54.
5. Wallace DV, Dykewicz MS, Bernstein DI, Blessing-Moore J, Cox L, Khan DA, et al. The diagnosis and management of rhinitis: an updated practice parameter. J Allergy Clin Immunol. 2008;122(2 Suppl):S1-84.

CHAPTER 21

Patch Test in Contact Dermatitis

Dipti Pujari

INTRODUCTION

Contact dermatitis is characterized by maculopapular rash with or without exfoliation of the skin with varying degrees of dryness and itchiness when the skin comes in contact with an offending allergen or irritant. If an allergen comes in contact with the skin for a longer duration and repeatedly, it can lead to scaling and lichenification of the skin called "chronic allergic contact dermatitis (ACD)." ACD is a T-cell-mediated delayed type IV reaction, which is detected by placing the allergens on the skin, in small wells, and occluding them for 48 hours, thereby creating a minireaction due to the offending agent. The reaction is then read after removing the covering occlusion at 48, 72, or 96 hours and finally after 7 days. This whole process of detecting the allergen-causing ACD is called "patch testing."

TABLE 21.1: Standard Footwear Series.

S. No.	*Patch test allergen*
1.	Formaldehyde
2.	Mercaptobenzothiazole
3.	Potassium dichromate
4.	Nickel sulfate
5.	Colophony
6.	Epoxy resins
7.	Neomycin sulfate
8.	Hydroquinone
9.	Thiuram mix
10.	Black rubber
11.	Glutaraldehyde
12.	Dioctyl phthalate
13.	Disperse orange
14.	Disperse blue
15.	Kathon CG

METHOD OF PATCH TESTING

Which allergens to choose?

With the increasing use of cosmetics, dyes, tattoos, artificial colors, synthetic materials, and perfumes, ACD cases are on the rise. It becomes extremely difficult to pinpoint the exact allergen. So, a detailed history and a thorough clinical examination are a must before starting a patch test. The timing and distribution of rash help one to decide which allergens need to be tested. But due to the complexity of the products and multiple products used in day-to-day life, it becomes difficult to decide on the allergens. In such cases, a panel of allergens is used for testing. Some commonly used panels are "Standard Footwear Series," as shown in **Table 21.1**, "Standard Cosmetic Series," as shown in **Table 21.2**, or a combination of the above two, called "Indian Standard Series," as shown in **Table 21.3**.

METHOD

After a detailed history and thorough examination, allergens to be tested are placed

TABLE 21.2: Standard cosmetic and fragrance series.

S. No.	Patch test allergen
1.	Vaseline
2.	Ethylenediamine
3.	Benzyl alcohol
4.	Benzyl salicylate
5.	Bronopol
6.	Butylated hydroxyanisole (BHA)
7.	Butylated hydroxytoluene (BHT)
8.	Cetyl alcohol
9.	Chloroacetamide
10.	Geranium oil
11.	2-Hydroxy-4-Methyl Benzotriazole
12.	2-Hydroxy-5-Methyl Benzotriazole
13.	Imidazolidinyl urea (Germall 115)
14.	Isopropyl myristate
15.	Jasmine absolute
16.	Lavender absolute
17.	Musk mix
18.	Benzyl salicylate
19.	Polyoxyethylene oleate (Tween 80)
20.	Rose oil
21.	Sorbitan Sesquioleate (Arlacel 80)
22.	Thiomersal
23.	Triclosan
24.	Triethanolamine
25.	Vanillin
26.	Cetrimide
27.	Hexamine
28.	Chlorhexidine digluconate
29.	Diazolidinyl urea (Germall II)
30.	Propylene glycol
31.	Kathon CG
32.	Sorbic acid

in allergen chambers or wells. These wells are made up of either aluminum or plastic, as shown in **Figure 21.1**. One test strip contains 10 such wells **(Fig. 21.2)**. Allergens are present in syringes in petrolatum or in liquid form

TABLE 21.3: Indian standard series.

S. No.	Patch test allergen
1.	Vaseline (Control)
2.	Peru balsam
3.	Formaldehyde
4.	Mercaptobenzothiazole
5.	Potassium dichromate
6.	Nickel sulfate
7.	Cobalt sulfate
8.	Colophony
9.	Epoxy resins
10.	Parabens mix
11.	Paraphenylenediamine
12.	Parthenium
13.	Neomycin sulfate
14.	Benzocaine
15.	Wool alcohols
16.	Chlorocresol
17.	Fragrance mix
18.	Thiuram mix
19.	Nitrofurazone
20.	Black rubber mix

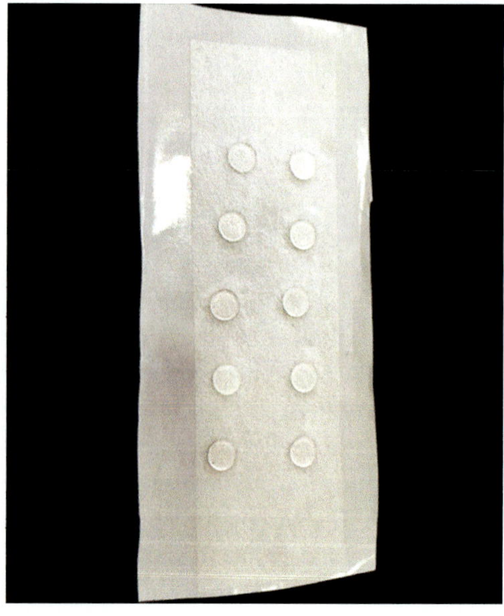

Fig. 21.1: Test strip with allergen chambers.

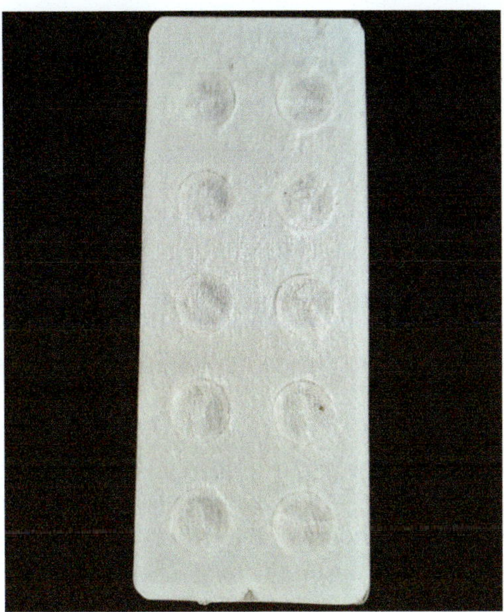

Fig. 21.2: Test strip with 10 wells.

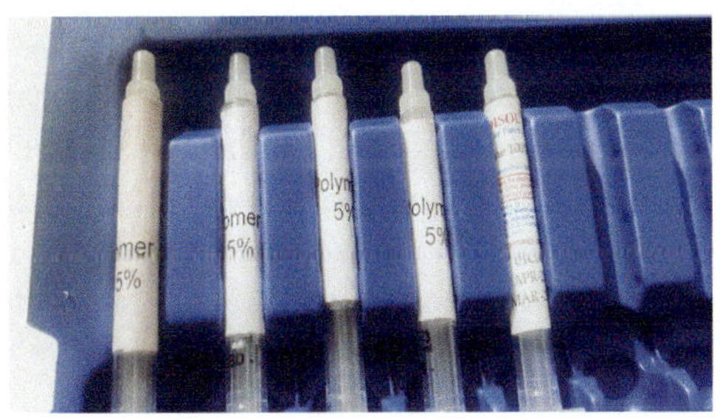

Fig. 21.3: Allergens present in syringes.

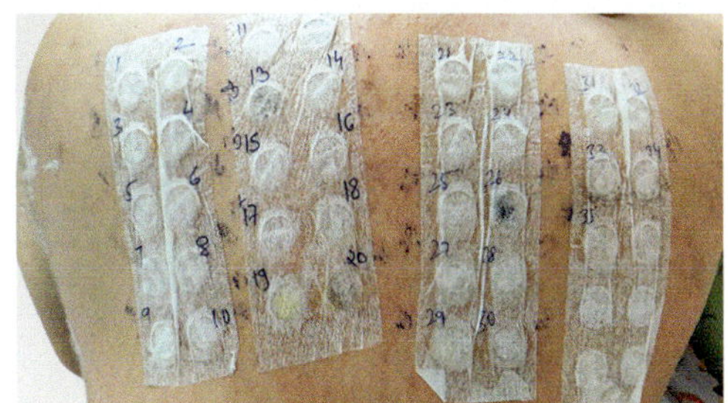

Fig. 21.4: Allergen strips placed on the back of a patient.

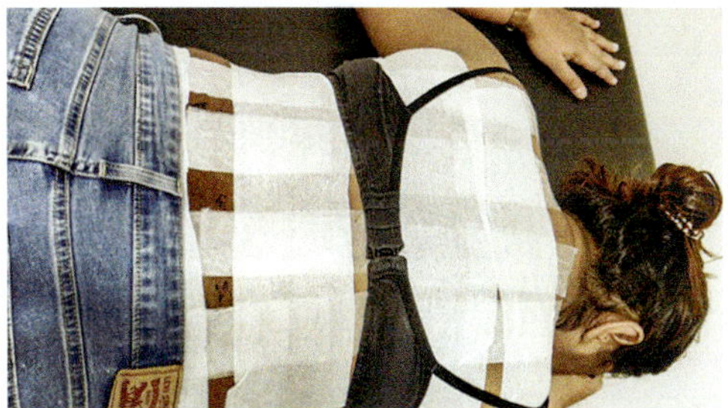

Fig. 21.5: Allergen strips secured on the back of a patient with adhesive tape.

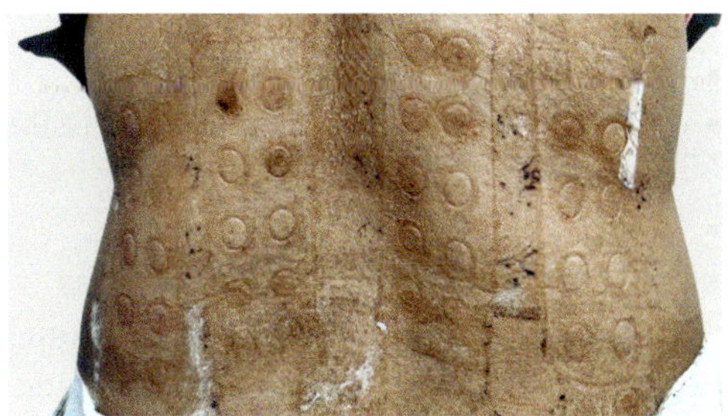

Fig. 21.6: Occlusion removed after 48 hours.

(Fig. 21.3). Once the allergens are placed in the wells, they are then carefully placed on the back of the patient **(Fig. 21.4)** and then secured properly in place with adhesive tape **(Fig. 21.5)**. These strips can be applied on the thighs or arms also. The outline of the strips is marked with a waterproof marker on patient's skin. A proper record needs to be maintained about the sequence and the number of allergens applied to the back. Once the strips are secured on the back, the patient is advised to avoid a bath for the next 7 days. He/she should not run, sweat, or scratch the back. The patient is also asked to wear loose comfortable clothes and to sleep on his/her sides and not on the back. Occlusion is removed after 48 hours, and first reading is taken **(Fig. 21.6)**. Then, subsequent readings are taken at 72 or 96 hours, and the final reading is taken on the 7th day from the day of application.

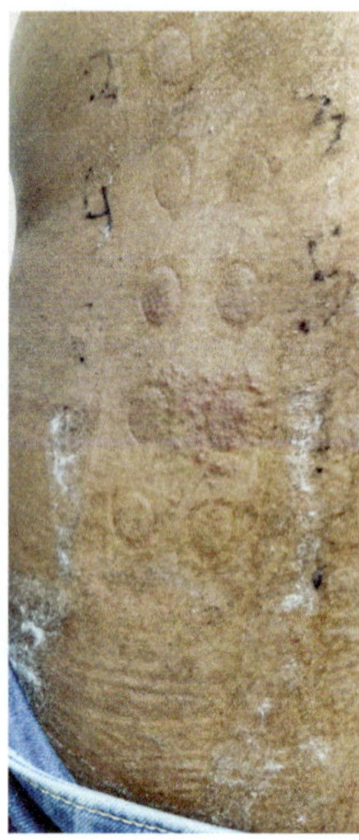

Fig. 21.7: Mild reaction seen in the form of "erythema and papules."

GRADING OF REACTION

Depending on the erythema, induration, and blistering, the positive reactions are graded as follows:

- *0:* Negative reaction
- *+:* Mild reaction—erythema and possibly papules **(Fig. 21.7)**
- *++:* Moderate reaction—vesicles
- *+++:* Severe reaction—bullous lesions

If a positive reaction at 48 hours becomes negative at 96 hours, it suggests local irritation and not ACD.

PITFALLS IN PATCH TESTING

- *False positive:* Many times, there is irritant contact dermatitis to the adhesive tape, which is used to occlude the allergen wells. The center of the well, where the allergen was placed, shows no reaction **(Fig. 21.8)**.
- If one is not careful while reading the reaction, then it can falsely be documented as positive ACD. The irritant reaction to the tape will disappear in the next 48 hours of removing the tape. It is also important that while performing the patch test, the back should not have active eczema. Otherwise, there could be many false-positive reactions due to adhesive tape or nearby allergens due to the "angry back syndrome."

  Sometimes, false-positive results can also be seen due to the pressure effect. The patient should be advised to stay in a comfortable environment. If there is excessive heat, then it might facilitate penetration of the allergen and give a false-positive reaction.

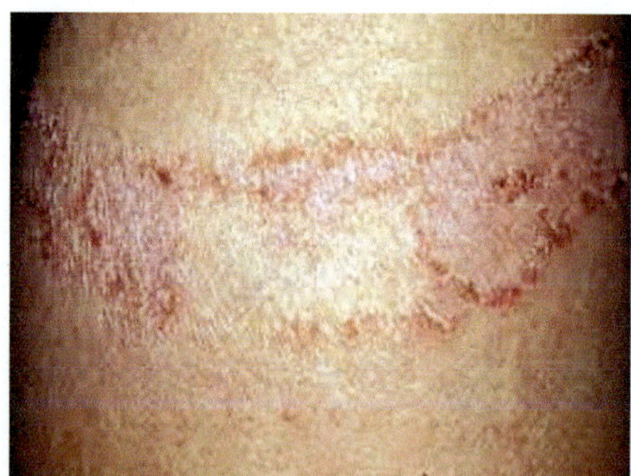

Fig. 21.8: False-positive reaction to adhesive tape.

- *False negative:* If the concentration of the allergen applied to the skin is not sufficient, the contact of the allergen with the skin is not correct, while applying the wells on the skin, the allergen gets displaced, or a wrong allergen is chosen, then all these might give false-negative reactions. So, one needs to be careful while applying the patches on the skin. Also, the importance of taking the final reading on the 7th day of the test cannot be undermined. Many allergens can show late positive reactions, especially if they have low penetrance in the skin or have long persistence on the skin. So, if the patient is not called on the

7th day, and the final reading is given only after 96 hours of patch application, then some late positive reactions could be missed. This is especially true with nickel, neomycin, isothiazolinone, and some cosmetic series allergens. So, the patient should always be called on the 7th day before the final reading is given.

- *Test circumstances:* It is important to advise patient to refrain from using topical steroids at the site of patch testing at least a week prior to the procedure. Also, the patient should avoid ultraviolet light exposure on the back. High-dose oral steroids should be avoided for at least a couple of weeks.

  Sometimes, false-positive results can also be seen due to the pressure effect. The patient should be advised to stay in a comfortable environment. If there is excessive heat, then it might facilitate penetration of the allergen and give a false-positive reaction.
- *Test methodology:* Allergens to be tested should be stored at 4–8°C. The chambers should be filled properly with the allergens, making sure that they come in contact with the skin. If the concentration of allergens to be tested is very high, then it might give a local irritant reaction. Sometimes, the liquid allergens tend to slip from the wells and leak into the neighboring skin area. This will result in a wrong interpretation of the test. So, one should be very careful while applying the patches on the skin.

REPEAT OPEN APPLICATION TEST

It is a simplified test to detect the offending allergen, useful in circumstances where patch testing is not possible. In this, the suspected allergen is placed on the antecubital fossa twice a day for 7 days. If no reaction occurs at the site of application, at the end of 7 days, then contact dermatitis is unlikely.

PATCH TEST IN SPECIAL CIRCUMSTANCES

In protein contact dermatitis, proteins when come in contact with previously affected skin give rise to eczema and wheals. It is a combination of types I and IV hypersensitivity reactions. So, a combination of noninvasive patch test, invasive skin prick test, and intradermal test is used to detect this type of contact dermatitis. The following steps need to be followed to detect allergens in protein contact dermatitis (PCD):

- *Noninvasive:*
  - *Open application:* Nonaffected (normal skin)
  - If negative
  - *Open application:* Slightly affected (or previously affected skin)
  - If negative
  - *Occlusive application (patch):* Nonaffected skin
  - If negative
  - *Occlusive application (patch):* Slightly/previously affected skin
  - If negative
- *Invasive:*
  - Skin prick test
  - If negative
  - Intradermal test

In PCD, there is a cutaneous reaction in response to a photoantigen applied to the skin in previously sensitized patients. It is a delayed type IV reaction. The agents are applied in duplicate on the midupper back skin on either side of the vertebrae. After 48 hours, one side of the patch test is removed, and the skin is irradiated with 5 J/cm^2 broad-spectrum ultraviolet A radiation (UVA). The other side remains unirradiated and serves as a control. These patches are then carefully reapplied and removed at 72 hours. Both sets of tests are then read at 96 hours. A photoallergy is confirmed if only the site exposed to UVA light shows a reaction. If both exposed and unexposed sites show equal reactions, a standard contact allergy is confirmed.

In drug allergy: For testing drugs, they are diluted at 10% in petrolatum. But the end product is of questionable stability, so it should be freshly made where possible. It is useful in maculopapular eruptions, fixed drug eruptions, symmetrical drug-related intertriginous and flexural exanthema (SDRIFE) (positive in 32–82%), drug reaction with eosinophilia and systemic symptoms (DRESS) (32–64%), Stevens-Johnson syndrome (SJS) (<30%), acute generalized exanthematous pustulosis (AGEP), and photosensitivity (with 5 J/cm^2 UVA).

DO'S AND DON'TS

- Oral steroids should be stopped at least 3 weeks before testing and topical steroids for at least 1 week prior to patch testing.
- Skin where patch testing needs to be done should not be exposed to ultraviolet light for at least a month prior to testing.
- Immunosuppressive drugs need to stop.
- Antihistamines do not interfere with the test as ACD is a type IV cell-mediated reaction.

Patch testing should be deferred in extensive active dermatitis/eczematous skin.

SUMMARY

Contact dermatitis cases are on the rise due to the increasing use of cosmetics and industrialization. Detailed history and examination, followed by a proper patch test with standardized allergens, will help in diagnosing the cases of ACD. The final reading of the patch test should always be taken on the 7th day, and the result should be correlated with the history. Improper testing conditions and interpretation might lead to many false-positive and false-negative reports. Once the diagnosis is confirmed, patient needs to be counseled to strictly avoid that ingredient in all the products, which he/she will be using in the future.

KEY POINTS

- Patch testing is the gold standard for diagnosing allergic contact dermatitis (ACD), which is a T-cell–mediated type IV hypersensitivity reaction.
- Allergen selection is guided by detailed history and examination; commonly used series include the Footwear, Cosmetic/Fragrance, and Indian Standard Series.
- Test procedure involves applying allergens in chambers on the skin (usually the back), with readings at 48, 72/96 hours, and a final mandatory reading on day 7 to detect late reactions.
- Reaction grading ranges from negative to severe (+++), based on erythema, papules, vesicles, or bullae. Day 7 reading is essential to avoid missing late positives (e.g., nickel, neomycin).
- Pitfalls include false positives (tape irritation, "angry back syndrome," excessive heat) and false negatives (inadequate concentration, poor technique, wrong allergen choice).
- Special situations such as protein contact dermatitis, photoallergic dermatitis, and drug allergy may require modified methods or additional tests; systemic steroids and immunosuppressants should be avoided before testing.

SUGGESTED READING

1. Fonacier L, Bernstein DI, Pacheco K, Holness DL, Blessing-Moore J, Khan D, et al. Contact dermatitis: a practice parameter-update 2015. J Allergy Clin Immunol Pract. 2015;3 (3 Suppl):S1-39.
2. Johansen JD, Aalto-Korte K, Agner T, Andersen KE, Bircher A, Bruze M, et al. European

Society of Contact Dermatitis guideline for diagnostic patch testing—recommendations on best practice. Contact Dermatitis. 2015;73: 195-221.

3. Lazzarini R, Duarte I, Ferreira AL. Patch tests. An Bras Dermatol. 2013;88(6):879-88.
4. Malajian DM, Belsito DV. Cutaneous delayed-type hypersensitivity in patient with atopic eczema. J Am Acad Dermatol. 2013;69(2): 232-7.
5. Mowad CM, Anderson B, Scheinman P, Pootongkam S, Nedorost S, Brod B. Allergic contact dermatitis: patient diagnosis and evaluation. J Am Acad Dermatol. 2016; 74:1029-40.
6. White JML. Patch testing: what allergists should know. Clin Exp Allergy. 2012;42:180-5.

CHAPTER

22

Tests in Chronic Urticaria

R Prasanna

INTRODUCTION

- Chronic urticaria is defined by the daily presence of wheals that are not always associated with angioedema, for over 6 weeks or with brief periods of well-being due to therapy.
- *Mechanism of action:* The dermal/submucosal mast cell serves as the primary effector cell. Upon degranulation, it releases prepared vasoactive mediators, including histamine, which is a significant mediator of urticaria and angioedema.
- Following the extravasation of fluid into the superficial tissues, cytokines, chemokines, and mediators generated from membranes (leukotrienes and prostaglandins) are produced, contributing to both early- and late-phase reactions.

CLASSIFICATION OF CHRONIC URTICARIA

Chronic urticaria can be classified into the following two groups:

1. *Chronic spontaneous urticaria (CSU)*: There is no identified trigger-inducing wheals and/or angioedema (autoimmune).
2. *Chronic inducible urticaria (CINDU)*: Wheals and/or angioedema appear after exposure to a certain trigger.

Table 22.1 compares the two types of CSU (autoimmune urticaria).

TABLE 22.1: Types of autoimmune urticaria.

Factors	*Type I autoimmune or autoallergy*	*Type II autoimmunity*
Mechanism	IgE against different autoantigens (TPO, TG, and IL-24)	IgG against IgE and FcεRI
Prognosis	• Moderate severity and activity • Short duration	• High severity and activity • Long duration
Other autoimmune comorbidities	Lower	Higher
Total IgE	Normal or high	Low
Basopenia and eosinopenia	Less	More

(IgE: immunoglobulin E; IgG: immunoglobulin G; IL-24: interleukin-24; TG: thyroglobulin; TPO: thyroid peroxidase)

Source: Adapted from Salman A, Porras NM, Gimenez-Arnau AM. Acute and Chronic Urticaria Diagnosis and Management Taking into Account Their Differences. Curr Treat Options Allergy. 2023;10:130-47.

TYPES OF CHRONIC-INDUCED URTICARIA

An overview of many kinds of chronic-induced urticaria is provided in **Table 22.2**.

Why do we need to evaluate chronic urticaria?

In chronic urticaria, the diagnostic workup has the following six major aims:

1. They are to confirm the diagnosis and exclude differential diagnoses.
2. To look for the underlying causes
3. To identify relevant conditions that modify disease activity
4. To check for comorbidities
5. To identify the consequences of chronic urticaria
6. To assess predictors of the course of disease and response to treatment and to monitor disease activity, impact, and control.

A comprehensive history; physical examination (which may involve looking through images of wheals and/or angioedema); standard testing; and an evaluation of the disease's impact, control, and activity are all part of the diagnostic workup.

HISTORY

Obtaining a thorough patient history is crucial when a patient is suspected of having chronic urticaria. This includes inquiring about the onset, course, and appearance of hives and/or angioedema; aggravating factors; length of illness; impact on daily life; and any prior diagnostic procedures or treatments **(Box 22.1)**.

Questions while an "allergic" cause is being considered?

- Might it be connected to any medications the patient has taken [nonsteroidal anti-inflammatory drug (NSAID), angiotensin converting enzyme (ACE) inhibitor, or aspirin]?
- Does it occur solely and reproducibly within 60 minutes (typically within 20 minutes) of consuming a certain food? Meat and crustaceans (e.g., prawns) are exceptions.
- Does it only happen after consuming a specific food—such as wheat—and exercising?
- Does it happen after the patient comes into contact with an allergen (food, latex, grass, animals, etc.) to which they are sensitized?

TABLE 22.2: Overview of chronic-induced urticaria.

CINDU type	*Trigger*
Symptomatic dermographism	Rubbing, scratching , scrubbing
• Cholinergic urticaria • Cold urticaria	• Sweating • Cold solids, liquids, or air
• Delayed pressure urticaria • Heat urticaria	• Vertical pressure • Hot solids, liquids, or air
Solar urticaria	UVA, UVB , Visible light
• Aquagenic urticaria • Vibratory angioedema • Contact urticaria	• Water, sweat, saliva, tears, ambiental humidity • Vibration (including laughing, applauses, machines) • Latex, animal products, vegetables /fruits, chemicals)

(CINDU: chronic inducible urticaria; UVA: ultraviolet A; UVB: ultraviolet B)
Source: Adapted from Salman A, Porras NM, Gimenez-Arnau AM. Acute and Chronic Urticaria Diagnosis and Management Taking into Account Their Differences. Curr Treat Options Allergy. 2023;10:130-47.

BOX 22.1: History-taking in suspected chronic urticaria.

Duration of disease:
- Time of onset
- Frequency/duration and provoking factors for hives
- Diurnal variation
- Occurrence in relation to weekends, holidays, and/or foreign travel

Physical symptoms:
- Shape, size, and distribution of hives
- Associated angioedema
- Associated subjective symptoms of lesions

Provoking factors:
- Induction by physical agents or exercise
- Observed correlation to food

Family history:
- Family and personal history regarding urticaria and atopy
- Previous or current allergies, infections, internal diseases, or other possible causes
- Psychosomatic and psychiatric diseases
- Surgical implantation and events during surgery, for example, after local anesthesia
- Gastric/intestinal problems
- Use of drugs (e.g., NSAIDs)
- Relationship to the menstrual cycle
- Smoking habits
- Type of work
- Hobbies
- Stress

Impact on everyday life: Quality of life related to urticaria and emotional impact

Previous diagnostic test/therapy:
- Previous therapy and response to therapy
- Previous diagnostic procedure/results

(NSAIDs: nonsteroidal anti-inflammatory drugs)
Source: Adapted from Weller K, Zuberbier T, Maurer M. Chronic urticaria: tools to aid the diagnosis and assessment of disease status in daily practice. J Eur Acad Dermatol Venereol. 2015;29(Suppl 3):38-44.

Is there a vasculitis process?

- Are the episodes of urticaria/angioedema persistent rather than evanescent and self-limiting?
- Do single lesions continue longer than a day?
- Rather than being itchy, are the urticarial lesions painful and tender?
- Is there any indication of purpura, bruises, or lingering petechial hemorrhage on the skin?
- Does the patient exhibit any indications or symptoms of an underlying medical condition, such as high fever, severe malaise, arthralgia, high blood pressure, or protein or blood in the urine?

PHYSICAL EXAMINATION

- Pink or white, well-defined, elevated wheals encircled by an erythematous base and central pallor are the hallmarks of urticaria.
- Urticarial lesions can vary in size and shape, ranging from millimeters to a few centimeters in size, and can have an annular to serpiginous outline.
- These wheals may confluence, generating huge plaques.
- The morphology of these wheals could be useful in differentiating between urticarias and other urticaria subgroups.
- Angioedema, a nonpitting, asymmetric swelling that can affect the lips, cheeks, limbs, genitalia, and periorbital area, can accompany wheals.

CONDITIONS THAT MAY MIMIC CHRONIC URTICARIA

Table 22.3 shows the conditions that mimic chronic urticaria, and how to differentiate from the same.

CLINICAL SCORING

International guidelines recommend the use of the Urticaria Activity Score (UAS) to measure disease activity and monitor

TABLE 22.3: Conditions that mimic chronic urticaria and their diagnosis.

Disease	***When to consider diagnosis***
Urticarial vasculitis	• Hives are painful (not pruritic) • Hives last >48 hours • Residual bruising or pigmentation occurs after resolution of hives • May have symptoms such as fever, chills, and arthralgias • May have previously another systemic inflammatory disease
Cryoglobulinemia	• Lesions over buttocks and lower extremities • May occur in patients with hepatitis B/C
Mastocytosis	Lesions occur with very mild physical trauma, for example, light touch
Polymorphic eruption of pregnancy	• Occur in pregnant patients • Presents within abdominal striae • Does not affect periumbilical area • Sparing of face, palms, and soles

Source: Adapted from Perera E, Sinclair R. Evaluation, diagnosis and management of chronic urticaria. Aust Fam Physician. 2014;43(9):621-5.

TABLE 22.4: Urticaria activity score.

Score	***Hives (wheals)***	***Score***	***Itch severity score***
0	None	0	None
1	Mild (<20 hives/24 h)	1	Mild (present but not annoying or troublesome)
2	Moderate (20–50 hives/24 h)	2	Moderate (troublesome but does not interfere with normal daily activity or sleep)
3	Intense (50 hives/24 h or large confluent areas of hives)	3	Intense (severe itch, which is sufficiently troublesome to interfere with normal daily activity or sleep)

Source: Adapted from Weller K, Zuberbier T, Maurer M. Chronic urticaria: tools to aid the diagnosis and assessment of disease status in daily practice. J Eur Acad Dermatol Venereol. 2015;29(Suppl 3):38-44.

response to treatment. **Table 22.4** gives an insight of the same.

DIAGNOSTIC APPROACH

In chronic urticaria, the following five factors are important in the diagnosis procedure:

1. To identify the elementary lesion that characterizes urticaria and urticarial rashes. Urticaria might present with hives (wheals) and/or angioedema, the latter involving the deeper mucocutaneous layers.
2. Among the possible differential diagnoses that we should take into account are autoinflammatory illnesses, cutaneous/systemic mastocytosis, urticaria vasculitis, and anaphylaxis.
3. Systemic symptoms as well as involvement of other organs have to be excluded.
4. To distinguish between CSU and CINDU, we need to determine whether there is a physical component causing the development of wheals or angioedema. Additionally, find out if a patient might have several urticaria at the same time.

5. Fifth, laboratory tests have a very limited role in the diagnosis. basophil histamine release assay/basophil activation test (BHRA/BAT), Western blot/enzyme-linked immunosorbent assay (WB/ELISA), and autologous serum skin test (ASST) can all be used to categorize chronic urticaria (CU) according to the autoimmune mechanism.

ALGORITHM FOR DIAGNOSIS OF CHRONIC URTICARIA (FLOWCHART 22.1)

- *Allergy testing:* Patients who think that their chronic urticaria is caused by food are frequently referred to hospitals. Excluding an atopic diathesis using skin prick testing (SPT) against a panel of aeroallergens and questionable meals is a feasible strategy. When a patient's SPT results are negative, it can reassure them that their symptoms are not caused by an allergy and possibly increase their adherence to long-term antihistamine treatment. If the symptoms of urticaria are associated with exertion or exercise, restricted specific immunoglobulin E (IgE) testing to dietary allergens such as lipid transfer proteins or omega-5-gliadin may be useful. It should be taken into consideration that eating raw fish can cause Anisakis simplex hypersensitivity in some Mediterranean regions.
- *Full blood count (FBC):* Infections with parasites and certain drug-induced responses might raise the eosinophil count. Urticarial vasculitis may be linked to an increased neutrophil count.
- *Urinalysis:* A screen for hematuria and proteinuria will help to detect the presence of urinary tract infection and renal involvement in vasculitis.
- *Acute phase response:* An underlying systemic illness such as persistent infection or vasculitis may be indicated by a raised erythrocyte sedimentation rate (ESR) and/or C-reactive protein (CRP), while paraproteinemia may be indicated by a high ESR with a normal CRP.
- *Thyroid function and autoantibodies:* Thyroid autoantibodies are linked to autoimmune urticaria diagnosis and are connected with chronic urticaria in both adults and children.
- *Complement studies:* Since urticaria and C1 inhibitor deficiency are unrelated, measuring C1 inhibitor is not necessary if urticaria is present. C4 and C1 inhibitors should be included in the initial complement investigations for patients with angioedema who do not have wheals. Even in between attacks, the C4 level will often be low in types I and II hereditary angioedema (HAE) instances. Quantitation of functional C1 inhibitors should be saved for ambiguous individuals with a suggestive history and normal levels of antigenic C1 inhibitor but low C4 levels. When urticarial vasculitis is suspected, it is important to assess C3 and C4, and if these levels are decreased, it may be helpful to measure anti-C1q antibodies.
- *Hematinics and vitamins:* If clinically indicated, measurement of serum iron and vitamin B_{12} levels can be useful.
- *Immunoglobulins:* Serum immunoglobulins and electrophoresis should be performed in individuals with CU who are typically older than 40 years old and who exhibit systemic symptoms such as fever, polyarthralgia, leukocytosis, malaise, or lymphadenopathy in order to look for an IgM paraprotein that may be suggestive of Schnitzler syndrome. Secondary cold urticaria may be linked to cryoglobulins

Flowchart 22.1: Diagnosis of chronic urticaria.

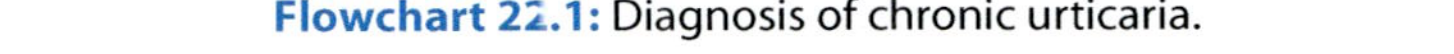

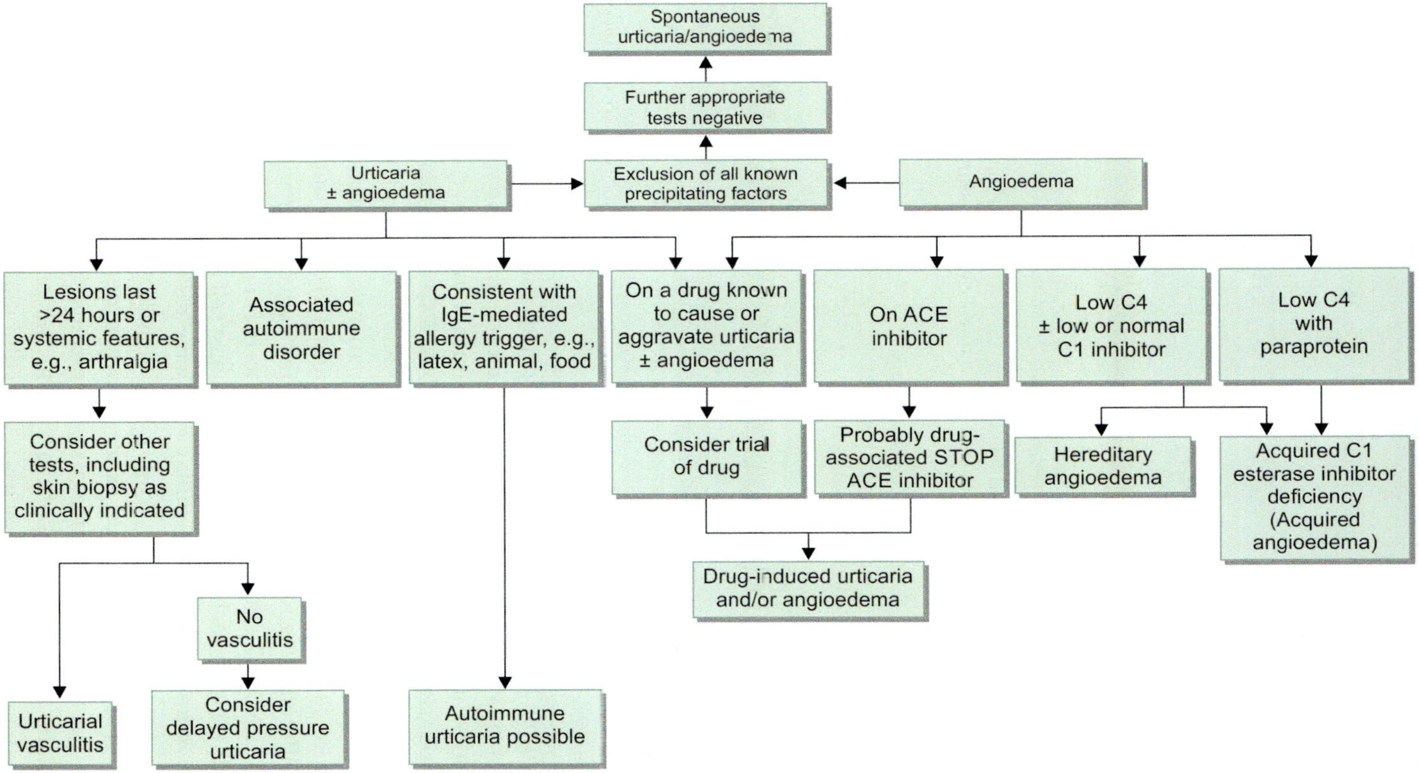

(ACE: angiotensin converting enzyme; IgE: immunoglobulin E)

Source: Adapted from Powell RJ, Leech SC, Till S, Huber PA, Nasser SM, Clark AT. BSACI guideline for the management of chronic urticaria and angioedema. Clin Exp Allergy. 2015;45(3):547-65.

TABLE 22.5: Diagnosis tools for CINDU.

CINDU type	*Trigger*	*Diagnostic tools*
Symptomatic dermographism	Rubbing, scratching, and scrubbing	*Moderate scratching of the skin with:* • Blunt smooth object • Fric test (four pins) • Dermographic tester (36g/mm square
• Cholinergic urticaria • Cold urticaria	Sweating Cold solids, liquids, or air	*Exercise machines* • Ice cubes test, assess critical stimulation time threshold (CsTT) • Temperature test, assess critical temperature threshold (CTT)
• Delayed pressure urticaria • Heat urticaria	• Vertical pressure • Hot solids, liquids, or air	• Suspension of weights over shoulder • Heat source, Temp test
Solar urticaria	UVA, UVB, and visible light	• UVA radiation • UVB radiation • Projector (Visible light)
• Aquagenic urticaria • Vibratory angioedema • Contact urticaria	• Water, sweat, saliva, tears, and ambiental humidity • Vibration (including laughing, applauses, and machines) • Latex, animal products, vegetables/fruits, chemicals)	• Soaked compressed or towel • Vortex vibrator • Skin prick test • Closed patch test • Open controlled application testing

(CINDU: chronic inducible urticaria; UVA: ultraviolet A; UVB: ultraviolet B)
Source: Adapted from Salman A, Porras NM, Gimenez-Arnau AM. Acute and Chronic Urticaria Diagnosis and Management Taking into Account Their Differences. Curr Treat Options Allergy. 2023;10:130-47.

(a clotted sample must be collected and sent to the lab at 37°C). B-cell lymphoma may be the cause of acquired angioedema without urticaria, in which case a paraprotein search may be necessary.

- *Challenges:* Chronic urticaria can be reproduced in labs using challenges. There are different diagnostic tools for each type of CINDU. **Table 22.5** depicts the diagnostic tools for each CINDU.
- *Skin biopsy:* When there is a peculiar pattern of presentation or when vasculitis is suspected, a lesional skin biopsy is suitable. Clinical indicators include lesions that last longer than 24 hours, systemic symptoms (such as fever, arthralgia, or arthritis), and skin discoloration that appears as the lesions recede. Excessive scratching is shown by linear bruises.
- *ASST and basophil release assay:* The ASST is an intradermal injection of the patient's own serum; a positive wheal-and-flare reaction is thought to be indicative of circulating autoantibodies to the high-affinity IgE receptor on the mast cell in CU patients; younger children have difficulty with the ASST because intradermal injections are uncomfortable when done without topical anesthetic creams. The clinical role of the BHRA in the management of CU patients is still unknown. The two assays currently available for autoimmunity in CU (BHRA

and ASST) do not consistently help clinicians understand the pathogenesis of spontaneous CU patients.

- *Nasal endoscopy:* If a patient has an unexplained pharyngeal blockage, nasal endoscopy may be investigated. This procedure can be particularly helpful during an attack as it allows direct sight of the pharynx and larynx, which can help determine or rule out the presence of throat angioedema. The differential diagnosis of "swelling, lump, or discomfort in the throat" includes vocal cord dysfunction, globus, and gastroesophageal reflux disease.

SUMMARY

- Chronic urticaria is a long-lasting skin condition with recurrent wheals and/or angioedema caused by mast cell activation.
- It is divided into spontaneous and inducible forms, with autoimmune mechanisms often contributing.
- Diagnosis requires a careful history, physical examination, and exclusion of conditions that mimic CU.
- Laboratory and provocation tests are used selectively, while clinical scoring systems help monitor disease activity.
- A structured diagnostic algorithm ensures accurate classification, assessment of comorbidities, and effective management.

KEY POINTS

- Chronic urticaria is wheals with or without angioedema for >6 weeks, caused by mast cell degranulation (histamine, cytokines, leukotrienes).
- Classified into CSU (spontaneous, autoimmune—Types I and II) and CINDU (inducible—cold, cholinergic, dermographism, solar, aquagenic, etc.).
- Evaluation needed to confirm diagnosis, rule out mimics, find triggers and comorbidities, assess prognosis, and monitor activity.
- Workup includes detailed history and examination, UAS scoring, and labs to include CBC, ESR/CRP, urinalysis, thyroid antibodies, and complements.
- Special tests are ASST, BHRA/BAT (autoimmune CSU), provocation tests (CINDU), skin biopsy (vasculitis) and allergy testing when indicated.

SUGGESTED READING

1. Perera E, Sinclair R. Evaluation, diagnosis and management of chronic urticaria. Aust Fam Physician. 2014;43(9):621-5.
2. Powell RJ, Leech SC, Till S, Huber PA, Nasser SM, Clark AT. BSACI guideline for the management of chronic urticaria and angioedema. Clin Exp Allergy. 2015;45(3): 547-65.
3. Salman A, Porras NM, Gimenez-Arnau AM. Acute and chronic urticaria diagnosis and management taking into account their differences. Curr Treat Options Allergy. 2023;10:130-47.
4. Weller K, Zuberbier T, Maurer M. Chronic urticaria: tools to aid the diagnosis and assessment of disease status in daily practice. J Eur Acad Dermatol Venereol. 2015;29(Suppl 3):38-44.
5. Zuberbier T, Latiff AHA, Abuzakouk M, Aquilina S, Asero R, Baker D, et al. The international EAACI/GA^{2}LEN/EuroGuiDerm/APAAACI guideline for the definition, classification, diagnosis, and management of urticaria. Allergy. 2022;77(3): 734-66.

CHAPTER 23

Wet Wrap Therapy and Bleach Bath

Rahima Saleem

WET WRAP THERAPY

INTRODUCTION

It is the application of bandages or dressings with a moist inner layer and a dry second outer layer to treat pruritic conditions such as refractory atopic dermatitis. Dampened bandages or water dressings were used as an ancient remedy by the Babylonians and Egyptians to reduce inflammation.

MECHANISM

It keeps the skin hydrated, thereby maintaining better penetration of medication, especially penetration of lipid-soluble nonpolar molecules. It may trigger increased lamellar body secretion, allowing the recovery of damaged lipid laminar structure. By occlusion, skin moisture content is increased, and transepidermal water loss is increased. By wet occlusion, stratum corneum can expand vertically to four to five times its breadth. Stimulation of DNA synthesis by occlusion causes epidermal proliferation, which further repairs the defects in the barrier.

PROCEDURE

Child is first bathed in lukewarm water and dried pat, and then mild topical steroid is applied to the affected areas and emollients to the unaffected areas. Soak the wraps in warm water and wring out the excess water; cover the area with wet dressing and then apply a dry clothing. Remove the wet dressing after 2–3 hours and apply moisturizer to entire body.

TYPES OF WRAPS

Wet wraps could be clean cotton wrap dressings, tubular dressings, or gauze or cotton socks with toe ends cutoff, and the dry dressing could be gauze or nighttime clothes/pajamas. Wraps made of a special nanopolyester were found to be just as effective and more comfortable than cotton wraps. For feet and hands, cotton socks or cotton gloves can be used as a wet wrap and vinyl gloves or plastic wrap for the dry layer. For face, gauze and surgical nets can be used.

EFFICACY

It is found to be very effective when used with emollients but more effective when used with topical steroids. González-López et al. systematically reviewed six trials of wet wrap therapy (WWT) with topical steroids. According to them, the overall grade of quality of evidence and safety outcomes were low and had more chances for infection. Density of bacterial colonization was also increased.

CONTRAINDICATIONS

Occlusive therapy should be avoided if there is maceration, infection, or allergy to occlusive material.

ADVERSE EFFECTS

Most common adverse effect is discomfort due to limited mobility caused by the bandages. Shivering can occur due to moist inner bandages, which can be decreased by using warm water. Occlusion itself will cause maceration and superadded bacterial and candidal infection. Topical steroid when used under occlusion causes atrophy, telangiectasia, depigmentation, striae, systemic absorption, and suppression of adrenal gland. Allergic contact dermatitis to the dressing material can occur.

BENEFITS

It can hydrate the skin and thereby better penetration of drugs. They have a cooling effect and can relieve itch. It also prevents the children from scratching, thus breaking the itch-scratch cycle of atopic dermatitis and also reduces secondary infection. Lesser topical medication will be required. It can be done at home giving quick relief during flares. Also, it is helpful during traveling.

SUMMARY

Wet wrap therapy plays a role as an acute therapeutic intervention in the management of moderate-to-severe atopic dermatitis. It could be costly and time-consuming for families and requires special training on the method of application. But by using clothing instead of bandages, it can be made simpler, less time-consuming, and inexpensive. If properly done, this simple measure can add significantly to the management of atopic dermatitis and minimize the need for more powerful medications.

BLEACH BATH

INTRODUCTION

Bleach baths are baths with diluted household bleach in bathing water. Bleach or sodium hypochlorite (NaOCl) solution decreases bacteria and reduces inflammation and itching in eczematous conditions. It reduces severity of atopic dermatitis and dose of topical and systemic medications.

Bleach contains 3–6% available chlorine (Cl_2) with 0.5–1.5% sodium hydroxide (NaOH) as a stabilizer, surfactant, and perfume. NaOCl is the active ingredient of household bleach. It is a clear, yellowish alkaline (pH 11–13) solution with potent oxidizing properties and antimicrobial action. It was used in the 17th century by surgeons for the treatment of burns, operating wounds, and ulcers and was also reported by Koch in 1880. Dakin then developed a buffered solution with a lower concentration (0.45–0.55% NaOCl) but retaining antiseptic properties.

MECHANISM OF ACTION

Sodium hypochlorite when mixed with water dissociates to form HOCl and NaOH. It has been shown to reduce colonization of bacteria, especially *Staphylococcus aureus*. HOCl as low as 0.005% can decolonize *S. aureus*. It is also effective against other gram-positive and gram-negative infections, viruses, fungus, and spores. In atopic dermatitis, there is a high prevalence of colonization with *S. aureus*, which produces exotoxins acting as superantigens that increase Th2-dominant inflammatory response and increased immunoglobulin E (IgE) production. Reduction in *S. aureus* levels on skin has been shown to improve atopic dermatitis. HOCl is not shelf-stable; so, to stabilize a pure form of HOCl (NVC-101), Wang et al. prepared a stable HOCl by minimizing Cl_2 formation, thereby increasing the antimicrobial activity.

Apart from antimicrobial action, bleach has an anti-inflammatory action in atopic dermatitis. It reduces Th2-Th1 shift by reducing interleukin-2 (IL-2) response, thereby reducing the chronicity of atopic dermatitis. It decreases proinflammatory cytokines such as IL-1A, 4, 6, 13; tumor necrosis factor-alpha (TNF-α); and pruritogenic cytokines. It also decreases IgE production, mast cell activation, and histamine release, thereby having a significant role in reducing atopic dermatitis.

PROCEDURE

Plain bleach (6%), which has no fragrance and is not concentrated, is used. Half cup of bleach (160 mL) is required for a full bathtub of water (100–150 L/40 gallons) and is poured while tub is filling. For baby bath, 30 mL or two tablespoonfuls of 2.2% bleach can be added to 15 L of water. Soak down in the tub below neck for 10 minutes and then gently rinse with lukewarm water. Do not use soap. Pat dry, do not rub, and then apply moisturizer. It can be done twice a week. Do not submerge head and face. Do not soak for >15 minutes. Do not add any other products in bleach bath.

ADVERSE EFFECTS

It can cause dryness, irritation of the skin and nose, and allergic contact dermatitis. It is due to the added perfumes or surfactants. It should be kept out of reach of children in a tight container with a child-protective top. Ingestion can lead to burning and irritation of the mouth and oropharynx, nausea, vomiting, and hematemesis. If ingested in excess, it can cause corrosion of mucous membrane, perforation of esophagus or stomach, melena and chest pain, delirium, and finally hemorrhage and shock. NaOCl has shown mutagenicity, but there are no data in humans regarding its carcinogenicity. When exposed to chlorine, there are reports of exacerbation of asthma.

SUMMARY

Bleach bath is widely available and inexpensive. It restores surface microbiome and reduces the need for topical and systemic medications. It has antipruritic and anti-inflammatory actions, thus playing a significant role in reducing atopic dermatitis. But there is a dearth of evidence regarding safety and efficacy of bleach baths, so that it can be implemented as a documented therapy in eczematous conditions, especially atopic dermatitis. There is no microbial resistance reported with NaOCl and has a wide range of antimicrobial spectrum, thus favoring its significant contribution to the therapeutic armamentarium.

SUGGESTED READING

1. Anderson RM, Thyssen JP, Maibach HI. The role of wet wrap therapy in skin disorders—a literature review. Acta Derm Venereol. 2015;95(8):933-9.
2. Barnes TM, Grieve KA. Use of bleach baths for the treatment of infected atopic eczema. Australas J Dermatol. 2013;54:251-8.
3. Dhanani S, Shah M, Nair P. Occlusive therapy in dermatology. Indian J Dermatol Venereol Leprol. 2025;91:132-5.
4. González-López G, Ceballos-Rodríguez RM, González-López JJ, Fieto Rodríguez M, Herranz-Pinto P. Efficacy and safety of wet wrap therapy for patients with atopic dermatitis: a systematic review and meta-analysis. Br J Dermatol. 2017;177(3):688-95.
5. Maarouf M, Shi VY. Bleach for atopic dermatitis. Dermatitis. 2018;29(3):120-6.

6. Mc Kenna PJ, Lehr GS, Leist P, Welling RE. Antiseptic effectiveness with fibroblast preservation. Ann Plast Surg. 1991;27:265-8.
7. Nicol NH, Boguniewicz M. Wet wrap therapy in moderate to severe atopic dermatitis. Immunol Allergy Clinic North Am. 2017; 37:123-39.
8. Sharma N, Dhar S, De A, Godse K, Krupa Shankar DS, Zawar V, et al. Use of bleach baths for atopic dermatitis: an Indian perspective. Indian J Dermatol. 2022;67(3):273-8.
9. Smith CH, Goldman RD. Staphylococcus aureus decolonisation for recurrent skin and soft tissue infections in children. Can Fam Physician. 2012;58(12):1350-2.
10. Wang L, Bassiri M, Najafi R, Najafi K, Yang J, Khosrovi B, et al. Hypochlorous acid as a potential wound care agent: part I. Stabilized hypochlorous acid: a component of the inorganic armamentarium of innate immunity. J Burns Wounds. 2007; 6:e5.

CHAPTER 24

Clothing, Bathing, and Moisturizer Use in Atopic Dermatitis: Recommendations and Practice Tips

Althea Valeen Pinto

INTRODUCTION

The mainstay in the control of atopic dermatitis (AD) flares is the protection of a dysfunctional skin barrier from further insults of the itch–scratch cycle. The decrease in the itch threshold causes skin in AD to be easily prone to itch due to mechanical stimuli, such as rubbing of clothing, and chemical stimuli from itch mediators. This discomfort severely impacts a child's quality of life, sleep, and overall well-being. Being a lifelong skin condition, medical treatment of flares must closely coexist with care of the skin during periods of remission for effective control. These strategies include appropriate fabric selection, gentle bathing practices, and regular application of moisturizers to support skin barrier healing. Sound knowledge of these basics can equip health care professionals and caregivers to teach the atopic child early on how to manage their condition effectively. This ultimately lays the foundation for a healthier, more manageable relationship with AD throughout their lives.

ROLE OF CLOTHING IN ATOPIC DERMATITIS

Fabric choices are crucial for skin health in AD. It is the fabric ends of clothing that stimulate low-grade activity in the C-tactile neurons, causing a mechanically evoked itch sensation. An appropriate selection of clothing for patients with AD should aim to improve skin barrier function by decreasing transepidermal water loss (TEWL), increasing hydration, and improving moisturizer and topical medication penetration, thereby decreasing skin inflammation.

Garment selection is influenced by the type of fabric (natural vs. manufactured) and the diameter of the fibers, as these factors affect comfort, sweat absorbency, and potential for irritation. Theoretically, an ideal fabric should be smooth, nonocclusive, absorbent (moisture-wicking material), bioactive, lightweight, and comfortable. It should also be easy to clean and able to withstand cycles of laundering. The textile industry broadly classifies fabrics into natural and man-made fibers. Natural fibers can be further divided into vegetable (cotton, hemp, bamboo, etc.), mineral (asbestos), and animal or protein (wool and silk). Man-made fibers can be classified as regenerated fibers from natural polymers (viscose, lyocell, modal, etc.), synthetic fibers (polyester, nylon, etc.), and inorganic fibers. Of these, all except mineral and inorganic fibers have been in use for regular daily apparel. There are a few fundamentals to be mindful of when selecting clothing in AD:

- *Fiber diameter:* Smaller diameter fibers <19–21 μm are generally soothing for the skin. Traditionally, it is for this reason that natural fibers of cotton and silk were deemed safe for AD due to their low itch potential. Among the woolen fabrics, those with large-diameter fibers are highly pruritic and rough. Linen fabrics also have a tendency to irritate due to their rough texture.

- *Occlusive properties:* Fabric weave patterns determine their occlusive properties, as well as influencing breathability, durability, and texture. Tightly woven and highly occlusive fabrics such as filamentous polyester and nylon initially promote moisture retention; however, their quick removal in a low-humid environment results in rapid evaporation of moisture from the skin, which leads to an increased loss in TEWL, upregulation of inflammatory cytokines, and minute skin fissures in AD skin. These fabrics have been the mainstay in many athletic equipment and potentially worsen AD. Therefore, a switch to cotton, 100% lyocell, bamboo, and clothes made from hemp is advisable. Besides being softer and breathable, their "moisture-wicking" abilities help draw sweat away from the skin and move it to the surface of the material, where it can evaporate, thereby helping the wearer feel dry and comfortable.
- *Allergenic potential:* Sometimes, the atopic flare may be experienced even with natural animal fibers such as silk, as they contain a protein called sericin. The synthetic fibers run through chemical processes to increase their pigment stability and durability and pose a risk for flare. Cost cutting and consumerism have allowed for the mass production of combination fibers. These are blended fabrics that are created by combining two or more types of fibers, such as cotton and polyester or wool and acrylic. This may serve to enhance their durability, stretch, and moisture-wicking abilities but carry a risk to atopic individuals as they are commonly treated with dyes or finishes. Hypoallergenic and preferably dye-free fabrics are preferred such as cotton and bamboo. If combination fibers are chosen, it is also advisable to opt for those that have a higher percentage of natural fibers. With regard to bedding material, recent studies have shown that polyurethane-encased (PE) bedding is highly occlusive and has been proposed to decrease allergen sensitization from bed mattresses and house dust mites.
- *Antimicrobial properties:* The skin in AD, besides having a defective skin barrier, is prone to frequent colonization with *Staphylococcus aureus*. Hence, the emergence of "functional textiles" which are fabrics imparted with antimicrobial treatments. These include silver nanoparticles, zinc oxide, citric acid, chitosan derived from crustacean shells, borage seed oil, ethylene vinyl alcohol (EVOH) fibers, bamboo charcoal, and copper. It is important to consider that while these newer additions can be beneficial, they should be individual based as some may tend to experience a flare even with these fabrics.
- *Fit and comfort:* Loose-fitting clothes are preferred to minimize friction. Even when using ideal fabrics, tight-fitting garments can raise body temperature and lead to excessive perspiration and discomfort, further promoting the itch–scratch cycle.
- *Layering and seasonal requirements:* Clothing requirements and styles change during the seasons. For the harsh summers with high humidity, lightweight, breathable, moisture-wicking, and loose-fitting garments are recommended.

For the colder seasons, including the monsoons, it is best to layer fabric. Layering starts with a soft base layer such as cotton or bamboo. This is followed by the addition of warm, nonirritating outer layers such as fleece or soft jackets. Though traditional woolens have high itch potential, superfine merino wool is certainly a softer alternative that can provide warmth without much irritation. Fleece and synthetic insulation materials are some other options. Again, it is advised to test materials as these are individual based, and certain synthetics, wool, and dyed fibers can trigger flares. Using removable layers is also another tip, as these add-on layers can be easily added or removed to manage temperature fluctuations and reduce the risk of overheating.

- *Laundering:* Consider using hypoallergenic, fragrance-free, plant-based laundry detergents to minimize skin irritation. Most fabric softeners have added fragrance; hence, they are best avoided. Traditional alternatives to modern-day detergents include soap nuts, sodium carbonate, baking soda, castile soap, borax, and coconut oil soap, used singly or in combination. Additionally, essential oils such as tea tree oil or lavender can be added instead of artificial fragrances. The practice of washing new clothes before wearing them helps to eliminate manufacturing chemicals, residues, dyes and any dust mites that may be present. Washing clothes in hot water helps eliminate allergens, bacteria, and irritants. A second rinse cycle would be more effective in removing all the detergents. Avoid overloading the washer to allow for thorough rinsing. Air drying is advised. Store clothes in a dry, clean place to prevent mold and dust mites.

Regular washing of bedding material and towels further reduces allergens and irritants.

RECOMMENDATIONS FOR BATHING IN ATOPIC DERMATITIS

Effective cleansing of the skin remains the primary aim of topical treatment as long as it is carried out properly to avoid further disruption of the skin barrier process. It facilitates the removal of scale, crust, dust, sweat, allergens, and irritants that can further cutaneous bacterial colonization. The following are a few things to be mindful of when instructing caregivers:

- *Soap:* A hypoallergenic, soap-free cleanser and shampoo that have low to neutral pH should be used. Direct usage of essential oils in soaps such as tree tea oil, lavender, or jasmine during bathing is superior in comparison to artificial fragrance additives in bubble baths; however, this is individual based and should be tested prior.
- *Bath water temperature:* The European guidelines have suggested drawing baths of 27–30°C, while the Japanese guidelines recommend a temperature of 36–40°C. The rationale is that pruritus is induced at a cutaneous temperature of 42°C or higher, while 36–40°C is the optimum range for the recovery of skin barrier functions.
- *Bathing duration and frequency:* Most international guidelines recommend bathing daily for about 5–10 minutes with warm water; however, there are a few variations to the frequency. The European guidelines recommend the use of bath oils in the last 2 minutes of bath. The Korean consensus guidelines specify that bathing should not exceed once per day, though emerging research challenges that the frequency of bathing does not impact the severity of AD significantly.

- *Bathing methods:* The "soak and seal" method of treating eczema involves having a warm quick bath within 5–10 minutes followed by sealing or hydrating the skin with liberal usage of moisturizers after gently patting dry. The "3-minute rule" encourages the application of moisturizers within 3 minutes of drying the skin. Scrubbing and loofahs must be avoided. Care should be taken to thoroughly dry all areas, including skin folds.
- *Bath additives:* The Japanese Task Force (JTF) and Asia Pacific groups suggest that bath additives have beneficial effects. However, the American Academy of Dermatology (AAD) and the European guidelines have either negative views or deferred from commenting. The following are some of the bathing additives mentioned in the literature:
  - *Bleach baths:* Recommended for moderate and severe AD. Diluted sodium hypochlorite 0.005% is obtained by adding 120 mL of 6% bleach in a full bathtub (40 gallons or 150 L) of lukewarm water or one scant teaspoon of bleach in 4 L of lukewarm water. This is anti-inflammatory and modulates the surface microbiome without causing antibiotic resistance.
  - Baby cleansers such as hypoallergenic, fragrance-free syndets (nonsoap cleansers) with neutral or low pH are recommended by the AAD, European, and JTF guidelines.
  - Bath oils create a lipid film on the skin after the bath, which normalizes the increased TEWL and reduces the loss of natural moisturizing factors.
  - Bath salts such as the Dead Sea water salt are rich in magnesium chloride ($MgCl_2$), which helps in removing dead keratin and improving the condition of impetiginized or ichthyotic skin.
  - *Cereal baths:* Rice water starch prepared by adding rice starch to bath water (10 g/L, 15 minutes twice-daily exposure for 4 consecutive days) has been shown to improve acutely inflamed pruritic skin and areas of chronic lichenification. Alternatively, the addition of colloidal oatmeal during bath or its application directly in the form of a paste provides relief.
  - New additives such as citric acid, acetic acid (vinegar), green tea extract, tannic acid, and sodium bicarbonate baths currently lack studies in the pediatric population.
- Deodorants, perfumes, and antiperspirants must be avoided, especially on inflamed skin.

MOISTURIZER USE IN ATOPIC DERMATITIS

Moisturization is the cornerstone of AD management and forms the basis of all maintenance therapy, both in mild-to-severe cases (reducing the duration of topical medical treatments) and during periods of remission. The main purpose is to increase skin hydration, prevent TEWL, prevent flare, as well as prolong the time to flare. Good moisturizer use also reduces the duration of topical steroid treatment. The following are some considerations:

- *Type of moisturizer:* Moisturizers may contain occlusives, humectants, and/or emollients. Occlusives such as petrolatum, mineral oil, lanolin, olive oil, and jojoba oil coat the upper layers of the skin and decrease TEWL. Humectants such as glycerin, urea, and hyaluronic acid aid in improving skin hydration but can dry out the skin in arid weather. Hence, they should be combined to receive the advantages of both.

Thick creams and ointments, which have low to nil water content, are also preferred; however, their greasiness is a disadvantage. Emollient creams, lotions, and oils such as coconut and sunflower oil are alternatives, though these may result in folliculitis in a humid environment. These oils when used singly may cause an increase in TEWL, and it is best to use them in an emulsion form.

Moisturizers that mimic stratum corneum-type lipids such as ceramides, fatty acids, cetyl stearate, and cholesterol soften the skin, and those containing glycyrrhetinic acid act as natural anti-inflammatory agents.

Overall, moisturizers have been successful in monotherapy for mild-to-moderate AD. Using gentle cleansers and moisturizers with barrier lipids from birth can help maintain the skin's barrier homeostasis, improve dryness, and potentially delay or reduce the onset of AD in predisposed infants.

- *Frequency of application:* Apply moisturizer daily from head to toe for all infants, increasing frequency for those with dry or fissured skin. It is best to use the moisturizer right after a quick bath, and it can be reapplied twice daily if necessary.
- *Hygiene:* Good hygiene must be maintained by using a specific container and applicator for the child to avoid cross-contamination.
- *Other considerations:* When choosing a moisturizer, it is important to account for seasonal changes. Hydrophilic moisturizers are ideal for summer, while lipophilic ones are better for winter. Lipophilic moisturizers are particularly beneficial for chronic eczema. "Emollient plus" are emollients that contain non-medicated active ingredients such as flavonoids, saponins, and riboflavins that offer extra anti-inflammatory and antipruritic benefits. These ingredients also support the skin microbiome and aid in restoring the skin barrier function.

SUMMARY

Managing AD effectively involves careful attention to clothing, bathing practices, and consistent moisturizer use. By selecting appropriate fabrics, optimizing bathing routines, and applying moisturizers regularly, caregivers can significantly enhance skin health and minimize flare-ups. These minor yet cornerstone basics enable children affected by AD to learn self-care tips from a young age, empowering them to take an active role in managing their condition. By fostering good habits early on, they can build resilience and confidence, leading to improved skin health and overall well-being as they grow.

KEY POINTS

- For patients with AD, smooth, breathable fabrics with moisture-wicking properties are recommended, avoiding rough materials and synthetic blends.
- Loose-fitting clothing helps minimize friction and overheating, while layering soft materials is ideal for temperature regulation in colder weather.
- Daily bathing for 5–10 minutes is beneficial, and while additives such as bleach baths may help, more research is needed.
- Effective moisturizers should contain occlusives, humectants, and emollients, with the 3-minute rule for application enhancing their effectiveness.

SUGGESTED READING

1. Appiah MM, Haft MA, Kleinman E, Laborada J, Lee S, Loop L, et al. Atopic dermatitis review of comorbidities and therapeutics. Ann Allergy Asthma Immunol. 2022;129(2):142-9.
2. Chu DK, Schneider L, Asiniwasis RN, Boguniewicz M, De Benedetto A, Ellison K, et al. Atopic dermatitis (eczema) guidelines: 2023 American Academy of Allergy, Asthma

and Immunology/American College of Allergy, Asthma and Immunology Joint Task Force on Practice Parameters GRADE- and Institute of Medicine-based recommendations. Ann Allergy Asthma Immunol. 2024;132(3):274-312.

3. Jaros J, Wilson C, Shi VY. Fabric selection in atopic dermatitis: an evidence-based review. Am J Clin Dermatol. 2020;21(4):467-82.
4. Mobolaji-Lawal M, Nedorost S. The role of textiles in dermatitis: an update. Curr Allergy Asthma Rep. 2015;15:17.
5. Pagliaro M, Pecoraro L, Stefani C, Pieropan S, Piacentini G, Pietrobelli A. Bathing in atopic dermatitis in pediatric age: why, how and when. Pediatr Rep. 2024;16(1):57-68.
6. Wollenberg A, Kinberger M, Arents B, Aszodi N, Valle GA, Barbarot S, et al. European guideline (EuroGuiDerm) on atopic eczema—part II: non-systemic treatments and treatment recommendations for special AE patient populations. J Eur Acad Dermatol Venereol. 2022;36(11):1904-26.

CHAPTER 25

Topical Corticosteroids in Atopic Dermatitis: Recommendations and Practice Tips

Rahima Saleem

INTRODUCTION

Atopic dermatitis (AD) is one of the most difficult-to-treat conditions, which is both challenging to the treating physician and the patient and their parents. There is no cure for AD; hence, the aim should be to control the inflammation, symptom management, avoid complications, and improve quality of life. Evidence is well established for topical corticosteroids (TCSs), which still continue to be the first-line anti-inflammatory therapy despite their well-known adverse effects.

HISTORY

Sulzberger and Witten in 1952 were the first ones to introduce topical steroids in the treatment of various dermatoses, which marked a cornerstone in the history of dermatology.

MECHANISM OF ACTION

Topical corticosteroids bind to glucocorticoid intracellular receptors in cytoplasm, which then traverse nuclear envelope and bind to DNA, thereby causing gene regulation and transcription of various mRNA. It produces an anti-inflammatory action by inducing proteins such as lipocortins, which inhibit phospholipase A2 activity, resulting in reduced production of arachidonic acid. It also inhibits mast cells and release of mast cell mediators, thereby decreasing pruritus and causing vasoconstriction. It also causes decreased prostaglandin production by inhibiting cyclooxygenase. It inhibits cytokine production and nitric oxide synthase causing suppression of inflammation. Thus, TCS is used for both controlling active inflammatory disease, decreasing pruritus and preventing relapses.

GUIDELINES ON TOPICAL STEROID USAGE

The choice of potency to be used is based on age, body site to be treated, and severity of eczema **(Table 25.1)**. Low-to-moderate potency TCS is used for mild eczema mainly on sensitive areas such as face, neck, scrotum, diaper areas, and flexures. Potent steroids are used for severe thick plaques and areas with thicker skin such as limbs and palmoplantar areas.

Quantity of Steroids

The finger-tip unit (FTU) is measured as the quantity of drug that can be expressed out of

TABLE 25.1: Topical steroids chosen according to age, site, and severity of eczema.

Age	*Face, genitalia, and body flexures*	*Trunk and limbs*
Up to 1 year	Mild	Mild
2–5 years	Mild	Moderate
5–10 years	Mild or moderate	Potent
10–15 years	Moderate	Potent

a tube with a nozzle of 5 mm diameter, where the length of the drug extends from distal crease to the tip of index finger, which equates to 0.5 g of the drug and covers both palms.

Frequency of Application

Once daily application is as effective as more frequent application but with lesser side effects. Proactive approach is to apply TCS to sites of possible relapse once or twice weekly even when the lesion is quiescent. This weekend therapy resulted in a large decrease in relapse from 25% to 58% in 1,149 patients from seven trials (moderate-certainty evidence). Proactive therapy is better than no topical steroid or reactive approach to prevent eczema flare-ups.

Potency of Steroids

Potency is measured using vasoconstrictor assay in the United Kingdom as mild, moderate, potent, and very potent and in the United States as class 1 (most potent) to class 7 (least potent). Chemically, halogenation, side chain substitutions, and pharmacologically active breakdown products can increase the potency. Also, type of formulation such as ointment base and longer duration of application also increase the unintended effects. Age limit for safe use of various TCS has been depicted in **Table 25.2**. Potent and moderate potent TCSs are probably more effective than mild in moderate-to-severe eczema. But there is no evidence of added benefit of high-potency steroids over potent steroids. The current National Health Service (NHS) guidelines are to apply emollients and then after 30 minutes, apply topical steroids. Applying steroids to wet skin soon after bathing or using wet wraps can also increase penetration and drug delivery, thereby increasing efficacy of topical steroids.

TABLE 25.2: Safety of topical corticosteroids in children.

Topical corticosteroids	*Age group*
Clobetasol propionate 0.05% foam	Above 12 years
Fluocinonide 0.1% cream	Above 12 years
Fluocinolone acetonide 0.01% oil	Above 2 years
Mometasone furoate 0.1% cream/ointment	Above 2 years
Fluticasone propionate 0.05% cream/lotion	Above 1 year
Alclometasone 0.05% cream/ointment	Above 1 year
Prednicarbate 0.1% cream/ointment	Above 1 year
Desonide 0.05% foam/gel	Above 3 months
Hydrocortisone butyrate 0.1% cream	Above 3 months

Combination Therapies

Avoid using antibiotics and antifungals as they can cause resistance and sensitization. Topical calcineurin inhibitors such as tacrolimus or pimecrolimus when used alternating with topical steroids can reduce the dose of TCS and decrease adverse effects, especially atrophy of the skin. Formulations with keratolytics and penetration enhancers increase drug penetration.

ADVERSE EFFECTS

Infants and children are more prone to adverse effects due to risk of absorption due to high body surface area-to-weight ratio. The risk is higher when high potency steroids are applied on thinner skin (younger age, flexures, and face) for prolonged duration and if given under occlusion. Adverse events include infection, skin atrophy, telangiectasia, easy bruisability, hypopigmentation, hypertrichosis, pustular eruptions, and striae.

Thinning was more with the use of high-potent steroids. It has been reported that skin can recover once topical steroids are stopped. An early sign of skin atrophy is to look for horizontally oriented dilated subcapillary plexus. Striae are linear scars due to a decline in collagen synthesis and fibroblast function by the topical steroids, thereby weakening the structural support of the skin. Topical steroids can also prolong anagen phase and can cause hypertrichosis. When applied over eyelid, it can cause cataracts and glaucoma. Creams and lotions need preservatives to maintain shelf life, which can also cause hypersensitivity reactions. Systemic absorption of TCS is rare but can cause hypothalamic–pituitary–adrenal axis suppression and retardation of growth due to premature closure of the epiphysis. Allergic contact dermatitis to TCS can occur, which is difficult to diagnose and is suspected if there is no response or exacerbation after TCS. Patch testing with tixocortol pivalate, budesonide, triamcinolone, and a delayed reading after 7–10 days may be taken as positive to prove allergic contact dermatitis to steroids. Use of topical, nasal, inhaled steroids can lead to perioral dermatitis presenting as scaling, papules, and pustules, which are caused by changes in microflora involving the perioral area and sparing the lip. It can be treated using topical metronidazole and calcineurin inhibitors. They can also develop steroid acne in adolescents. Continuous use of topical steroid on face can cause persistent erythema, thinning, burning, unpleasant sensation, and steroid dependence known as topical steroid damaged face (TSDF), which can be managed by slowly tapering steroids and trying to replace steroids by emollients and topical calcineurin inhibitors. Red face syndrome and red scrotum syndrome characterized by persistent erythema occur after prolonged use of TCS. It can also cause exacerbation of infections and alter its morphology when inadvertently used on infective conditions. When applied to dermatophytic infection, it loses its annularity and develops bizarre, pustular, and nodular lesions, known as tinea incognito. Due to impairment in immune response to *Candida* due to topical steroids, they can develop papules and nodular lesions over the gluteal area known as granuloma gluteal inguinale.

REVIEWING THE RECOMMENDATIONS

There is overwhelming literature and high certainty evidence to support the use of TCS in treatment of AD, making the working group strongly recommending their use. When compared with pimecrolimus 1% cream, moderate-potency steroids were more effective in changing the severity and reducing itching without a difference in infection risk. But tacrolimus 0.1% was found to be better efficacious than fluticasone 0.05% ointment in reducing severity score and local eczema flares. Van Halewijn et al. reviewed various recommendations and concluded that guidelines differ in the initial type of TCS recommended. They either used a short burst of high-potency TCS or a lowest possible potent TCS or TCS type tailored to severity or the suggestion that a short treatment with a potent TCS is as effective as a longer treatment. Two guidelines based these recommendations on a randomized controlled trial by Thomas et al., which was conducted among children with AD. Nine guidelines do not mention safety or side effects. Regarding area and age, guidelines advise using only mild and moderate TCS in children and on areas prone to adverse effects such as genital, facial, or intertriginous skin areas regardless of age.

Last, one guideline emphasizes that the risk of adverse events is low when TCS is used properly, and the harm associated with undertreatment is generally greater than the potential for adverse effects to moderate eczema in children. It was concluded that a short burst of a potent topical corticosteroid is just as effective as prolonged use of a milder preparation. Proactive approach or weekend therapy can reduce the flares. Few guidelines recommend that "the least potent preparation that adequately controls the disease process should be selected" and that "higher potency TCS is generally preferred in the acute phases."

SUMMARY

Though a wonder drug when used judiciously, its use has to be tailored to decrease its adverse events, and there is a need for better quality research trials regarding adverse effects. Strategies for withdrawal of steroids by substituting with emollients or alternating with nonsteroidal agents should be in place for all children on prolonged treatment. Prescription sharing and misuse of steroids for skin whitening have to be discouraged.

KEY POINTS

- *Topical corticosteroids (TCSs)* remain the first-line treatment for atopic dermatitis (AD), with potency chosen based on age, site, and severity of eczema.
- *Once-daily application* is generally effective and safer; proactive "weekend therapy" helps prevent relapses better than reactive use.
- *Potency classifications* vary globally; higher potency is not always more effective and carries increased risk of side effects, especially in children.
- *Adverse effects* include skin atrophy, striae, perioral dermatitis, tinea incognito, and rare systemic effects like HPA axis suppression.
- *Combination therapies* with calcineurin inhibitors help minimize steroid use and related skin damage; antibiotics and antifungals should be avoided unless clearly indicated.

SUGGESTED READING

1. Ahluwalia A. Topical glucocorticoids and the skin—mechanisms of action: an update. Mediators Inflamm. 1998;7(3):183-93.
2. Caloe J, Zirwas MJ. Allergens in corticosteroid vehicles. Dermatitis. 2008;19:38-42.
3. Eichenfield LF, Tom WL, Berger TG, Krol A, Paller AS, Schwarzenberger K, et al. Guidelines for care of the management of atopic dermatitis: section 2. Management and treatment of atopic dermatitis with topical therapies. J Am Acad Dermatol. 2014;71(1):116-32.
4. Galli E, Neri I, Ricci G, Baldo E, Barone M, Fortina AB, et al. Consensus conference on clinical management of pediatric atopic dermatitis. Ital J Pediatr. 2016;42:26.
5. González-López G, Ceballos-Ródriguez RM, González-López JJ, Fieto-Ródriguez M, Herranz-Pinto P. Efficacy and safety of wet wrap therapy for patients with atopic dermatitis: a systematic review and meta-analysis. Br J Dermatol. 2017;177(3):688-95.
6. Katz HI, Prawer SE, Mooney JJ, Samson CR. Preatrophy: covert sign of thinned skin. J Am Acad Dermatol. 1989;20:731-5.
7. Lax SJ, Harvey J, Axon E, Howells L, Santer M, Ridd MJ, et al. Strategies for using topical corticosteroids in children and adults with eczema. Cochrane Database Syst Rev. 2022;2022(3):CD013356.
8. Saraswat A. Topical corticosteroid use in children: adverse effects and how to minimize them. Indian J Dermatol Venereol Leprol. 2010;76:225-8.
9. Sathishkumar D, Moss C. Topical therapy in atopic dermatitis in children. Indian J Dermatol. 2016;61(6):656-61.
10. Schmitt J, von Kobyletzki L, Svensson A, Apfelbacher C. Efficacy and tolerability of proactive treatment with topical

corticosteroids and calcineurin inhibitors for atopic eczema: systematic review and meta-analysis of randomized controlled trials. Br J Dermatol. 2011;164(2):415-28.

11. Sidbury R, Alikhan A, Bercovitch L, Cohen DE, Darr JM, Drucker AM, et al. Guidelines of care for the management of atopic dermatitis in adults with topical therapies. J Am Acad Dermatol. 2023;89(1):e1-20.
12. Thomas KS, Armstrong S, Avery A, Po ALW, O'Neill C, Young S, et al. Randomised controlled trial of short bursts of a potent topical corticosteroid versus prolonged use of a mild preparation for children with mild or moderate atopic eczema. BMJ. 2002;324:768.
13. Van Halewijn KF, Lahnstein T, Bohnen AM, Van Den Berg PJ, Gma Pasmans S, Je Bindels P, et al. Recommendations for emollients, bathing and topical corticosteroids for the treatment of atopic dermatitis: a systematic review of guidelines. Eur J Dermatol. 2022;32(1):113-23.
14. West DP, Worobec S, Solomon LM. Pharmacology and toxicology of infant skin. J Invest Dermatol. 1981;76:147-50.

CHAPTER 26

History Taking in Food Allergy

R Prasanna

INTRODUCTION

An unfavorable immunological reaction to a food is known as a food allergy. Reactions that are immunoglobulin E (IgE) mediated or non-IgE mediated can be distinguished. T cells are thought to be involved in a large number of non-IgE responses, which are poorly understood in both clinical and scientific contexts. Mixed IgE and non-IgE allergic reactions are defined as reactions that exhibit a combination of both IgE and non-IgE responses.

FOOD-INDUCED ALLERGIC DISORDERS

Table 26.1 depicts in a nutshell about food-induced allergic disorders, manifestation, and prognosis.

DIVERSITY OF CONDITIONS ASSOCIATED WITH IMMUNOGLOBULIN E-MEDIATED REACTIONS TO FOOD

One of this IgE-mediated reactions to food itself has diverse associated conditions, as depicted in **Box 26.1**.

A detailed history is necessary for identifying food allergies. Let us see the important details in history taking that is essential to identify an etiology.

HISTORY TAKING IN FOOD ALLERGY

Was the child breastfed?

- Duration/partial—exclusive
- If exclusively breastfed, maternal dietary intake/food avoided
- Age when formula/milk introduced
- Which formula (soya/hypoallergenic)/milk
- Changes in formula milk/subsequent reactions
- Took feeds well or seemed uncomfortable
- Problems weaning

Weight Gain

- History of failure to gain weight
- Appetite/do they eat well/enjoy food

Dietary History from Birth

What food groups are eaten and any reaction (s)? Ask about the age of onset of symptoms/frequency/consistency of reaction(s). Make sure the big eight is included in this given as follows:

- Cow's milk
- Egg
- Peanuts
- Tree nuts (walnuts/hazelnuts/almonds/Brazil nuts/cashew nuts)
- Sesame/hummus (Sesame + Chickpea)
- Wheat
- Fish
- Shellfish
- Legumes and pulses (soya, chickpea, kidney bean, lupin, and baked beans)
- Fruits/vegetables (banana/kiwi fruit/potato/chestnut/tomato/avocado)
- Any food(s) avoided

TABLE 26.1: Summary of food-induced allergic disorders, manifestation, and prognosis.

Immunopathology	***Disorder***	***Clinical features***	***Typical age group***	***Prognosis***
IgE mediated	• Pollen food allergy syndrome	• Pruritus and mild edema confined to oral cavity	• Onset after pollen allergy established (adult > young child)	• May be persistent and may vary by season
	• Urticaria/ angioedema	• Triggered by ingestion or direct contact	• Children > Adult	• Depends on food
	• Rhinoconjunctivitis/ asthma	• Accompanies food-induced allergic reaction but rarely isolated symptoms • May be triggered by the inhalation of aerosolized food protein	• Infant/child > Adult except for occupational disease	• Depends on food
	• Gastrointestinal symptoms	• Symptoms such as nausea, emesis, abdominal pain, and diarrhea triggered by food ingestion	• Any age	• Depends on food
	• Anaphylaxis	• Rapid progressive, multisystem reaction	• Any age	
	• Food-dependent, exercise-induced anaphylaxis	• Food triggers anaphylaxis only if ingestion is followed temporally by exercise	• Onset in late childhood/ adulthoo	• Depends on food presumed persistent
Mixed IgE and cell mediated	• Atopic eczema/ dermatitis	• Associated with food in 30–40% of children with moderate/severe eczema	• Infant > Child > Adult	• Usually resolves
	• Eosinophilic gastrointestinal disorders	• Symptoms vary depending on the site of the intestinal tract involved and degree of eosinophilic inflammation	• Any age	• Likely persistent
Cell mediated	• Dietary protein-induced proctitis/ proctocolitis	• Mucus-laden, bloody stool in infants	• Infancy	• Usually resolves
	• Food protein-induced enterocolitis syndrome	• Chronic exposure, emesis, diarrhea, poor growth, and lethargy • Re-exposure after restriction, emesis, diarrhea, and hypotension a couple of hour after ingestion	• Infancy	• Usually resolves

(IgE: immunoglobulin E)

Source: Adapted from Muraro A, Werfel T, Hoffmann-Sommergruber K, Roberts G, Beyer K, Bindslev-Jensen C, et al. EAACI food allergy and anaphylaxis guidelines: diagnosis and management of food allergy. Allergy. 2014;69:1008-25.

BOX 26.1: Immunoglobulin E (IgE)-mediated reactions to food.

- Systemic IgE-mediated reactions (anaphylaxis):
  - Immediate-onset reactions
  - Late-onset reactions
- IgE-mediated gastrointestinal reactions:
  - Oral allergy syndrome
  - Immediate gastrointestinal allergy
- IgE-mediated respiratory reactions:
  - Asthma and rhinitis secondary to ingestion of food
  - Asthma and rhinitis secondary to inhalation of food (e.g., occupational asthma)
- IgE-mediated cutaneous reactions:
  - Immediate-onset reactions:
    - Acute urticaria or angioedema
    - Contact urticaria
  - Late-onset reactions:
    - Atopic dermatitis

Source: Adapted from American College of Allergy, Asthma, & Immunology. Food allergy: a practice parameter. Ann Allergy Asthma Immunol. 2006; 96(3 Suppl 2):S1-68.

Family History, Ask if

Either parent avoids certain food/detailed history in them

- Symptoms and Signs in an Infant
- Irritability
- Problem in sleeping
- Persistent crying
- Back arching
- Colic
- Vomiting/reflux (small amount of milk but not vomiting)
- Constipation/straining
- Crying when their bowels are opened
- Eczema, age of onset

Symptoms and Signs in Children

- Blocked runny nose
- Respiratory symptoms/cough/wheeze
- Blood or mucus in motions
- Redness around bottom/soreness
- Difficulty in swallowing/food sticking
- Sleep patterns
- Late manifestations of allergy, especially gastrointestinal and eczema

SYMPTOMS AND REACTIONS

What are the symptoms of concern? What is their severity? Ask for a thorough description of the most recent reaction. Ask about age of onset of symptoms/frequency/consistency of reaction(s).

- Clinical manifestation/duration (e.g., skin, gastrointestinal, respiratory, and cardiovascular)
- In relation to exposure to a given food (up to 6 hours)/more than one factor (e.g., food plus exercise)
- Food ever be eaten without these symptoms occurring
- First reaction to that food; if answer is "no," then severity of previous reaction
- Quantity/type (e.g., raw/cooked)
- Reaction on skin contact (e.g., parent eating peanut, kissing child)
- Symptoms present at times other than after exposure to a given food

Management of Previous Reactions to Food

- Symptoms resolved without specific/ medical intervention
- Medication given/which route/time from treatment to recovery

Take into account the potential for a food allergy in children whose symptoms do not go away after receiving treatment for:

- Atopic eczema
- Gastroesophageal reflux disease
- Chronic gastrointestinal symptoms, including chronic constipation

RECOMMENDATIONS TO PREVENT FOOD ALLERGY IN INFANTS AT HIGH RISK OF DEVELOPING ALLERGY

- Mothers who are nursing their babies ought to do so for at least the first year of life. Breastfeeding can be supplemented with hypoallergenic formulae during this period for infants who are at risk. While breastfeeding, mothers should avoid eating peanuts and tree nuts (such as walnuts), as well as eggs, cow's milk, fish, and may be other food. High-risk infants should not be fed solid food until they are 6 months old. Dairy products should be given up to a year old; eggs to 2 years old; and fish, peanuts, and nuts to 3 years old.
- Pregnant women do not need to follow any dietary restrictions, possibly with the exception of not eating peanuts.
- Breastfeeding mothers on a restricted diet should consider the use of supplemental minerals (calcium) and vitamins.
- It is not recommended to offer supplemental nutrients before the fifth month of life.
- Dietary products utilized in infancy for preventative reasons should be thoroughly assessed in suitable clinical studies for their nutritional and preventive effects.
- Because it can lower the incidence of adverse food responses, particularly to cow's milk protein, exclusive feeding of a formula with a verified reduced allergenicity is advised for bottle-fed infants with an established hereditary atopic risk (affected parent or sibling).

CROSS-REACTIVITY AMONG SPECIFIC FOOD FAMILIES

The food family, overall risk of cross-reactivity, and specific considerations are shown in **Table 26.2**.

- Every patient and family should receive recommendations based on the likelihood of a true allergy and the significance of the food to the individual's diet; for example, a thorough investigation of potential allergies to fish, tree nuts, and legumes may be crucial for a family that follows a vegetarian diet but less significant for another family.
- The evaluation should always start with a thorough history. No testing should be done to food the patient has clearly tolerated due to cross-sensitization in skin and IgE tests. If the history is unclear or the patient has never eaten the food, testing should be based on the likelihood of true cross-reactivity.
- An extensive and thorough checklist is sometimes needed to analyze the causative food. We provide with one chart for both animal and plant sources.

CLASSIFICATION OF FOOD FROM ANIMAL SOURCES

The categorization of foods derived from animal sources is outlined in **Box 26.2**.

CLASSIFICATION OF FOOD FROM PLANT SOURCES

Box 26.3 depicts in a nutshell about classification of food derived from plant sources.

FOOD ALLERGY DIARY

Directions for Keeping Diet Diary (Table 26.3)

- Note everything that goes into your stomach in your diet journal. This include, in addition to, meals, medications, vitamins, supplements, snacks, and coffee.
- Enumerate the ingredients of mixed dishes and culinary combinations. Not even writing down "ham sandwich" will do. Additionally, you should specify the type

TABLE 26.2: Cross-reactivity among specific food families.

Food family	*Overall risk of cross-reactivity*	*Specific considerations*
Mammalian milk	High	Very high rate of CR between cow, goat, and sheep's milk; very low rate with mare, camel, and donkey's milk
Mammalian milk and meat	Low	10–20% rate of CR between cow's milk and beef
Hen's egg and avian meats	Low	Estimated 5–10% CR between egg and chicken
Fish	High	High frequency of CR among different species; OFCs to specific fish may be indicated based upon testing and importance to diet
Shellfish	Variable	High (>50%) CR between different crustaceans and different mollusks; low between crustaceans and mollusks
Tree nuts	High	Most patients are allergic to more than one nut; nearly 100% CR between walnut and pecan and between cashew and pistachio
• Legumes	• Variable	• Low CR between peanut and other legumes except possibly lupine; higher CR between lentil and other legumes such as pea and chickpea
• Wheat and cereal grains	• Variable	• High CR between wheat and rye, less between wheat and barley, and low between wheat and other grains

Source: Adapted from Kazatsky AM, Wood RA. Classification of food allergens and cross-reactivity. Curr Allergy Asthma Rep. 2016;16(3):22.

BOX 26.2: Classification of food from animal sources.

Mollusks
- Abalone
- Mussel
- Oyster
- Scallop
- Clam
- Squid

Amphibians
- Frog

Mammals
- Beef
- Pork
- Goat
- Mutton (lamb)
- Venison
- Horsemeat
- Rabbit
- Squirrel

Crustaceans
- Crab
- Crawfish
- Lobster
- Shrimp

Reptiles
- Turtle

Birds
- Chicken
- Duck
- Goose
- Turkey
- Guinea hen
- Squab
- Pheasant
- Partridge
- Grouse

Fish
- Sturgeon
- Hake
- Anchovy
- Sardine
- Herring
- Haddock
- Bass
- Pompano
- Salmon
- Whitefish
- Scrod
- Shad
- Eel
- Carp
- Codfish
- Halibut
- Catfish
- Sole
- Pike
- Flounder
- Drum
- Mullet
- Trout
- Mackerel
- Tuna
- Bluefish
- Snapper
- Sunfish
- Swordfish
- Grouper
- Plaice

Source: Adapted from American College of Allergy, Asthma, & Immunology. Food allergy: a practice parameter. Ann Allergy Asthma Immunol. 2006;96(3 Suppl 2):S1-68.

BOX 26.3: Classification of food from plant sources.

Grain family
- Wheat
- Graham flour
- Gluten flour
- Bran
- Wheat germ
- Rye
- Marley
- Malt
- Corn
- Oats
- Corn
- Rice
- Wild rice
- Sorghum
- Cane

Mustard family
- Mustard
- Cabbage
- Cauliflower
- Broccoli
- Brussels sprouts
- Turnip
- Rutabaga
- Kale
- Collard
- Celery cabbage
- Kohlrabi
- Radish
- Horseradish
- Watercress

Ginger family
- Ginger
- Turmeric
- Cardamom

Pine family
- Juniper
- Pine nut

Tea family
- Tea

Pedalium family
- Sesame seeds

Mallow family
- Okra
- Cottonseed

Spurge family
- Tapioca

Arrowroot family
- Arrowroot

Arum family
- Taro

Buckwheat family
- Buckwheat
- Rhubarb

Potato/nightshade family
- Potato
- Tomato
- Eggplant
- Red pepper
- Green pepper

Chili pepper

Gooseberry family
- Gooseberry
- Currant

Honeysuckle family
- Elderberry
- Citrus family
- Orange
- Grapefruit
- Lemon
- Lime
- Tangerine
- Kumquat

Birch family
- Hazelnut

Mulberry family
- Mulberry
- Fig
- Hop
- Breadfruit

Maple family
- Maple syrup

Palm family
- Coconut
- Date
- Sago

Pomegranate family
- Pomegranate

Ebony family
- Persimmon

Rose family
- Raspberry
- Blackberry
- Loganberry
- Boysenberry
- Dewberry
- Strawberry

Banana family
- Banana
- Plantain

Grape family
- Grape
- Raisin

Mint family
- Mint
- Peppermint
- Spearmint
- Thyme
- Sage
- Marjoram
- Savory

Gourd family
- Pumpkin
- Squash
- Cucumber
- Cantaloupe
- Muskmelon
- Honeydew melon
- Persian melon
- Casaba
- Watermelon

Rosaceae/apple family
- Apple
- Pear
- Quince

Poppy family
- Poppy seed

Rosaceae/plum family
- Plum
- Prune
- Cherry
- Peach
- Apricot
- Nectarine
- Almond

Orchid family
- Vanilla

Madder family
- Coffee

Olive family
- Green olive
- Ripe olive
- Red pepper
- Green pepper
- Bell pepper
- Chili
- Tabasco

Pimento

Lily family
- Asparagus
- Onion
- Garlic
- Leek
- Chive
- Aloe

Goosefoot family
- Beet
- Spinach
- Swiss chard

Pineapple family
- Pineapple

Papaw family
- Papaya

Parsley family
- Parsley
- Parsnip
- Carrot
- Celery
- Celeriac
- Caraway
- Anise
- Coriander
- Fennel
- Cumin

Heath family
- Cranberry
- Blueberry

Lecythis family
- Brazil nut

Composite family
- Leaf lettuce
- Head lettuce
- Endive
- Escarole
- Artichoke
- Dandelion
- Chicory
- Guava

Myrtle family
- Allspice
- Cloves

Contd...

Contd...

Legume family
- Navy bean
- Kidney
- Lima bean
- String bean
- Soybean
- Lentil
- Black-eyed peas
- Pea
- Peanut
- Licorice
- Acacia
- Senna

Morning glory family
- Sweet potato
- Yam

Sunflower family
- Jerusalem artichoke
- Sunflower seed

Pepper family
- Black pepper

Nutmeg family
- Nutmeg

Laurel family
- Avocado
- Cinnamon
- Bay leaf

Walnut family
- English walnut
- Black walnut
- Butternut
- Hickory nut
- Pecan

Cashew family
- Cashew
- Pistachio
- Mango

Beech family
- Beechnut
- Chestnut

Fungi family
- Mushroom
- Yeast

Sterculia family
- Cacao
- Chocolate (processed from cacao)

Source: Adapted from Spector SL. The diagnosis of food allergy: theory and practice. In: Spector SL (Ed). Provocative Challenge Procedures: Background and Methodology. Mt Kisco, NY: Wiley-Blackwell; 1993.

TABLE 26.3: Example of a diet diary chart.

Time	***Food/drink/medication***	***Time of symptoms***	***Symptoms (0–4)***
		12:00–7:30	• Up twice during night • Coughing and sneezing
7:30 AM	Awakened	7:30 AM	No symptoms
8.30 AM	• Milk/coffee/tea/juice/sugar • Idli/dosa/bread/chapati		
		9:00 AM	Runny nose 2+, sneezing 2+
		10:00 AM	No symptoms
		12:00 PM	No symptoms
12:30 PM	Vegetable soup/cooked rice/cooked dhal/egg/vegetables (potato, carrot, peas, beetroot) mutton/chicken		
		1:00 PM	Trouble breathing 4+, felt faint lasted 10 minutes
3:00 PM	One glass of milk		
		3:10 PM	Abdominal pain 4+
3:30 PM	Vitamin supplements		
		4:00 PM	No symptoms
		5:30 PM	Stuffy nose 1+
6:30 PM	Coffee		
7:30 PM	Dosa/idli/chapati/cooked rice/cooked dhal		
		8:00 PM	Belching + Nausea+
10:00 PM	One glass of milk		
		10:30 PM	Hives on neck for 1 hour 4+
11.00 PM	Went to bed		

of bread, spread, and dressing (e.g., "ham sandwich—whole wheat bread, butter, and mustard"). In a same vein, "salad" leaves out important details. The salad's ingredients (e.g., salad-lettuce, tomato, carrot, peppers, artichoke, and bleu-cheese dressing) should be listed in the entry. Every time you record something in your diary, ask yourself, "Have I provided enough information about what's in this food?"

- Write down every symptom you experience, including when it started, how long it lasted, and how severe it was. Common allergic symptoms include running or congested noses, wheezing, shortness of breath, sneezing, coughing, itching, cramps, gas, hives, headaches, migraines, fatigue, and so on. This is not an exhaustive list, so please write down any additional symptoms you may be experiencing.
- List symptoms on a basis of 0-4+ to indicate the severity.
- Make sure to note your symptoms before every meal and snack, as well as 30-60 minutes afterward.
- Record whenever a symptom gets better or worse.

SUMMARY

Food allergy history-taking is a vital step in diagnosing and managing food allergies, which may be IgE-mediated, non-IgE-mediated, or mixed.

A comprehensive clinical history includes feeding patterns (breastfeeding, formula), dietary introduction timelines, and symptom patterns related to food intake.

Assessment should focus on the "big eight" allergens, symptom timing, severity, and consistency, alongside growth parameters and family allergy history.

The food allergy diary is a crucial tool for tracking intake and correlating symptoms, requiring detailed entries on food components and reaction severity. History should explore exposure routes, tolerance, and cross- reactivity risks among food groups.

KEY POINTS

- *Feeding and weaning history:* Assess breastfeeding duration, formula types, weaning challenges, and the introduction of solids to identify early exposure to allergens.
- *Dietary recall/family and atopy history:* Document all foods eaten since birth, with emphasis on common allergens along with any observed reactions and family history of allergies.
- *Detailed symptom timeline:* Record all symptoms (gastrointestinal, skin, respiratory), their onset after food intake, and any triggers like exercise or skin contact.
- *This will help determine whether the food-induced allergy is IgE-mediated, non-IgE-mediated or mixed.*

SUGGESTED READING

1. American College of Allergy, Asthma, & Immunology. Food allergy: a practice parameter. Ann Allergy Asthma Immunol. 2006;96(3 Suppl 2):S1-68.
2. Fox AT, Lloyd K, Arkwright PD, Bhattacharya D, Brown T, Chetcuti P, et al. The RCPCH care pathway for food allergy in children: an evidence and consensus based national approach. Arch Dis Child. 2011;96 (Suppl 2): i25-9.
3. Kazatsky AM, Wood RA. Classification of food allergens and cross-reactivity. Curr Allergy Asthma Rep. 2016;16(3):22.
4. Muraro A, Werfel T, Hoffmann-Sommergruber K, Roberts G, Beyer K, Bindslev-Jensen C, et al. EAACI food allergy and anaphylaxis guidelines: diagnosis and management of food allergy. Allergy. 2014;69:1008-25.
5. Walsh J, O'Flynn N. Diagnosis and assessment of food allergy in children and young people in primary care and community settings: NICE clinical guideline. Br J Gen Pract. 2011;61(588):473-5.

CHAPTER 27

Elimination Diets in Food Allergy

Sowmya Arudi Nagarajan, Sushma C

INTRODUCTION

An elimination diet involves removing specific foods or groups of foods from one's diet to identify and manage food intolerances, allergies, and various health disorders, such as urticarial disease, eosinophilic esophagitis, irritable bowel syndrome (IBS), or migraine headaches.

The specific protocol for each elimination diet depends on the symptoms presented or the diagnosed disease. The elimination can be guided by food allergen tests or implemented empirically. Strict elimination diets, such as the gluten-free diet and the low FODMAPs (fermentable oligosaccharides, disaccharides, monosaccharides, and polyols) diet, are highly regimented. For severe reactions, such as anaphylaxis, the patient must be evaluated and individualized avoidance strategy designed based on patient history, the allergen involved, and diagnostic methods such as skin prick tests, serum-specific immunoglobulin E (IgE) measurements, or component-resolved diagnostics outcome.

Elimination diets have shown efficacy in controlling symptoms and enhancing patient satisfaction across various disease processes, supported by several randomized controlled trials and observational studies. This review covers commonly used elimination diets, the diseases they can help identify and treat, their limitations, and the best practices for optimizing patient outcomes through their implementation.

Elimination diets have demonstrated both diagnostic and therapeutic values for patients with food allergies or intolerances. They also offer benefits for individuals with functional gastrointestinal (GI) disorders, such as IBS, which are often triggered by specific foods.

Elimination diets can be complex for patients, making it difficult for them to follow recommendations. Eating competence is also vitally important to the socialization of the child, and children with food allergies may have food aversions and self-limited diets beyond the elimination diet. Anxiety issues may even arise about eating and food in general, which will have a further impact on the child's ability to participate fully in activities. By employing an interprofessional team approach for each patient, treatment can be optimized, outcomes improved, and long-term symptom relief achieved.

SIGNIFICANCE

Using an elimination diet combined with oral food challenges in patients with allergies and intolerances can be an economical and noninvasive way to pinpoint trigger foods.

SIX-FOOD ELIMINATION DIET

A stepwise or six-food elimination diet (6FED) serves is a common, effective diagnostic, and therapeutic approach for identifying and removing triggering allergens, alleviating symptoms, and aiding in the overall management of eosinophilic esophagitis. The 6FED involves three key steps given as follows:

1. *Elimination phase*: Removes the six main food allergens—(1) milk, (2) eggs, (3) soy, (4) wheat, (5) nuts (tree nuts and peanuts), and (6) fish (including shellfish)
2. *Observation phase*: Avoid these foods for 4–6 weeks while monitoring for symptom improvement
3. *Reintroduction phase*: Gradually reintroduce each food group to identify which ones trigger symptoms and then eliminate only the problematic foods

Other diets, such as one-food, two-food, and four-food elimination diets, operate similarly. For instance, eliminating just animal milk has shown effectiveness comparable to the 6FED in treating eosinophilic esophagitis.

Specific elimination diets also target certain conditions. The low FODMAP diet addresses IBS, and a gluten-free diet is used for celiac disease.

In general, elimination diets work by removing suspected foods, identifying triggers through reintroduction, and then avoiding those triggers to manage symptoms effectively.

Elimination diets require careful attention to detail and face several obstacles to full adherence. Factors such as limited medical knowledge, socioeconomic challenges, a lack of diverse food options, and concerns about the diets can all lead to less-than-optimal compliance. It is, therefore, necessary to provide extensive education and empower the family and eventually the child/patient to participate in all the daily activities while avoiding the food to which the child is allergic.

Patients with bowel disease often eliminate major food groups based on the belief that these foods worsen their condition. Those adhering strictly to a gluten-free diet tend to have lower intake levels of iron, fiber, and carbohydrates compared to their prior diet that included gluten.

Individuals on a low FODMAP diet have been found to have lower calcium intake compared to those on a regular diet, likely due to reduced consumption of lactose-containing dairy products, which are high in calcium. This may lead to nutritional deficiencies in the longer run. Therefore, nutritional education is crucial when following an elimination diet to prevent deficiencies in vitamins and minerals, depending on which foods are excluded.

Achieving optimal outcomes with an elimination diet is most effective through an interprofessional approach. Patients with food allergies or gastrointestinal issues often consult their primary care practitioner, who should take a thorough medical history and perform a comprehensive physical examination. This history should encompass the current illness, past medical and surgical history, family history, current medications, and social determinants of health. Care should be tailored to each patient's needs according to established guidelines. Before diagnosing a food allergy or intolerance, clinicians should rule out other conditions that mimic similar symptoms. While an elimination diet can be a valuable diagnostic and therapeutic tool, it should not replace a complete, guideline-directed evaluation. Clinicians must recognize the limitations and appropriate use of elimination diets and be aware of potential pitfalls that could lead to unsuccessful outcomes.

When prescribing an elimination diet, it is crucial to ensure the patient fully understands the specific instructions and goals of the regimen. Registered dietitians play a key role in enhancing patient education by assessing their comprehension and providing detailed dietary guidelines. This includes teaching patients how to read food labels, identify foods to avoid, and prevent nutritional deficiencies. Clinical nurses and support staff are also vital for the success of an elimination diet, as they gather important information about patient compliance, current elimination or reintroduction stages, and any changes in symptoms. An interprofessional team approach can optimize treatment, improve outcomes, and offer long-term symptom relief.

EATING COMPETENCES

Eating competence is vitally important to the socialization of the child, and children with food allergies may have food aversions and self-limited diets beyond the elimination diet. Eating competence describes the child's ability to eat and enjoy a wide variety of foods of varying flavors and textures that will support adequate nutrition for growth and development. Assessment of eating competences will help to provide an effective nutrition care plan and avoid picky eating and nutritional deficiencies.

FOOD LABELING

Food labeling legislation applies to the country or region in which the product is sold. In the United States, the Food Allergen Labeling and Consumer Protection Act (FALCPA) mandates clear, plain language labeling of all ingredients derived from the foods considered major allergens. Those foods considered major allergens in the United States are milk, egg, wheat, soy, peanut, tree nuts, fish, and crustacean shellfish. In 2021, the United States added sesame as the ninth major food allergen. However, the FALCPA does not cover fresh fruits and vegetables in their natural state. The FALCPA also does not cover any highly refined oil derived for a food specified in the major allergen group.

It is noteworthy that an unintentional cross-contact of the allergen with the manufactured food cannot be prevented, and this need not to be mentioned on the food labels. Hence, the patients with history of severe food reactions must always carry an adrenaline autoinjectors with them in schools, restaurants, and while traveling.

FOOD DIARY

It is a record of what the child eats and what symptoms they feel. It is used as part of the diagnosis process to narrow down a food allergy trigger. It is helpful when patient is having symptoms but parents are unaware what is causing them.

It is not needed when patient has already been diagnosed with a food allergy, has history of anaphylaxis, if there is a temporal correlation with food consumed, or the symptoms of the suspected food allergy are nonspecific or suggestive of food intolerance.

The food diary asks to specify what the child ate in the day, number of servings, and ingredients in the food/dish, including the fluids consumed. It further asks to specify what was the time of food consumption, symptoms of food allergy experienced, and whether child performed any exercise/activity soon after consumption. This detailed record has to be maintained at least for a period of 2 weeks, including weekends. It is also helpful to carry the food packaging that contained the food item while showing the food diary to the doctor.

It is important to convey to the parents/patients that the food diary is not diagnostic of a food allergy. Instead, it helps in suggesting the possibility of food allergy. This, in turn, will help the clinician to diagnose the food allergy by planning the further investigations. Other uses of this food diary are to ensure that the child is receiving nutrition and caloric intake as per the recommended daily allowance (RDA).

SUMMARY

Current management of food allergy entails dietary avoidance of the identified allergen, requiring extensive education. Allergen elimination diets should not be prescribed lightly, and the global impact of these diets should be considered. In theory, these elimination diets seem an easy task, but avoidance issues are complex, and accidental ingestions are not uncommon. Thus, food allergy management must also include comprehensive education on how to recognize and treat a food allergic reaction.

KEY POINTS

Elimination diets in food allergy:

- *Core management strategy:* Involves strict dietary avoidance of the identified allergen.
- *Need for education:* Requires extensive patient and caregiver education on food labels, hidden ingredients, and safe alternatives.
  - *Caution in use:* Elimination diets should not be prescribed lightly due to potential nutritional and social impacts.
  - *Complexity of avoidance:* Although seemingly simple, complete avoidance is difficult and prone to accidental exposures.
  - *Risk of accidental ingestion:* Cross-contamination and mislabeled foods make unintentional allergen intake common.
- *Comprehensive management:*
  - Must include education on:
    - Recognizing allergic reactions
    - Emergency response, including use of epinephrine
- *Global Impact:* The psychosocial and nutritional consequences of long-term elimination must be considered.

SUGGESTED READING

1. Food and Drug Administration. (2022). FASTER Act Video for Food Industry and Other Stakeholders. [online] Available from https://www.fda.gov/food/cfsan-constituent-updates/faster-act-video-food-industry-and-other-stakeholders. [Last accessed April, 2025].
2. Food and Drug Administration. (2022). Food Allergen Labeling and Consumer Protection Act of 2004 (FALCPA). [online] Available from https://www.fda.gov/food/food-allergensgluten-free-guidance-documents-regulatory-information/food-allergen-labeling-and-consumer-protection-act-2004-falcpa. [Last accessed April, 2025].
3. FPIES Foundation. (2015). FPIES Tools: Food Journal's for Food Allergies! [online] Available from https://fpiesfoundation.org/fpies-tools-food-journals-for-food-allergies. [Last accessed April, 2025].
4. Kliewer KL, Cassin AM, Venter C. Dietary therapy for eosinophilic esophagitis: elimination and reintroduction. Clin Rev Allergy Immunol. 2018;55(1):70-87.
5. Kliewer KL, Gonsalves N, Dellon ES, Katzka DA, Abonia JP, Aceves SS, et al. One-food versus six-food elimination diet therapy for the treatment of eosinophilic oesophagitis: a multicentre, randomised, open-label trial. Lancet Gastroenterol Hepatol. 2023;8(5): 408-21.
6. Navarrete-Rodríguez EM, Del Río-Navarro BE, García-Aranda JA, Medeiros M, Enciso Peláez S, García Hernández HR, et al. Nutritional implications of elimination diets. Bol Med Hosp Infant Mex. 2015;72(2): 112-7.
7. Wood RA. Diagnostic elimination diets and oral food provocation. Chem Immunol Allergy. 2015;101:87.
8. Zalewski A, Doerfler B, Krause A, Hirano I, Gonsalves N. Long-term outcomes of the six-food elimination diet and food reintroduction in a large cohort of adults with eosinophilic esophagitis. Am J Gastroenterol. 2022;117(12):1963-70.

CHAPTER 28

Oral Food Challenges

Sowmya Arudi Nagarajan

INTRODUCTION

Food allergies have been seeing an increasing trend in the last few decades. Self-reported food allergies prevalence has been shown to be around 0.1–6% in a systematic review in Europe. Self-reported rates of food allergies are far higher than true food allergy. Not all children reported actually had food allergy. One in seven children reported food allergies, but only two among them were confirmed by history, skin prick testing (SPT), and oral food challenge (OFC).

Approach to a diagnosis of food allergy is not very straightforward; clinical history suggests the probability, and the laboratory tests for the diagnosis of true food allergy have a poor specificity. Therefore, OFC remains the gold standard for the diagnosis of food allergy. It is usually conducted to make diagnosis, monitor for resolution of a food allergy, or identify the threshold of responsiveness.

The basic methodology underlying all OFCs is administration of the suspect food in gradually increasing doses under close observation in a medical setting. Variations in challenge methodology include the inclusion of placebo controls, blinding, and different dosing strategies. It is carried out under careful supervision of healthcare professionals trained in handling the adverse allergic reactions that may occur in the OFCs.

METHODOLOGY

Inclusion Criteria

Patients of any age with history of adverse reaction to a food:

- *For establishment or exclusion of the diagnosis of food allergy:*
    - Eating regularly but possible recent reaction
    - Non-immunoglobulin E (IgE)-mediated food allergy
- For scientific reasons in clinical studies
- *For assessment of tolerance*:
    - Some food allergies are usually outgrown.
    - Falling specific IgE (sIgE) levels and smaller or negative skin tests—though not an essential criterion for tolerance assessment

Exclusion Criteria

When a challenge is not necessary for diagnosing food allergy:

- Repeated reactions
- *Recent anaphylaxis*: It is recommended to wait for at least for 4 weeks from the episode of anaphylaxis before scheduling for an OFC.
- In *selected* cases where positive test results make challenges unnecessary:
    - *Skin prick test/sIgE:* Results above the 95% predictive value for positive reaction

BOON OR BANE

- *Advantages:*
  - Lessen fear and stress
  - Allows a more varied diet
  - Determination of threshold level
  - Promotes tolerance
- *Disadvantages:*
  - Possibility of a severe reaction
  - Time-consuming

WHEN CAN WE DECIDE ON ELIMINATION DIET WITHOUT ORAL FOOD CHALLENGE?

French guidelines on food allergy in 2009 suggested that *a suggestive clinical history* if cutaneous signs (eczema, rash, urticaria, and angioedema), gastrointestinal signs (nausea, vomiting, diarrhea, and abdominal pain), respiratory signs (rhino conjunctivitis, cough, respiratory distress, and bronchospasm), and/or arterial hypotension occur shortly after ingesting the food (and positive IgE test results).

In the last decade, Sampson et al. have defined convincing symptoms as a relative immediate reaction to a food within few minutes to 2 hours of ingestion in the last 2 years and required medical care for the same.

Sensitization on SPT/serum-specific IgE can be associated with a probability of an allergy, which can be considered in the context of clinical history. This determines the food allergy prevalence in the specific patient in whom it is being tested. It is imperative that always the results of sensitization on SPT or serum-specific IgE should be interpreted in the context of the clinical history.

CHALLENGE SETTINGS AND PROCEDURES

Factors to be Considered During Oral Food Challenge

- Risk of a reaction
- Patient/family preference
- Nutritional importance of a food in question
- Impact of a positive challenge on the patient and the family
- The probability of an allergic reaction and the severity of an allergic reaction if it was to occur are two separate and important considerations when deciding the risks, benefits, protocol, and location of an OFC.
- OFCs to baked milk and baked egg have been implemented clinically in varied ways, with some physicians aiming to demonstrate tolerance to full servings and others intending to put a small amount in the diet.
- The protocol and clinical assessment of symptoms or signs of a positive reaction during an OFC are influenced by age.

The OFC procedure is tailored to the type of expected reactions [immediate, delayed, and cofactors (e.g., nonsteroidal anti-inflammatories and exercise)].

Types of Challenges

- *Double blind:* In a double-blinded OFC, both the doctors and the patient are blinded to the food being offered in the OFC to reduce the confounding factors and the bias. It is generally done in prospective studies and tolerance assessments. It is quite expensive and requires the OFC being done in a healthcare setting equipped to manage allergic reactions.
- *Single blind:* In a single-blinded OFC, usually the patient is blinded to the food being offered in the OFC. Negative open OFC generally excludes a reaction to the food, a positive result with subjective symptoms, such as itching of the mouth area, sickness, or abdominal pain, is not conclusive for a firm diagnosis of a food allergy and should be confirmed by a blind OFC.

- *Open:* In the open OFC, both the doctor and the patient (and the family members) are aware of the food being offered. It is the simplest OFC, the least expensive in terms of time and costs, and, therefore, the most frequently used. On the other hand, it can cause psychogenic symptoms, which may result in a false-positive OFC.
- *Double-blind placebo-controlled food challenge (DBPCFC):* It is the gold standard for the diagnosis of food allergy, followed in many research studies and quite extensive in the protocol. It is difficult to follow this practically; single blinded or open challenges are being preferred for the ease of the procedure.
- *Exercise + Oral challenge:* This procedure is relevant in food-dependent exercise-induced anaphylaxis patients to confirm the diagnosis and the exercise tolerance.

The OFC procedure is tailored to the type of expected reactions [immediate, delayed, and cofactors (e.g., nonsteroidal anti-inflammatories and exercise)].

Points that Require Consideration

Before we proceed for an OFC, it is important to cover few basic areas given as follows:

- It is essential to go through the clinical history, which can indicate the type of reaction—IgE- or non-IgE-mediated reactions, severity of the reactions, food diary correlation, and any concurrent atopic diseases such as asthma control.
- Consent must be taken from the patients/parents with detailed description and discussion on the risk-benefit ratio, benefits, and hindrances about possible outcome of a positive OFC.
- Food to be challenged must be discussed with the patient and the family and the relevance of the negative OFC following which the patient can include the same food in their diet.
- Nutritional value of the foods being considered for the OFC is also of primary importance.
- It is important to discuss with the patient and the family whether to do the challenge in the in-patient setting or in the outpatient department taking into consideration about the severity of a previous reaction and the current sensitization profile of the patient.

DOSING STRATEGIES AND OUTCOMES

The starting doses vary widely from the low microgram level for studies aimed at determinations such as lowest observable adverse event levels (LOAELs) and no observable adverse event levels (NOAELs) to doses from the low milligram level to several 100 mg in schedules used for other purposes. For patients deemed to be at higher risk for a severe reaction, it may be prudent to begin with one or more smaller doses, as shown in **Figure 28.1**. This may be appropriate for challenges conducted in the research setting, such as for a treatment study enrolling more sensitive patients compared with the clinical setting, in which less sensitive patients are undergoing challenges.

Incremental scales vary from 10-fold increase to fivefold, doubling dose, or even smaller increase, with the latter being associated with schedules aiming to deliver cumulative doses. Usually, the dosing intervals between doses are typically 20–30 minutes.

In patients for consideration of oral immunotherapy for foods, where the threshold dose being considered to start OIT, longer intervals may be required between each dose. Observation must be done at least for 2 hours after the last step of the OFC.

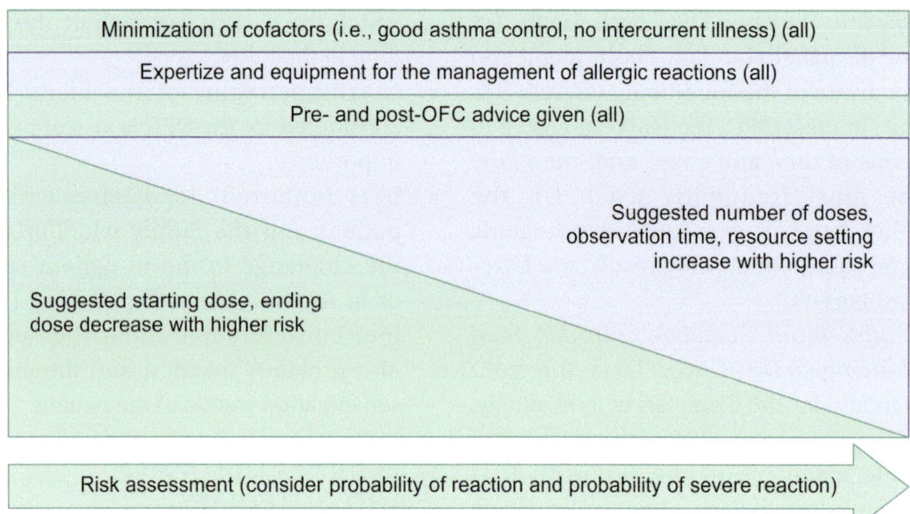

Fig. 28.1: The risk assessment of the OFC influences the protocol of the OFC. (OFC: oral food challenge). *Source:* Upton JEM, Bird JA. Oral food challenges: special considerations. Ann Allergy Asthma Immunol. 2020;124(5):451-8.

EXPECTED FOOD-INDUCED REACTIONS

The expected food-induced reactions involve some combination of cutaneous, gastrointestinal, respiratory, and cardiovascular reactions. Skin and gastrointestinal reactions are most common, and severe or life-threatening reactions are rare. If a patient experiences a severe reaction, observation for a minimum of 4 hours is recommended, and some patients need to be hospitalized for continued treatment or more prolonged observation in the event of more severe or persistent symptoms. These risks can be minimized by appropriate dosing and by performing challenges in a controlled setting with experienced personnel trained for emergency preparedness.

CONTRAINDICATIONS

There are certain times when an OFC may need to be rescheduled or delayed. These indications include concurrent illness such as a viral/bacterial infection, poorly controlled associated atopic disease, uncontrolled cardiovascular diseases, on antihistamines (may need to be stopped atleast 5–7 days prior to testing), patient on beta-blockers, and pregnancy (relative contraindications).

OUTCOMES

Oral food challenge must be initiated with small dose (especially with previous anaphylaxis) and followed by incremental doses with interval of 15–30 minutes depending on the food being challenged, protocol being followed, and the severity of the previous reactions. In patients for consideration of oral immunotherapy for foods, where the threshold dose being considered to start OIT, longer intervals may be required between each doses. Observation must be done at least for 2 hours after the last step of the OFC.

SUMMARY

Although all OFCs carry risk, they remain an essential tool in the management of patients with suspected food allergy. Given the enormous nutritional and social benefits that can result from a negative challenge, these risks are reasonable when the risk-to-benefit ratio is carefully considered for each patient and challenges conducted in a location that is well equipped to deal with anaphylactic reactions by physicians and staff who are well trained in dealing with such reactions. This does not exclude practicing allergists' offices because most allergists administering immunotherapy are fully equipped to deal with anaphylactic reactions.

KEY POINTS

- *Gold Standard Test:* OFC is the definitive method to diagnose or exclude food allergy.
- *Indications:* Uncertain diagnosis, assessing allergy resolution, determining reaction threshold.
- *Types:* Open, single-blind, and double-blind placebo-controlled (DBPCFC—rigorous).
- *Preparation:* Review history, stop antihistamines, ensure stable health, and obtain informed consent.
- *Procedure:* Administer increasing doses under close medical supervision with emergency treatment ready.
- *Positive result:* Objective allergic reaction confirms food allergy.
- *Negative result:* No reaction indicates tolerance.
- *Risks:* Potential for anaphylaxis; contraindicated in uncontrolled asthma or severe prior reactions.
- *Follow-up:* Monitor for delayed reactions, provide dietary advice, and reinforce emergency plans.
- *Importance:* Prevents unnecessary food avoidance, reduces anxiety, and guides management.

SUGGESTED READING

1. Calvani M, Arasi S, Bianchi A, Caimmi D, Cuomo B, Dondi A, et al. Is it possible to make a diagnosis of raw, heated and baked egg allergy in children using cut-offs? A systematic review. Pediatr Allergy Immunol. 2015;26:509-21.
2. Calvani M, Bianchi A, Reginelli C, Peresso M, Testa A. Oral food challenge. Medicina (Kaunas). 2019;55(10):651.
3. Crevel RW, Ballmer-Weber BK, Holzhauser T, Hourihane JO, Knulst AC, Mackie AR, et al. Thresholds for food allergens and their value to different stakeholders. Allergy. 2008;63:597-609.
4. Koutlas N, Stallings A, Hall G, Zhou C, Kim-Chang J, Mousallem T. Pediatric oral food challenges in the outpatient setting: a single-center experience. J Allergy Clin Immunol Glob. 2023;3(1):100187.
5. Patel N, Shreffler WG, Custovic A, Santos AF. Will oral food challenges still be part of allergy care in 10 years' time? J Allergy Clin Immunol Pract. 2023;11(4):988-96.
6. Perry TT, Matsui EC, Connover-Walker MK, Wood RA. The relationship of allergen-specific IgE levels and oral food challenge outcome. J Allergy Clin Immunol. 2004;114:144-9.
7. Sampson HA, Aceves S, Bock SA, James J, Jones S, Lang D, et al. Food allergy: a practice parameter update—2014. J Allergy Clin Immunol. 2014;134:1016-25.
8. Sampson HA, Gerth van Wijk R, Bindslev-Jensen C, Sicherer S, Teuber SS, Burks AW, et al. Standardizing double-blind, placebo-controlled oral food challenges: American Academy of Allergy, Asthma & Immunology-European Academy of Allergy and Clinical Immunology PRACTALL consensus report. J Allergy Clin Immunol. 2012;130(6):1260-74.
9. Vlieg-Boerstra BJ, van der Heide S, Bijleveld CM, Kukler J, Duiverman EJ, Du bois AE. Placebo reactions in double-blind, placebo-controlled food challenges in children. Allergy. 2007;62:905-12.

CHAPTER

29

Radiology in Pediatric Allergic Diseases

S Elayaraja

INTRODUCTION

Pediatric allergic diseases are a widespread health concern, affecting millions of children worldwide. Common allergies in children include asthma, allergic rhinitis, food allergies, eczema, and systemic anaphylactic responses. Given the early onset and potential complications associated with untreated allergies, early diagnosis and management are essential. While clinical assessment remains foundational, radiology serves as an invaluable adjunct, especially in cases where anatomical visualization is necessary for diagnosis or management. By providing critical insights into the structural and sometimes functional alterations caused by these conditions, radiology aids healthcare providers in delivering timely and targeted care.

TYPES OF ALLERGIC DISEASES IN CHILDREN AND RELEVANT IMAGING

Respiratory Allergies

Asthma

Pediatric asthma presents in various forms, from mild, episodic wheezing to chronic, severe cases. Chest X-ray usually shows hyperinflation and bronchial wall thickening **(Fig. 29.1)**. Imaging, particularly high-resolution computed tomography (HRCT), can reveal early structural changes that may not be evident clinically. HRCT is useful in detecting airway remodeling, bronchial wall thickening, and mucus plugging. Early detection of these structural changes can help in tailoring management approaches, especially in severe cases where standard treatments may not suffice.

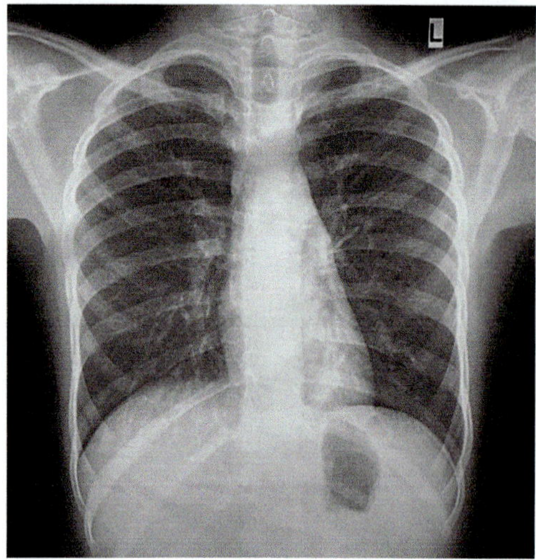

Fig. 29.1: Chest X-ray shows hyperinflation in an asthmatic child.

Allergic Rhinitis and Sinusitis

Chronic sinusitis is a frequent complication of allergic rhinitis. CT scans are routinely used for assessing sinus involvement, revealing findings such as mucosal thickening, sinus opacification, and air-fluid levels **(Fig. 29.2)**. In cases of allergic fungal sinusitis, MRI may be more advantageous as it can differentiate

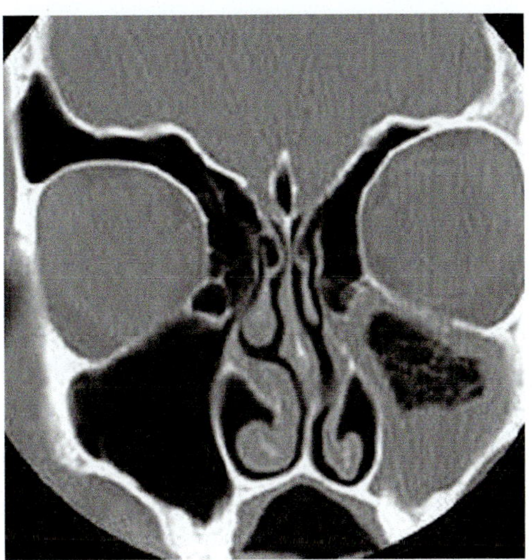

Fig. 29.2: CT PNS shows air-fluid levels with opacification of the left maxillary sinus.

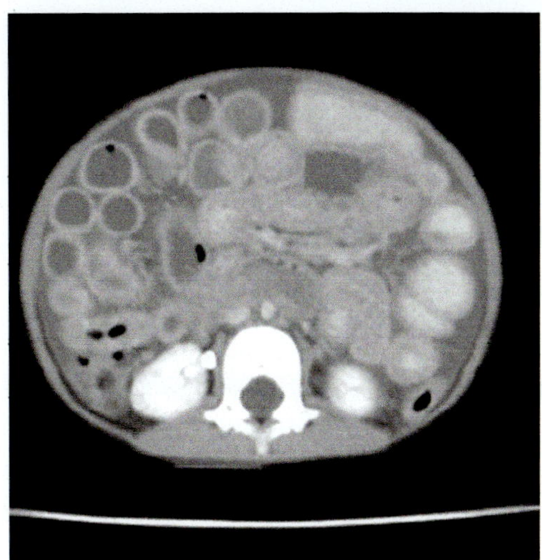

Fig. 29.3: CT of the abdomen shows gross ascites, dilated bowel loops with bowel wall thickening, in eosinophilic gastroenteritis.

fungal material from other tissue types, aiding in precise diagnosis and treatment planning.

Gastrointestinal Allergies

Food Allergies and Eosinophilic Gastroenteritis

Food allergies in children can manifest as gastrointestinal symptoms, often necessitating imaging to identify or rule out related structural or inflammatory conditions. Abdominal ultrasound and MRI are commonly employed to examine the bowel for signs of thickening, fluid accumulation, and lymphadenopathy. In eosinophilic gastroenteritis, imaging findings may include bowel wall thickening and localized edema, which are significant for differential diagnosis and management **(Fig. 29.3)**.

Systemic Allergic Reactions

Anaphylaxis and Allergic Vasculitis

Systemic allergic reactions, such as anaphylaxis, can involve multiple organs, warranting comprehensive imaging to assess the extent of involvement. Whole-body MRI or CT is often indicated in severe cases to identify manifestations such as organ edema, effusions, and potential vascular involvement in cases of allergic vasculitis. These imaging modalities provide an overall picture of the allergic reaction's systemic impact and help clinicians devise suitable interventions.

ADVANCED IMAGING TECHNIQUES IN PEDIATRIC ALLERGIC DISEASES

Magnetic resonance imaging's lack of radiation makes it particularly valuable for repeat imaging in children. Recent advancements, such as diffusion-weighted imaging (DWI), allow for enhanced visualization of inflamed tissues, such as those in sinus and airway allergies, without the need for contrast agents. Additionally, functional MRI techniques are being explored to assess inflammatory activity in allergic diseases, further broadening MRI's applications in pediatrics.

Functional Imaging and Nuclear Medicine

Functional imaging modalities such as positron emission tomography (PET)-CT and single-photon emission computed tomography (SPECT) can help in understanding the molecular underpinnings of chronic inflammatory and allergic conditions. PET-CT, for instance, can assess metabolic activity in inflamed tissues, providing insights into the severity and distribution of allergic inflammation. This approach is especially useful in complex cases where systemic involvement is suspected.

BENEFITS, RISKS, AND ETHICAL CONSIDERATIONS IN PEDIATRIC IMAGING

While radiology is indispensable in diagnosing pediatric allergic diseases, it comes with inherent risks, particularly from radiation exposure. Low-dose imaging protocols and the judicious use of CT scans are essential in minimizing these risks. Sedation, often required in pediatric MRI, also presents challenges. Ethically, it is crucial to weigh the diagnostic benefits against potential risks, ensuring that imaging is used appropriately and only when necessary.

CASE STUDIES

Case Study 1: Asthma Complicated by Fungal Infection

An 8-year-old boy with bronchial asthma presents with recurrent episodes of wheezing. He has been on inhaler therapy with poor compliance and frequent exacerbations. Blood investigations showed eosinophilia with markedly elevated immunoglobulin E (IgE) levels. CT of the chest showed multiple areas of air trapping, mosaic attenuation, and mucus plugging **(Fig. 29.4)**. He was diagnosed with allergic bronchopulmonary aspergillosis (ABPA) and started on antifungal treatment. This case highlights HRCT's role in assessing complications in chronic asthma.

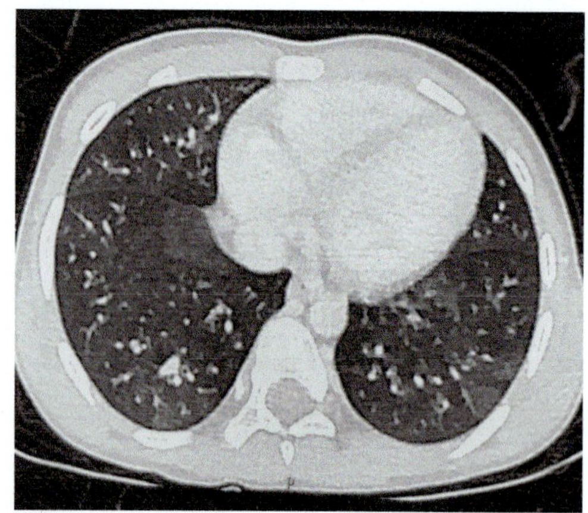

Fig. 29.4: CT of the chest shows mucus plugs, air trapping, and mosaic attenuation in ABPA. (ABPA: allergic bronchopulmonary aspergillosis)

Case Study 2: Eosinophilic Esophagitis Mimicking Gastroesophageal Reflux Disease

A 10-year-old girl with suspected gastroesophageal reflux disease (GERD) underwent fluoroscopy, which revealed esophageal mucosal thickening and ring formation, indicative of eosinophilic esophagitis **(Fig. 29.5)**. This case underscores the utility of radiology in distinguishing between eosinophilic esophagitis and other conditions presenting with similar symptoms.

SUMMARY

Radiology provides a comprehensive framework for diagnosing and managing pediatric allergic diseases. Advanced imaging techniques, when used judiciously, offer detailed insights into disease progression and complications. Future research and technological innovations will likely further

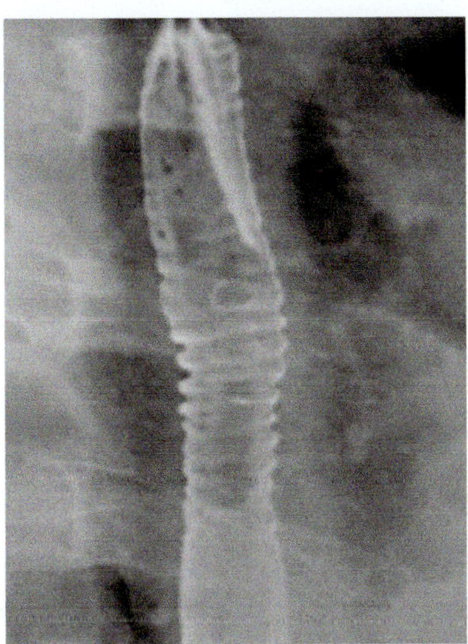

Fig. 29.5: Fluoroscopy shows ringed esophagus in eosinophilic esophagitis.

enhance radiology's diagnostic power, supporting even more targeted and effective management of allergic conditions in children.

KEY POINTS

- Radiology can be a valuable adjunct to clinical diagnosis in children with allergic diseases.
- Computed tomography is a useful imaging technique to detect complications in conditions like uncontrolled asthma and allergic rhinitis.
- Newer advancements like functional MRI, and PET-CT while offering better insights in the disease severity, must be considered after carefully analyzing risks vs benefits.

SUGGESTED READING

1. Ma L, Li W, Xiao M, Liu W, Liu J, Zhou W, et al. Eosinophilic gastroenteritis: Imaging spectrum on intestinal ultrasonography and CT enterography. Eur J Radiol. 2024;181: 111820.
2. Nurko S, Teitelbaum JE, Husain K, Buonomo C, Fox VL, Antonioli D, et al. Association of Schatzki ring with eosinophilic esophagitis in children. J Pediatr Gastroenterol Nutr. 2004;38(4):436-41.
3. Sung A, Naidich D, Belinskaya I, Raoof S. The role of chest radiography and computed tomography in the diagnosis and management of asthma. Curr Opin Pulm Med. 2007;13(1):31-6.
4. Triulzi F, Zirpoli S. Imaging techniques in the diagnosis and management of rhinosinusitis in children. Pediatr Allergy Immunol. 2007;18 (Suppl 18):46-9.

CHAPTER 30

Allergy and Sleep Studies

Nihala Tarannum H

INTRODUCTION

Allergic diseases such as allergic rhinitis, asthma, atopic dermatitis, and food allergy are serious public and medical concerns due to their high prevalence. Allergic diseases are characterized by epithelial dysfunction and dysregulated immune response (allergic immune response). Sleep is very important for all in promoting physical and mental health. High-quality sleep is crucial for learning and effective development in children. Deprivation of sleep can alter immune function in healthy subjects. Patients with chronic diseases are vulnerable to sleep disruptions caused by the presence of illness-related symptoms at night and potential for poor illness control, both of which can affect sleep quality. Asthma and allergic conditions are common chronic conditions if not treated adequately and can affect sleep in many ways. Asthma and allergic diseases can affect sleep through various levels of influence involving pathophysiologic (e.g., inflammatory mediators), environmental (e.g., poor trigger control in the home), individual (e.g., nonadherence to medications), and family/cultural (e.g., cultural beliefs) factors.

The connection between pediatric allergies and sleep disturbances is multifaceted, involving both direct and indirect interactions. Direct impact of allergies on sleep can be due to (1) nasal congestion and rhinitis, making it difficult for children to breathe through their nose while sleeping. This congestion often leads to mouth breathing, which can contribute to snoring and fragmented sleep. It can also increase the risk of developing obstructive sleep apnea (OSA). Sleep-disordered breathing (SDB) disrupts both sleep quality and cardiorespiratory physiology. (2) Allergies can cause chronic coughing or throat irritation, which may worsen at night. Persistent coughing can lead to frequent awakenings, thereby reducing sleep quality and total sleep duration. (3) Allergic conditions such as eczema can cause intense itching and discomfort, especially during the night. Itching can lead to frequent awakenings and difficulty falling asleep, resulting in fragmented sleep.

Indirect impact of allergies on sleep can affect (1) sleep quality and immune response. Allergies can trigger inflammation and immune responses that might be exacerbated by poor sleep. Poor sleep can further compromise the immune system, potentially leading to more severe allergic reactions or increased susceptibility to other illnesses. (2) Behavioral and psychological effects: Chronic sleep disturbances can affect a child's mood, behavior, and cognitive function. Behavioral issues and irritability caused by a lack of sleep can complicate the management of allergies and overall health.

In most cases of pediatric obstructive sleep apnea syndrome (OSAS), children present with signs or symptoms of obstructive breathing patterns during sleep, including snoring, labored breathing, witnessed apnea, gasping, mouth breathing, or sleeping in unusual positions (such as with the neck hyperextended). Failure to thrive or signs of right-sided heart failure may be present in severe cases. Associated daytime symptoms can be difficult to elicit. Unlike adults in whom excessive daytime sleepiness is often the presenting complaint, younger children tend to manifest daytime sleepiness as hyperactivity or inability to concentrate, leading to poor school performance or behavioral issues. Most children with OSA have a normal physical examination. However, physical findings of retrognathia, oropharyngeal crowding, high-arched palate, adenotonsillar hypertrophy, mouth breathing, or stertor at rest suggest the need for further evaluation for OSAS. Prematurity, hypotonia (e.g., children with cerebral palsy or muscular dystrophy, Down syndrome), or craniofacial anomalies are the risk factors for OSAS. Polysomnography (PSG) is indicated in any child who snores and has labored breathing during sleep and who has any predisposing physical examination findings or daytime symptoms. PSG is the gold standard for the diagnosis of OSAS.

SLEEP STUDY

Pediatric PSG, also called a sleep study, is the noninvasive, diagnostic study of choice to evaluate for OSA in children and to evaluate cardiorespiratory function in infants and children with chronic lung disease or neuromuscular disease when indicated. It is helpful to investigate atypical cases of parasomnias. It is important to understand that children are not just small adults when being studied in a sleep laboratory. They require a child-friendly atmosphere, and the approach needs smaller and more specialized equipment, and because of developmental and physiologic differences from adults, they have age-adjusted rules for the scoring and interpretation of polysomnograms.

Polysomnography consists of an all-night recording performed in a dedicated sleep laboratory to characterize sleep architecture and identify sleep pathology. Depending on the number of sensors and channels used and whether the study is done at a sleep study center or at home, a sleep study is of four types **(Table 30.1)**.

TABLE 30.1: Types of polysomnography (PSG).

Level I PSG—gold standard • Done in sleep laboratory and observed in real time by a sleep technologist • *Level I study monitors:* Brainwaves, electrocardiogram (ECG), breathing activity, limb movement, and oxygen saturation. Pediatric patients also include CO_2 monitoring	*Level II PSG:* • Can be completed in a sleep laboratory or the home but is an unattended study • Same setup and monitoring as a level I
Level III PSG—often referred to as a home sleep testing (HST) or a limited sleep study • Level III study monitors breathing activity, oxygen saturation, and heart rate	*Level IV PSG:* • Often referred to as an overnight pulse oximetry test and completed at home • Level IV study monitors oxygen saturation and heart rate

RESPIRATORY INDICATIONS OF POLYSOMNOGRAPHY

- To assess sleep-related breathing disorders (e.g., OSA)
- *Before adenotonsillectomy (AT):* It helps identify which children are at greatest risk for persistent OSA following AT. Children with mild OSAS preoperatively should have clinical evaluation following AT to assess for residual symptoms. If there are residual symptoms of OSAS, PSG should be performed.
- *Following AT:* To assess for residual OSAS in children with preoperative evidence for moderate-to-severe OSAS, obesity, craniofacial anomalies that obstruct the upper airway, and neurologic disorders (e.g., Down syndrome, Prader-Willi syndrome, and myelomeningocele).
- Positive airway pressure (PAP) titration in children with OSAS
- Congenital central alveolar hypoventilation syndrome or sleep-related hypoventilation due to neuromuscular disorders or chest wall deformities.
- After treatment of children for OSAS with rapid maxillary expansion to assess the level of residual disease and to determine whether additional treatment is necessary.
- For noninvasive positive pressure ventilation (NIPPV) titration in children with other sleep-related breathing disorders

NONRESPIRATORY INDICATIONS OF POLYSOMNOGRAPHY

- In the case of hypersomnolence (e.g., narcolepsy), a multiple sleep latency test (MSLT) is followed by PSG.
- In suspected periodic limb movement disorder (PLMD)
- To confirm the diagnosis of an atypical or potentially injurious parasomnia or differentiate a parasomnia from sleep-related epilepsy using extended electroencephalogram (EEG) montages.
- Suspected of having restless legs syndrome (RLS) who require supportive data for diagnosing RLS.

How to set up a polysomnography?
Polysomnography can be challenging in pediatrics because children have a limited ability to cooperate with the setup and may have trouble sleeping in a strange environment.

PREPARATION

Children are advised to come to the sleep study center a few hours before starting the study, as they need some time to get accustomed to the place. Dedicated sleep technologists with pediatric experience are present at all times to monitor the patient and ensure a high-quality recording. They play an important role in getting an appropriate sleep study. They connect the sensors, record the audio and video, and help the child if any of the sensor is disconnected. Typical pediatric sleep study is conducted from 9 PM to 6 AM. A good sleep study should have a total sleep time of at least 6 hours.

CONNECTING THE POLYSOMNOGRAPHY SENSORS

Electrodes and sensors are attached to various body parts **(Fig. 30.1)**.

Table 30.2 shows the various sensors in level I PSG.

Once the leads are setup, biocalibration is done. This helps us to determine baseline information, and it aids in troubleshooting electrode placement. Sleep technician now continuously monitors the live recording of

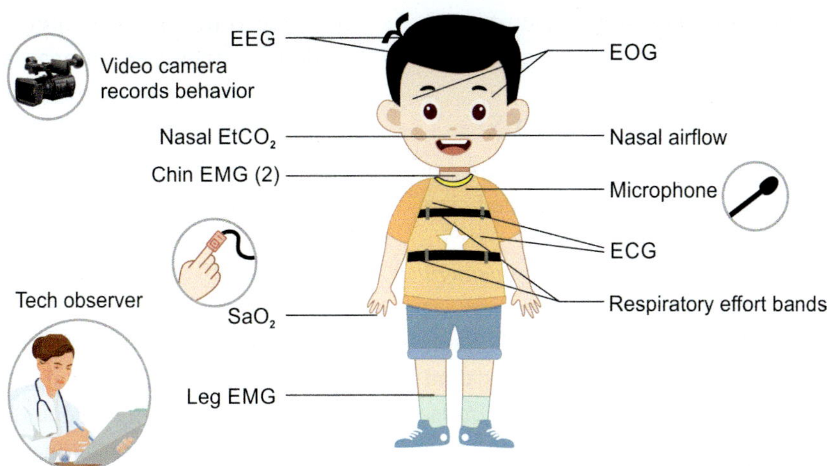

Fig. 30.1: Connecting the various leads of PSG. (ECG: electrocardiogram; EEG: electroencephalogram; EMG: electromyogram; EOG: electro-oculogram; $EtCO_2$: end-tidal carbon dioxide; PSG: polysomnography; SaO_2: oxygen saturation)

TABLE 30.2: Twenty-eight sensors for a typical level I PSG.

Channels	***What it measures***
Fifteen sensors on the head and face: • Six EEG channels (F3, F4, C3, C4, O1, and O2) • Two eye leads • Three chin leads • Four referencing channels (Cz, Fpz, M1, and M2)	Useful in sleep staging
One snore sensor/microphone	Detects snoring
Two-lead ECG	Measures cardiac rhythm
Two effort belts (chest and abdomen)	Measures respiratory efforts
Four leg sensors (two on each leg)	Detects the leg movements (PLMD)
One pulse oximeter	Detects desaturations
One $TcCO_2$ monitor	Detects CO_2 level (hypoventilation)
One nasal cannula (nasal flow and $EtCO_2$)	Detects changes in nasal pressure
One oronasal thermosensor	

(ECG: electrocardiogram; EEG: electroencephalogram; $EtCO_2$: end-tidal carbon dioxide; PLMD: periodic limb movement disorder; PSG: polysomnography)

the sleep study, including audio and video. Concurrent audio and video recordings allow clinical correlation with events. They troubleshoot equipment issues, fix electrodes, and attend to patient needs. They provide documentation and summary of sleep study.

REPORTING A POLYSOMNOGRAPHY

After completing the sleep study, all the electrodes are disconnected in the morning. Child is sent home. Overnight study computer data are generated, and manual scoring is done by a pediatric pulmonologist or sleep specialist.

SCORING OF SLEEP STUDIES

- *Scoring of sleep stages:* It is done as per the American Academy of Sleep Medicine (AASM) guidelines.
  - *Identification of rapid eye movement (REM) and nonrapid eye movement (NREM) (N1, N2, and N3)*: Each screenshot of the recording is called an epoch. Each epoch is 30 seconds. There are typically 1,080 epochs in a single night sleep study. EEG recordings show different brain wave patterns during different stages of sleep: (1) *Wakefulness:* Beta waves are present, with the highest frequency and lowest amplitude. (2) *Stage N1 (light sleep):* Theta waves are present, with low voltage. (3) *Stage N2 (deeper sleep):* Sleep spindles and K complexes are present. Sleep spindles are symmetric bursts of activity that usually occur at 12–14 Hz. (4) *Stage N3 (deepest NREM sleep):* Delta waves are present, with the lowest frequency and highest amplitude. (5) *REM sleep:* Beta waves are present, similar to brain waves during wakefulness.
  - *Identify arousal based on EEG, electro-oculogram (EOG), and chin electromyogram (EMG)*: The AASM Scoring Manual endorses scoring of arousals during all stages of sleep if an abrupt shift of EEG frequency occurs, including alpha, theta, or frequencies >16 Hz (but not spindles). The disruption should last at least 3 seconds, with at least 10 seconds of preceding stable sleep.
- *Scoring of respiratory events:* Depending on the age of the patient and respiratory rate, respiratory events are observed in 30–90-second screen. As per the AASM guidelines definition, apnea, hypopnea, and hypoventilation are identified. Apnea is defined as cessation of flow >90% of the baseline for more than two breaths or >10 seconds. Hypopnea is defined as a flow reduction by ≥30% for more than two breaths or >10 seconds with either a ≥3% oxygen desaturation or arousal (on EEG). Apnea is divided into obstructive, central, or mixed apnea. Additional information is available from video and audio such as snoring, gasps, pauses, apneas, work of breathing, and sleep posture.
- *Criteria for hypopnea on PSG (AASM scoring rule):* The peak signal excursions drop by ≥30% of the pre-event baseline using the nasal pressure signal. The duration of the event lasts for more than or equal to two breaths. There is a ≥3% oxygen desaturation from pre-event baseline or event associated with arousal **(Fig. 30.2)**.
- *Criteria for obstructive apnea:* There is a drop in the peak signal excursion by ≥90% of pre-event baseline airflow. The duration of the event is at least two breaths during baseline breathing. It is associated with the presence of respiratory effort throughout the entire period of absent airflow. There is no oxygen desaturation requirement for obstructive apnea **(Fig. 30.3)**.
- *Criteria for central apnea:* Absent inspiratory effort throughout the entire duration of the event, and at least one of the following is met:
  - The event lasts ≥20 seconds.
  - The event lasts at least the duration of two breaths during baseline breathing and is associated with an arousal or a ≥3% oxygen desaturation.

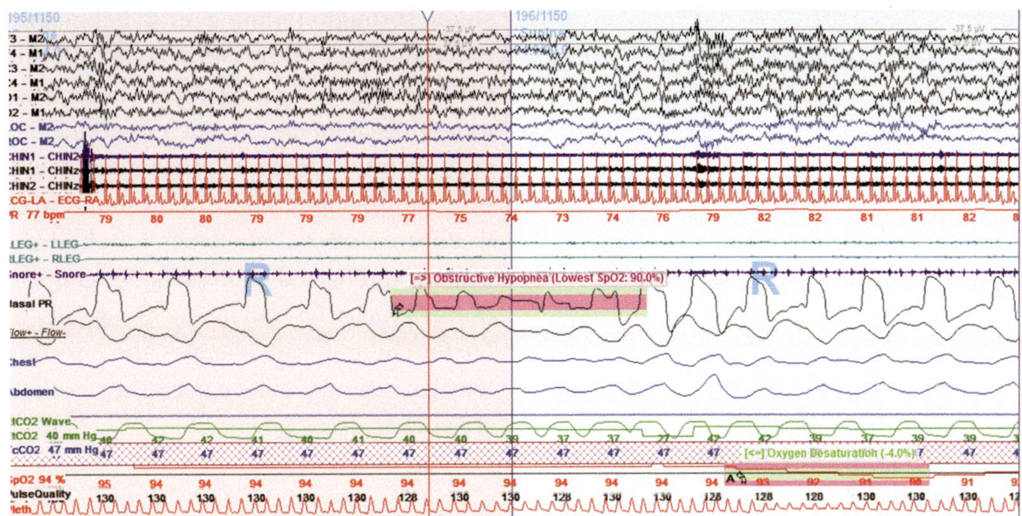

Fig. 30.2: Epoch of obstructive hypopnea (check nasal PR). (Nasal PR: nasal pressure recording channel; SpO_2: peripheral oxygen saturation)

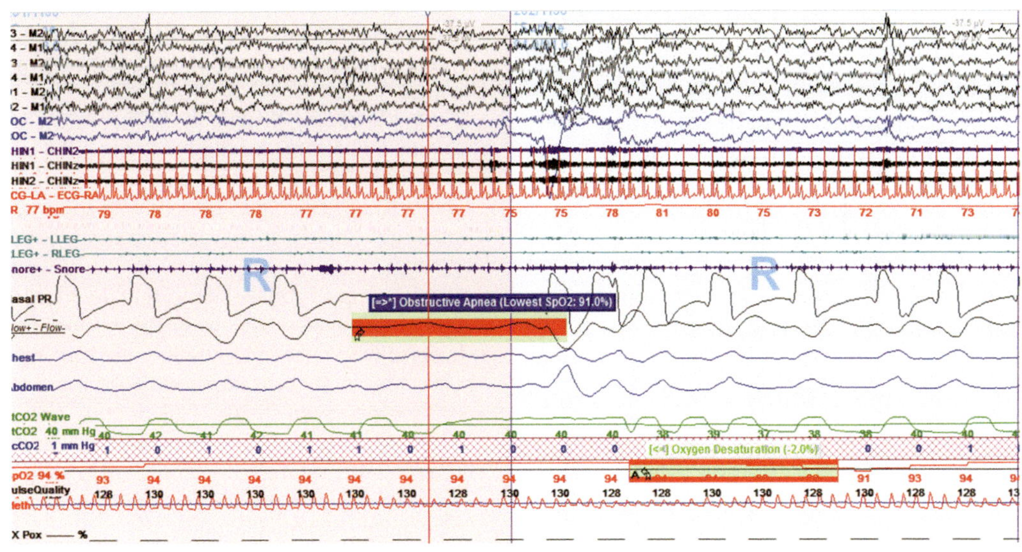

Fig. 30.3: Epoch of obstructive apnea (check oronasal thermal airflow sensor). (SpO_2: peripheral oxygen saturation)

- The event lasts at least the duration of two breaths during baseline breathing and is associated with a decrease in heart rate to <50 beats per minute for at least 5 seconds or <60 beats per minute for 15 seconds (infants under 1 year of age only).

- *Mixed apnea:* Duration of the event is at least two breaths from baseline breathing and is associated with absent respiratory effort during one portion of the event and the presence of inspiratory effort in another portion, regardless of which portion comes first.

TABLE 30.3: Classification of obstructive sleep apnea (OSA) severity based on the apnea–hypopnea index (AHI).

AHI	<1	Normal
OAHI	1–5	Mild OSA
OAHI	5–10	Moderate OSA
OAHI	>10	Severe OSA

(OAHI: obstructive apnea–hypopnea index)

OTHER PARAMETERS

- *Obstructive events:* If the events are associated with snoring, retractions, flattening of nasal flows, or thoracoabdominal paradox.
- The most important parameter defining SDB is the apnea-hypopnea index (AHI), which is defined as the number of apneas and hypopneas per hour of total sleep time. It is used to quantify the severity of sleep apnea. AHI can be scored separately as obstructive apnea-hypopnea index (OAHI) and central apnea-hypopnea index (CAHI) **(Table 30.3)**.

Total sleep time, sleep efficiency, sleep latency, REM latency, and oxygen desaturation index are also measured.

Hypnogram is a graphical representation of sleep study, which shows an overall summary of sleep stages, body position, peripheral oxygen saturation (SpO_2), carbon dioxide (CO_2), arousals, pulse rate, and limb movement.

Once the detailed report is generated and analyzed, depending on the severity, management of OSAS is planned.

SUMMARY

The connection between pediatric allergies and sleep is complex, with allergies directly affecting sleep quality through physical symptoms and indirectly influencing sleep through immune and behavioral mechanisms. Addressing both allergic conditions and sleep disturbances requires a multidisciplinary approach that includes appropriate allergy management, sleep hygiene practices, and careful monitoring to improve overall outcomes for children. Understanding and addressing this connection is crucial for enhancing the quality of life for children with allergies and ensuring they get restorative sleep necessary for their growth and development.

KEY POINTS

- *Allergies and sleep interaction:* Pediatric allergic diseases (asthma, rhinitis, eczema, food allergy) significantly impact sleep quality both directly (e.g., nasal congestion, cough, itching) and indirectly (immune dysfunction, behavioral issues).
- *Sleep-disordered breathing (SDB):* Allergic rhinitis and asthma increase the risk of sleep-disordered breathing and obstructive sleep apnea (OSA), which may present with snoring, labored breathing, or unusual sleep postures in children.
- *Daytime impact:* Unlike adults, children with OSA often manifest daytime symptoms such as hyperactivity, poor concentration, and learning difficulties rather than excessive sleepiness.
- *Polysomnography (PSG)*: PSG is the gold standard for diagnosing pediatric OSA and other sleep-related breathing disorders. Pediatric PSG requires age-specific scoring rules and a child-friendly setup.
- *Clinical applications of PSG:* PSG is indicated for both respiratory (e.g., OSA diagnosis, PAP titration, postadenotonsillectomy assessment) and nonrespiratory (e.g., narcolepsy, PLMD, parasomnias, restless legs syndrome) conditions.
- *Management approach:* Effective care requires a multidisciplinary strategy combining allergy control, sleep hygiene, and appropriate use of PSG to optimize sleep quality and overall health outcomes in children.

- *Therapeutic implications:*
  - Treating allergies (antihistamines, intranasal steroids, immunotherapy) improves sleep quality.
  - Addressing sleep-disordered breathing (e.g., adenotonsillectomy in children with allergic rhinitis + OSA) yields significant benefits.

SUGGESTED READING

1. Aurora RN, Lamm CI, Zak RS, Kristo DA, Bista SR, Rowley JA, et al. Practice parameters for the non-respiratory indications for polysomnography and multiple sleep latency testing for children. Sleep. 2012;35:1467-73.
2. Aurora RN, Zak RS, Karippot A, Lamm CI, Morgenthaler TI, Auerbach SH, et al. Practice parameters for the respiratory indications for polysomnography in children. Sleep. 2011;34:379-88.
3. Berry R, Quan S, Abreu A (2022). The AASM manual for the scoring of sleep and associated events: Rules, terminology and technical specifications, version 2.6. American Academy of Sleep Medicine, Darien.
4. Suzanne E, Beck MD, Carole L, Marcus MBB. Pediatric polysomnography. Sleep Med Clin. 2009;4(3):393-406.
5. Timothy F, Hoban MD. Polysomnography should be required both before and after adenotonsillectomy for childhood sleep disordered breathing. 2007;3(7):675-7.

CHAPTER 31

How to Read a Research Paper?

Priya Sreenivasan

INTRODUCTION

Reading a research paper involves critical appraisal; it is not possible with leisurely quick reading. It has to be critically appraised systematically in terms of its relevance, validity, precision, and trustworthiness. An understanding of the basics of research methodology would help the reader a lot. Attending journal clubs is recommended.

Critical appraisal of research paper is inevitable in evidence-based practice. The clinician faces lots of queries on a day-to-day basis; queries may be asked by patients, peers, students, or self. Questions may be related to the frequency, risk/prognostic factors, predictors, diagnosis, treatment, prevention, or screening of an illness. The clinician tries to formulate a specific answerable research question. He does a literature search and finds out the updated best available research evidence by critically appraising research papers. A decision is made based on this evidence, clinician experience, and patient perspective. Inculcating critical reading of articles is important in undergraduate and postgraduate students' curriculum.

The reader may be attracted to the conclusions of the research paper in the first instance. But the crux of an original research work lies in the study design and methodology. In the first instance, see whether the study design/methodology is apt and appropriate for the research question. Each study design has its own intricacies, possible biases, strengths, and limitations. Hence, a "one-size-fits-all" approach is not possible. A busy clinician may use design-specific detailed checklists published by the EQUATOR network for easy critical appraisal. The CONSORT checklist for allergen-specific immunotherapy (GA2LEN) and checklist for allergy and immunology survey research are also available.

A practical stepwise approach is given below.

TITLE

1. **Is the research question relevant to one's present interest and setting?**

   The research question may not be explicitly stated in all papers. It may be understood either from *title or objective.* Though methodologically sound, the research question addressed in the paper may not be relevant to the reader and his setting. If not relevant, the reader can go to the next research paper.

   If relevant, observe the *journal characteristics.* See whether it is peer-reviewed and indexed. Check the impact factor and number of citations. Go through the authors and the center where the research activity was conducted. Identifying the center gives the reader an idea about generalizability, and whether the findings are applicable in his setting or not. The date of publication gives the reader an idea about the novelty. Landmark articles may not be recent but may have influenced further developments in that particular field of research. Landmark articles have more citations to its credit.

2. **Is the research question clearly framed so that the reader can easily identify PICO?**
   PICO is an acronym: *P*opulation or participants, *I*ntervention (in experimental studies) or independent variables (e.g., risk factor, prognostic factor, and predictor), *C*omparison or control group (in analytical studies where two or more groups are involved), and *O*utcome. If not explicit in the title, PICO should at least be written clearly as objective of the study in the "Introduction." In some titles, PICOTS is stated; time frame and study design are also included. PICOC is the recent acronym; the second C stands for the context in which the study is conducted.

METHODOLOGY

1. **Is the study design appropriate for the research question?**
   The hierarchy of evidence is well known to all. Hierarchy is based on the strength of study designs; systematic reviews with meta-analysis of randomized controlled trials (RCTs) rank top, RCTs next, cohort and case-control study designs come still down, and so on.

   One research question may be answered by many *study designs*. The best study design may not be feasible in one's setting. The study design adopted should be able to address the research question **(Table 31.1)**. In an analytic study design where two or more groups are involved, the *study hypothesis* should be identified.

TABLE 31.1: Study designs appropriate for research questions.

Research questions	*Study design*
Burden of illness/prevalence	Cross-sectional
Incidence	Cohort
Explore an association	Cross-sectional
Risk factor	Case control/cohort
Prognosis	Cohort
Diagnosis	Diagnostic test evaluation
Efficacy/effectiveness of an intervention	Randomized controlled trials
In-depth understanding of perceptions	Qualitative

2. **Is the study population well described with explicit inclusion and exclusion criteria?**
   Description of the *study population* gives the reader an idea of the generalizability of the study results in his setting. In analytical studies where *study groups* are compared, the reader should be able to understand the methodology adopted for grouping.

   In case-control studies, see whether the case and the control have been defined explicitly. The source population from which cases and controls are identified should be mentioned clearly. In an RCT, participants are allocated to groups to receive or not receive an intervention by a disciplined process called randomization.

3. **Are the study procedures appropriate for the study design?**
   Study procedures include the exact blueprint of how the study was conducted. The procedures should be meticulously stated

in such a way that another researcher should be able to replicate the study in a similar setting if needed. Systematic bias creeps in and affects validity if study procedures are flawed.

For example, in a RCT, the reader should critically appraise procedures adopted for *selection of study population, ethical procedures*, randomization, maintenance of compliance, follow-up, and *ascertainment of outcome*.

The reader should make a note of *sample size* and *sampling technique*. Adequacy of sample size is important to minimize random error.

4. **Are potential sources of bias anticipated and addressed?**
Each study design is inherently prone to specific biases that may affect validity of the study. Broadly, biases are *selection bias, measurement bias, and confounding*. Observational study designs are more prone to bias than RCTs.

For example, a case-control study design is prone to selection bias. The reader should see whether cases and controls are selected from the same source population based on explicit diagnostic criteria and not based on the exposure under study. The reader should see whether recall bias, interviewer bias, and misclassification bias were anticipated, and how they were addressed. Matching is a procedure done in case-control studies in the design stage itself to address selected confounders such as age and sex.

Design-specific checklists published in the EQUATOR network give an idea of the biases that should be anticipated in each study design. Apart from methodological flaws specific to each design, each study may have its own clinical intricacies, which may yield biased results.

RESULTS

1. **Are all data relevant to the objectives summarized and reported in an easily understandable manner?**
Data should be organized and presented using *tables* and appropriate *figures*. See whether tables and figures are self-explanatory with titles, footnotes, and column and row headings for ease of understanding. *Baseline sociodemographic data* are presented in a table format. In analytical studies where two or more groups are involved, go through this table to see whether groups are comparable. Identify the *key summary measures. Univariate analysis and multivariate analysis* may be shown in tables with statistical test values, *p*-value, measures of disease frequency or association or effect (e.g., prevalence, odds ratio, relative risk, absolute risk reduction), and confidence intervals. In diagnostic test studies, see the sensitivity, specificity, predictive values, and likelihood ratios. In studies where two continuous variables are correlated, the summary measure is the correlation coefficient.

Study flowchart provided as a figure gives details of number of participants screened, enrolled, included, excluded, followed up, lost follow-up, died, number available for ascertainment of outcome, and so on. Figures appropriate for study designs may be published. Examples include receiver operating characteristic (ROC) curve in diagnostic test evaluation studies, scatter plot in correlation studies, and forest plot in meta-analysis.

2. **Is statistical analysis performed correctly?**
In analytical studies with a comparison group, we state and test the hypothesis using an appropriate statistical test. A discussion on the statistical test appropriate to each context is beyond the scope of this chapter; one may read reference textbooks or a Research Methodology Beginner's Manual edited by the author for a better understanding. Preset values of probabilities of types 1 and 2 errors (α, β) and power should be stated. The reader should focus not only on *p*-value but on the confidence interval as well. A confidence interval captures the population parameter and gives the reader an idea about statistical significance, and whether the sample size was adequate or not.

Statistical analysis may involve multivariate analysis in case-control studies and prediction modeling studies. The choice of regression analysis is based on the outcome. If the outcome is binary, logistic regression is appropriate. If the outcome is a continuous variable, linear regression is appropriate.

DISCUSSION

1. **Are the limitations discussed?**
Even the best study is not without limitations. See whether these are stated by the authors. The reader should know the limitations of the study and whether attempts were made to address the same. A well-informed reader can make decisions regarding the generalizability of study results and may help him in case he plans to replicate the study in his setting.

2. **Are conclusions drawn based on results obtained from the study?**
Conclusions should be based on study results only. Conclusions may have practice, policy, or research implications and can make a change in the respective realm.

Statements made outside the realm of study results as conclusions are totally baseless.

3. **Do the results hold true for my patients as well?**
Generalizability is a matter of informed and reasoned judgment made by the author. The reader should decide whether the results are applicable in his setting, which may differ in many ways from the study setting. The population to which results are generalizable is also a matter of scientifically reasoned judgment.

Randomized controlled trials are study designs high up in the hierarchy; stringent inclusion and exclusion criteria with maintenance of compliance confer validity. However, in reality, these criteria and compliance are difficult to meet, and generalizability is less.

4. **Are open disclosures made regarding possible conflicts of interest?**
The reader should check for the *possibility of vested interests* in study results that might have crept in during the study or in the process of publication. This compromises study objectivity. Common competing interests are financial, personal, intellectual, institutional loyalties, and career advancement. An effort to limit bias due to competing interests includes open disclosure.

KEY POINTS

- Research paper has to be critically appraised systematically in terms of its relevance, validity, precision, and trustworthiness.
- Stepwise approach starts with title, methodology, results, discussion, and, finally, conclusions.
- The study design adopted should address the research question.
- The reader should decide whether the study results are generalizable to his setting.
- Conclusions should be solely based on study results.

SUGGESTED READING

1. Bousquet PJ, Brozek J, Bachert C, Bieber T, Bonini S, Burney P, et al. The CONSORT statement checklist in allergen-specific immunotherapy: a GA2LEN paper. Allergy. 2009;64(12):1737-45.
2. EQUATOR Network. (2024). Reporting guidelines for main study types. [online] Available from equator-network.org/reporting-guidelines/. [Last accessed April, 2025].
3. Moore-Clingenpeel M, Greenhawt M, Shaker M. Reporting guidelines for allergy and immunology survey research. Ann Allergy Asthma Immunol. 2023;130(5):674-80.e1.
4. Norman GR, Streiner DL. Sections: the second, third and fourth. In: Norman GR, Streiner DL (Eds). The Bare Essentials, 3rd edition. India: BC Decker Inc.; 2008. pp. 70-274.
5. Ratnani I, Fatima S, Abid MM, Surani Z, Surani S. Evidence-based medicine: history, review, criticisms, and pitfalls. Cureus. 2023; 15(2):e35266.
6. Sreenivasan P. Statistical analysis. In: Sreenivasan P (Ed). Research Methodology: A Manual for Beginners, 1st edition. India: Paras Medical Books Pvt. Ltd.; 2021. pp. 85-98.

CHAPTER 32

Oxygen Delivery Devices

Abdul Rauf KK, Arunima Ashok

INTRODUCTION

Oxygen has rightfully asserted its prominence in clinical medicine since 1890s, when supplemental oxygen was first used for bacterial pneumonia. Subsequently, there were advancements in its delivery modalities evolving presently into our varied available oxygen delivery devices. Irrespective of the etiopathogenesis, indications for oxygen therapy are hypoxemia [partial pressure of oxygen in the arterial blood (PaO_2) <60 mm Hg/oxygen saturation in arterial blood (SpO_2) <92%] or an acute situation in which hypoxemia is suspected or in which suspected regional hypoxia may respond to an increase in PaO_2.

PRINCIPLE BEHIND OXYGEN THERAPY: PHYSIOLOGY

Regarding the physiological effects, the peripheral systemic vasodilatation and pulmonary vasoconstriction during hypoxia is reversed with oxygen. At cellular level, oxygen therapy results in the restoration of homeostatic intracellular environment with the use of adenosine triphosphate (ATP)-dependent ion pumping systems and reversal of inhibition of mitochondrial respiratory chain.

Arterial oxygen content (CaO_2) in mL/dL is calculated by:

$$CaO_2 = (1.34 \times Hb \times SaO_2) + (0.003 \times PaO_2)$$

Oxygen delivery (DO_2) is the product of CaO_2 in the blood and cardiac output (L/min)

$$DO_2 = CO\ [(Hb \times SaO_2 \times 1.34) + (PaO_2 \times 0.0031)]$$

Where DO_2: rate of oxygen delivery (mL/min); CO: cardiac output; Hb: hemoglobin concentration (g/dL); SaO_2: percentage of saturated hemoglobin with oxygen, and PaO_2: partial pressure of oxygen in the arterial blood (mm Hg).

OXYGEN DELIVERY SYSTEM AND DEVICES

An oxygen delivery system is a device used to administer, regulate, and supplement oxygen to increase the arterial oxygenation. The essential components include sources of oxygen supply, flowmeter, blender, tubing, humidifier, and a delivery device interface. The device to be selected depends on the age of patient, tolerance to the selected interface, disease pathology, treatment targets, and the humidification requirements.

Oxygen delivery systems are classified as low-flow and high-flow devices on comparing to peak inspiratory flow rates (PIFR) of the patient **(Table 32.1)**.

Low-flow Devices

Noncontact/"Wafting"/Blow-by Method

Free-flow oxygen is delivered usually by an oxygen tubing (typically large bore), which

TABLE 32.1: Comparison between low- and high-flow oxygen delivery devices.

	Low-flow device	*High-flow device*
Flow rate	< PIFR of patient	≥ PIFR of patient
FiO_2	Depends on PIFR, variable dilution with room air	Specified FiO_2 throughout with fixed entrainment of room air
Rebreathing of CO_2	Occurs with lower flow rates	Does not occur as CO_2 is washed out
Indication	Emergency, short term and intermittent uses	Controlled oxygen therapy with constant FiO_2 delivery for longer time
Examples	• Nasal prongs • Enclosure systems (oxygen hood and tents) • Simple nasal mask • Nonrebreathing masks	• Venturi mask • Air entrainment nebulizer • High-flow nasal cannula • NIV/NIPPV

(CO_2: carbon dioxide; FiO_2: fraction of inspired oxygen; NIPPV: noninvasive positive pressure ventilation; NIV: noninvasive ventilation; PIFR: peak inspiratory flow rate)

may or may not be connected to a simple facemask, which is directed toward patient's face, but not in contact. It is a crude way of oxygen therapy not guaranteeing a specific fraction of inspired oxygen (FiO_2) and is best for claustrophobic patients with minimal FiO_2 requirement, those needing occasional intermittent therapy (e.g., postsurgical during procedural anesthesia).

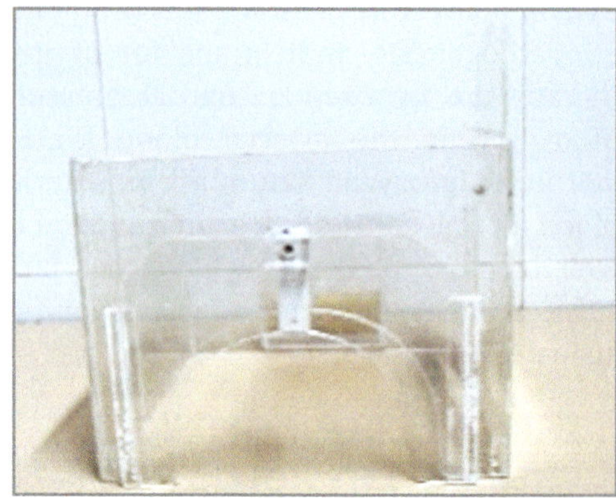

Fig. 32.1: Enclosure systems (oxygen hood).

Enclosure Systems: Oxygen Hood and Tents

Oxygen hood or tent is a plastic box or cylinder where the head of a neonate or infant is placed inside through a gap on the same **(Fig. 32.1)**. A continuous flow of humidified oxygen is ensured through the air entry portal into the hood or tent. The exhaled air is passively let out through the opening for the neck. A range of FiO_2 from 22 to 80% can be achieved with a minimum flow rate of 6–10 L/min oxygen into the hood and 21–50% FiO_2 using 15–30 L/min flow within a tent. It is always preferable to keep an oxygen analyzer to decipher the actual FiO_2 delivered. A minimum flow of 6 L/min should be used with enclosure systems, as the risk of rebreathing increases below that flow rate.

Nasal Cannula/Prongs

Nasal prong is a simple and commonly used oxygen delivery device that ends in two short, tapered tubes lying just within the nostrils **(Fig. 32.2)**. They deliver a constant flow of oxygen to nasopharynx and oropharynx, thereby utilizing one third of the anatomical

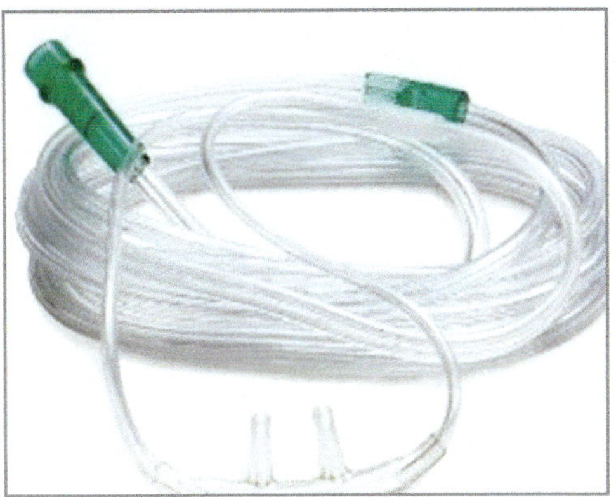

Fig. 32.2: Nasal prong.

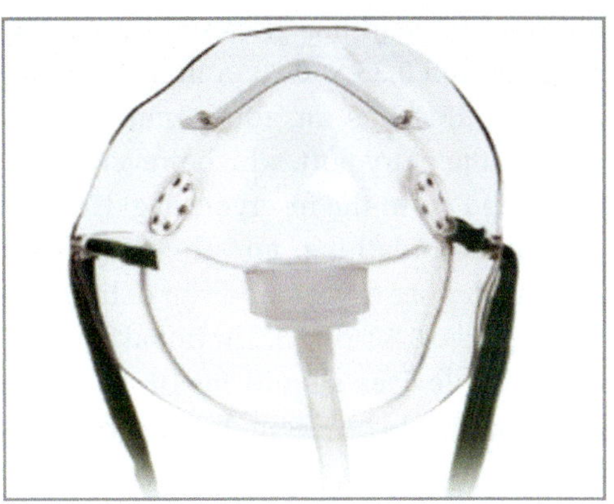

Fig. 32.3: Simple facemask.

dead space as the oxygen reservoir. It delivers a restricted range of FiO_2 starting from 0.22 to 0.40 with flow rates from 0.5 to 6 L/min though flow exceeding 3 L/min is not usually tolerated well. FiO_2 depends on the flow rate and ratio of prong and nasal diameters. It is effective only for low FiO_2 requirements, but is easy to use and tolerated, does not interfere with talking or feeding, and does not require humidification with standard oxygen flow rates. A simple and crude way to calculate the FiO_2 for proper size nasal cannula is addition of 3% FiO_2 to room air for each liter flow. For example, 1 L/min flow of nasal prong gives 24% FiO_2 and 3 L/min flow of nasal prong gives 30% FiO_2.

Simple Facemask

The Hudson facemask, being one of the common low-flow devices used in practice **(Fig. 32.3)** adds an extra 150–250 mL to the oxygen reservoir and can deliver a FiO_2 of 0.4–0.6 with a minimum flow rate of 6–10 L/min. Higher FiO_2 requires tight seal. All mask-based delivery devices require a minimum flow rate of 6 L/min flow to decrease rebreathing of expired carbon dioxide. The oxygen concentration delivered varies, depending on the patient's inspiratory flow rate and the oxygen flow into the system. Masks are best for short-term therapy for hypoxemic events, such as postoperative period and asthma.

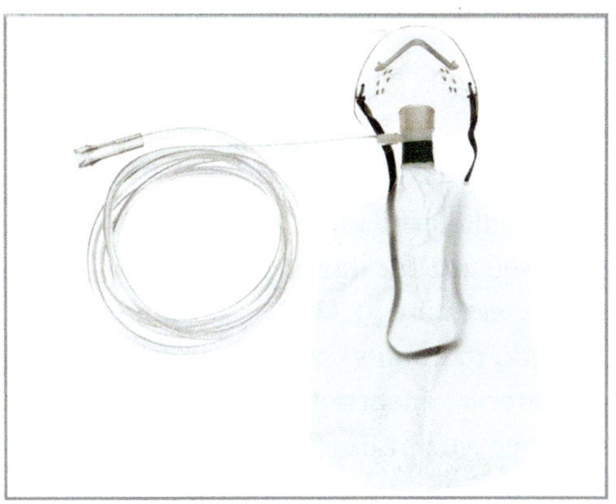

Fig. 32.4: Masks with reservoir bag (nonrebreathing mask).

Mask with Reservoir Bags: Partial Rebreathing and Nonrebreathing Masks

Masks with reservoir bags add additional volume by incorporating a bag below the chin, to increase FiO_2 **(Fig. 32.4)**. A partial rebreathing mask employs a single one-way valve at the exhalation port so that patient breaths only from the reservoir. However, the gas exhaled at the initial phase of expiration returns to the reservoir bag, which causes minimal rebreathing. It can deliver a FiO_2 ranging from 0.35 to 0.80. A nonrebreathing mask (NRM) has an additional one-way valve at the entry port, which prevents entry of expired air to the reservoir bag. Hence, it prevents rebreathing, and the reservoir is filled with pure oxygen and can deliver FiO_2 ranging from 0.40 to 0.95. The initial flow rates for these devices should be 10–15 L/min, tight seal should be ensured, and care should be taken to adjust the flow rate to prevent collapsing of the reservoir bag. Recently, open oxygen mask designs like Oxymask have come up, which claims higher FiO_2 delivery using diffuser technology though substantiating pediatric studies are lacking.

Nasal and Nasopharyngeal Catheters

Nasal catheter is a thin and flexible tube that is passed into the nose and ends with its tip in the nasal cavity (0.5 L/min for neonates and 1 L/min in infants), while a nasopharyngeal catheter is inserted more deeper to the nasopharynx (a depth of 1 cm less than the distance from nostril to tragus, usually 7 cm in infants, resting slightly behind the uvula). External humidification is mandatory to avoid drying of the pharyngeal mucosa and to reduce the likelihood of thickened secretions.

Tracheostomy Masks/Oxygen Adapters

Tracheostomy masks (while connected to oxygen reservoir) are specially designed to be placed over the tracheostomy stoma and secured round the neck. Tracheostomy adapter with an oxygen supply tube connected can also provide oxygen therapy with variable FiO_2 for short-term purposes.

High-flow Devices

High-flow devices provide flow rate, which meet or exceed the patient's minute volume/inspiratory demands, thereby avoiding variable room air entrainment and delivering fixed concentration of oxygen regardless of the inspiratory flow/breathing pattern.

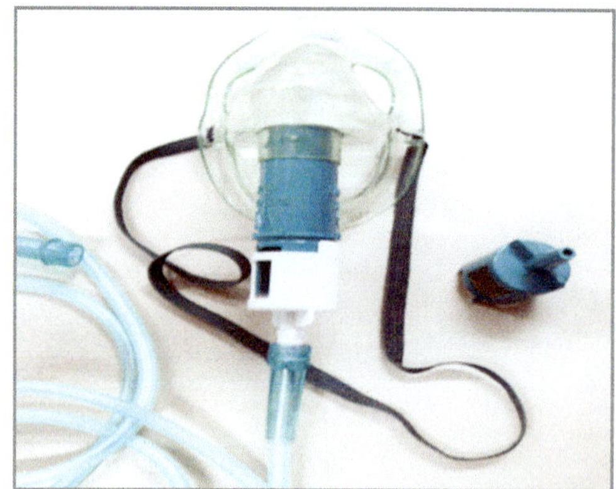

Fig. 32.5: Venturi mask.

Venturi Masks/Air Entrainment Masks

Venturi mask is a high-flow device, which is cone-shaped with entrainment ports of various sizes at its base, to adjust the oxygen concentrations **(Fig. 32.5)**. The FiO_2 can be adjusted by changing the size of the nozzle, the flow rates, and the ports. There are two types of Venturi masks available: A fixed FiO_2 model with color-coded jets (green 60%, red 40%, yellow 35%, orange 31%, white 28%, and blue 24%), which produce a known FiO_2 with a given flow and a variable FiO_2 model with graded adjustment of the air entrainment port, set to allow variation in delivered FiO_2. Venturi mask can deliver FiO_2 between 0.25 and 0.60, but a tight seal is imperative.

Air Entrainment Nebulizer

Air entrainment nebulizers, commonly used for aerosol can deliver constant FiO_2 **(Fig. 32.6)**. Along with particulate water with/without medication, heated nebulizers can deliver gas saturated with water vapor at

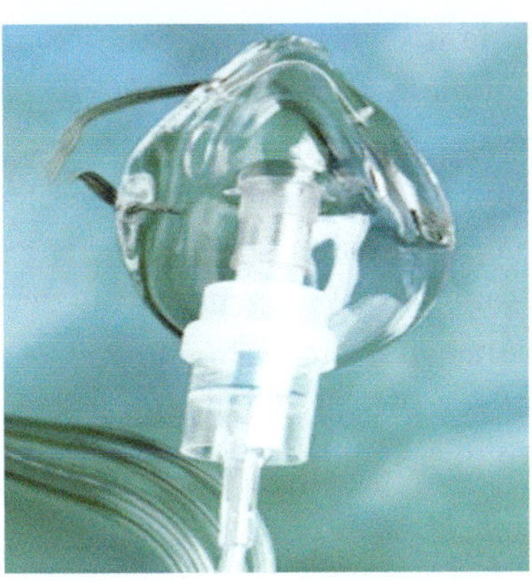

Fig. 32.6: Air entrainment nebulizer.

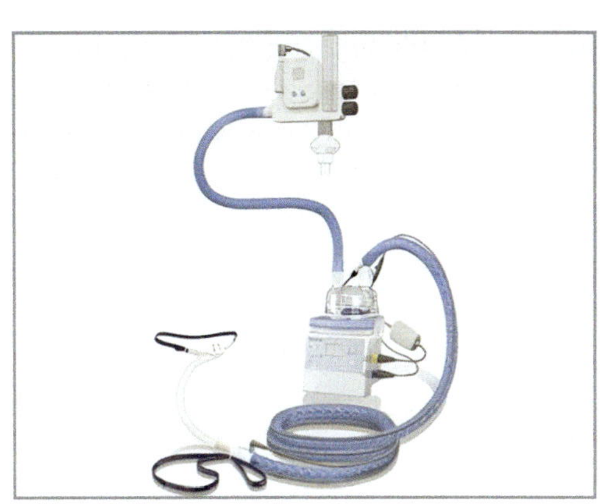

Fig. 32.7: High-flow nasal cannula.

body temperature. At 10–15 L/min, it provides a range of FiO_2 of 28–100%.

Heated Humidified High-flow Nasal Cannula

The basic components of heated humidified high-flow nasal cannula (HHHFNC)/high-flow nasal cannula (HFNC) are (1) a source of pressurized oxygen and air regulated by a flowmeter and blender, (2) sterile water reservoir attached to a heater humidifier, (3) insulated and/or heated circuit that maintains temperature and relative humidity, and (4) nonocclusive cannula interface **(Fig. 32.7)**. The mechanism of action is by reduction in work of breathing by decreasing inspiratory resistance at nasopharynx and washout of dead space, decreased energy expenditure due to humidification and provision of some positive end-expiratory pressure (PEEP). Recent data support the use of weight-based flow setting, such as 1 L/kg/min or 2 L/kg/min.

Successful use of HFNC has been well described in bronchiolitis, viral-induced wheeze, pneumonia, obstructive sleep apnea, asthma, and prevention of postextubation respiratory failure. HFNC is also used in neonates for conditions such as respiratory distress syndrome, apnea of prematurity, congenital cardiac lesions, and postextubation.

Continuous Positive Airway Pressure and Bilevel Positive Airway Pressure

Continuous positive airway pressure (CPAP) and bilevel positive airway pressure (BiPAP), both deliver positive pressure through a noninvasive interface such as a facemask/nasal mask/nasal pillows. The components include a continuous gas flow into the circuit, which is usually 5–10 L/min, an oxygen blender with an oxygen source, a nasal interface-short nasal prongs, an expiratory limb with the distal end submerged in water to generate end expiratory pressure (in case of bubble CPAP). CPAP is an effective intervention in neonates with preterm lungs presenting with issues such as respiratory distress syndrome, apnea of prematurity, and meconium aspiration syndromes. It has also been used as an adjunct to surfactant therapy, during resuscitation and indeed decreased the need for neonatal transfer, intubation, and ventilation. Noninvasive ventilation (NIV)/noninvasive positive pressure ventilation (NIPPV)/BiPAP provides an inspiratory positive airway pressure (IPAP: 10–12 cmH_2O) and an expiratory positive airway pressure (EPAP: 5–6 cmH_2O) setting contrary to CPAP, which has a uniform pressure throughout the respiratory cycle. The difference between IPAP and EPAP drives the tidal volume. Mode can be spontaneous, timed or spontaneous/timed depending on patient's status. Indications include pneumonia, asthma, mild acute respiratory distress syndrome (ARDS), obstructive sleep apnea, postextubation scenarios, and neuromuscular diseases.

A summary of oxygen delivery devices is mentioned in **Table 32.2**.

Oxygen therapy needs to be monitored and guided by target oxygen saturations as

TABLE 32.2: Comparison of common oxygen delivery devices.

Delivery device	***Flow rate (L/min)***	***FiO_2 delivered (%)***	***Design***	***Indications***	***Remarks***
Blow-by method	5–10	0.3–0.4	Low flow/ variable	Do not tolerate masks or cannula, minimal FiO_2 requirement	Unreliable FiO_2
Hood Tent	7–10 >15	0.25–0.9 0.25–0.5	Low flow	Hypoxemic neonates	Unreliable FiO_2, risk of hypercarbia with lower flows
Simple facemask	6–10	0.35–0.65	Low flow, variable	When low FiO_2 for short periods	Claustrophobia, risk of hypercarbia with low flows
Partial/ nonrebreathing mask	10–15	• 0.50–0.60 (partial) • 0.65–0.95 (non)	Low flow with reservoir	Hypoxemia in ED	Tight seal needed, not ideal for long periods
Nasal prongs/ cannula	1–6	0.25–0.45	Low flow, variable	Minimal FiO_2 requirements	Irritates with higher flows
Venturi mask	3–10	0.24–0.60	High flow, air entrainment system	Hypoxemia with targeted FiO_2 needed	Provides a constant preset level of FiO_2
CPAP	• 5–10 (b-CPAP) • 10–40 (BiPAP)	0.21–1.0	Low-to-high flow	ICUs for hours to days	b-CPAP gives PEEP BiPAP gives IPAP and EPAP
HFNC	2–60	0.21–1.0	Low-to-high flow, variable and fixed	Preoxygenation, postintubation, moderate-to-severe hypoxemia	Some PEEP, less interface-related problems

(BiPAP: bilevel positive airway pressure; b-CPAP: bubble continuous positive airway pressure; CPAP: continuous positive airway pressure; ED: emergency department; EPAP: expiratory positive airway pressure; FiO_2: fraction of inspired oxygen; HFNC: high-flow nasal cannula; ICUs: intensive care units; IPAP: inspiratory positive airway pressure; PEEP: positive end-expiratory pressure) hyperoxia is harmful. Pulmonary oxygen toxicity can lead to damage to alveolar membrane, atelectasis, and ARDS. Retinopathy of prematurity (ROP) results from alteration of the normal retinal vascular development, reversible constriction of peripheral field of vision, reversible myopia, and delayed cataract. Oxygen can deform red blood cells (RBCs) and cause osteonecrosis.

At the institutional level, Oxygen Monitoring Team and Oxygen Audit Committee may be formed to monitor and supervise the rational use of oxygen therapy.

SUMMARY

Oxygen delivery devices are divided into low-flow devices (wafting, hood/tent, nasal prongs, cannula, and simple and nonbreathing masks) and high-flow devices (Venturi masks, air entrainment nebulizers, HFNC, CPAP, and BiPAP). The oxygen delivery device to be selected depends on the age, tolerance to the interface, disease pathology, treatment targets, humidification requirements, etc.

KEY POINTS

- Oxygen delivery devices are classified into two types: low flow and high flow with comparison to peak inspiratory flow rate of the patient.
- Low flow devices are wafting, hood/tent, nasal prongs, cannula, and simple and nonbreathing masks.
- High-flow devices are Venturi masks, air entrainment nebulizers, HFNC, CPAP, and BiPAP.
- Delivery device selection should be done considering the age, tolerance to the interface, disease etiopathology, respiratory efforts of the patient, anticipated duration of treatment, targeted saturations and humidification requirements.
- Oxygen therapy needs to be guided and monitored by targeted oxygen saturations and discontinued whenever possible by the earliest.

SUGGESTED READING

1. Batool S, Garg R. Appropriate use of oxygen delivery devices. Open Anesth J. 2017;11: 35-8.
2. Hardavella G, Karampinis I, Frille A, Sreter K, Rousalova I. Oxygen devices and delivery systems. Breathe (Sheff). 2019;15(3):e108-16.
3. Napolitano N, Berlinski A, Walsh BK, Ginier E, Strickland SL. AARC clinical practice guideline: management of pediatric patients with oxygen in the acute care setting. Respir Care. 2021;66(7):1214-23.
4. Uygur P, Oktem S, Boran P, Tutar E, Tokuc G. Low- versus high-flow oxygen delivery systems in children with lower respiratory infection. Pediatr Int. 2016;58(1):49-52.
5. Walsh BK, Smallwood CD. Pediatric oxygen therapy: a review and update. Respir Care. 2017;62(6):645-61.
6. World Health Organization. (2016). Oxygen therapy for children: a manual for health workers. [online] Available from https://apps.who.int/iris/handle/10665/204584. [Last accessed April, 2025].

CHAPTER 33

Tests in Inborn Errors of Immunity and their Interpretation

Sagar Bhattad, Jyothi Janardhanan

INTRODUCTION

Inborn errors of immunity (IEI), previously known as primary immunodeficiencies, are a group of heterogeneous disorders characterized by increased susceptibility to infections, autoimmunity, atopy, and malignancy due to defects in the immune system with a majority of them, being monogenic. The International Union of Immunological Societies (IUIS) Expert Committee 2022 classification enlisted 485 diseases. The latest IUIS classification provides 10 classes of IEI. However, for clinical assessment, IEIs can be classified into four broad categories: (1) B-cell defect; (2) T-cell defect/combined immunodeficiencies; (3) Phagocytic defects; and (4) Complement defects.

An important aspect of diagnosing IEIs is clinical suspicion. The clinical profile and initial laboratory evaluation will guide the selection of appropriate immunological tests for each patient. The most valuable first-line investigations include a complete blood count (CBC) with differential counts, lymphocyte subset analysis, serum immunoglobulin (Ig) levels, nitroblue tetrazolium (NBT) test, and dihydrorhodamine (DHR) test. Genetic testing would confirm the diagnosis; however, it must be noted that a negative genetic test (exome sequencing) does exclude an IEI. This chapter aims to illustrate investigations carried out in patients with IEIs through case scenarios.

HINTS FROM A COMPLETE BLOOD COUNT

Case 1

A 6-month-old girl presented with fever and breathing difficulty. She also had a history of recurrent oral thrush from early life and failure to thrive.

- *Evaluation:* It showed CBC: Hemoglobin (Hb) 9.8 g/dL, total count (TC) 5,000/mm^3 ($N_{85\%}$, $L_{5\%}$), absolute lymphocyte count (ALC) 250, and platelet count (PC) 153,000/mm^3.
- All hemograms showed persistent lymphopenia. Further evaluation showed hypogammaglobulinemia with very low CD3 and CD19 cells with normal CD56 cells.
- *Diagnosis:* Severe combined immunodeficiency (SCID)

Lymphopenia

A simple CBC can provide valuable information for diagnosing a patient. It is important to note that the absolute lymphocyte count indicating lymphopenia differs significantly between infants (<3,000/mm^3) and adults (<1,000/mm^3). If an infant's lymphocyte count is <3,000/mm^3, it is important to consider SCID.

TABLE 33.1: Hematological parameters.

Hb (g/dL)	9.2	8.9
TLC (N/L/M) (mm^3)	7,200 ($N_{9\%}$ $L_{81\%}$ M_5)	5,600 ($N_{6\%}$ $L_{80\%}$ M_{10})
ANC (mm^3)	648	336
PC (mm^3)	500,000	489,000

(ANC: absolute neutrophil count; Hb: hemoglobin; PC: platelet count; TLC: total leukocyte count)

Flowchart 33.1: Approach to neutropenia.

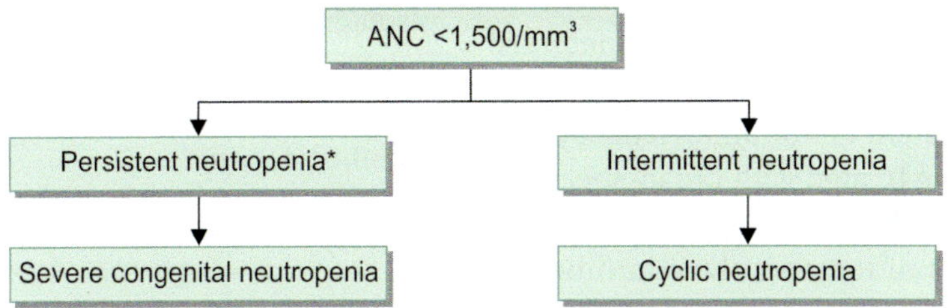

*Neutropenia in serial CBC done two times a week for 6 weeks.
(ANC: absolute neutrophil count; CBC: complete blood count)

Severe combined immunodeficiency is a medical emergency, and a timely diagnosis could be lifesaving. In young children with lymphopenia, human immunodeficiency virus (HIV) infection needs to be ruled out, usually through an HIV viral load assay, rather than serological testing for anti-HIV antibodies. Additionally, mechanical loss of lymphocytes, as observed in the cases of intestinal lymphangiectasia, should be considered, particularly when diarrhea is a prominent symptom. Chylous loss and circulation abnormalities can also result in T-cell lymphopenia.

Message: Persistent lymphopenia in infants
—Think of SCID

Case 2

A 5-month-old boy, a product of third-degree consanguinity, presented with two episodes of otitis media, and an episode of pneumonia. There was no significant family history. A review of his records showed persistent neutropenia (**Table 33.1**). Bone marrow showed maturation arrest in the myeloid lineage. The erythroid and megakaryocytic lineages were normal.

- *Genetic studies:* Pathogenic mutation in *ELANE* gene
- *Diagnosis:* Severe congenital neutropenia

Neutropenia

Neutropenia is defined as an absolute neutrophil count (ANC) of <1,500/mm^3 in children older than 1 year, and <2,000/mm^3 in children younger than 1 year. The approach to neutropenia is described in **Flowchart 33.1**.

Classification of Neutropenia

Classification of neutropenia is shown in **Table 33.2**.

Case 3

A 3-month-old girl, born of a third-degree consanguineous marriage, presented with pneumonia. On review of her medical

TABLE 33.2: Classification of neutropenia.

Classification	*ANC*
Mild neutropenia	1,000–1,500/mm^3
Moderate neutropenia	500–1,000/mm^3
Severe neutropenia	<500/mm^3
Cyclic neutropenia	ANC with periodic oscillations and nadir <1,000/mm^3

(ANC: absolute neutrophil count)

history, she had omphalitis in the neonatal period with delayed cord fall. She was noted to have persistent neutrophilic leukocytosis and was being treated with broad-spectrum antimicrobials. Though she became afebrile after 2 weeks of therapy, she continued to have marked neutrophilia.

- *Evaluation:* CBC: Hb 9.6 g/dL, TC 56,000/mm^3 ($N_{85\%}$, $L_{6\%}$), PC 253,000/mm^3, ANC 47,600/mm^3
- *Further investigations:* CD18 assay by flow cytometry: 0% (Control 99%)
- *Diagnosis:* Leukocyte adhesion deficiency (LAD)

> *Message:* Persistent neutrophilic leukocytosis with history of recurrent infections
>
> **—Think of LAD**

Case 4

A 1-year-old boy, presented with blood in stools and severe eczema. There was a significant family history, wherein two of his maternal uncles had expired at a young age. Thrombocytopenia was documented in several records.

- *Complete blood count:* Hb 9.8 g/dL, TC 10,000/mm^3 ($N_{65\%}$ $L_{20\%}$ M_6 E_9), PC 68,000/mm^3
- *Mean platelet volume (MPV):* 5 fL (7–11)
- *Genetic evaluation:* Pathogenic mutation in *WAS* gene
- *Diagnosis:* Wiskott-Aldrich syndrome (WAS)

Thrombocytopenia

The causes of thrombocytopenia in any child are numerous. However, in a male child with a history of recurrent infections, eczema, and colitis, the possibility of WAS should be borne in mind. A characteristic feature of WAS is a low MPV. A milder phenotype, X-linked thrombocytopenia (XLT) also presents with microthrombocytopenia and is often misdiagnosed as immunothrombocytopenic purpura (ITP). Hence, it is pertinent to look at MPV in every boy with persistent thrombocytopenia.

> *Message:* Male + Thrombocytopenia + Low MPV
>
> **—Think of WAS**

The above cases emphasize the importance of CBC in diagnosing IEIs. Therefore, it is crucial to spend significant time analyzing the differential white cell counts.

UTILITY OF IMMUNOGLOBULIN ASSAY

Case 5

A 2-year-old boy presented with a history of multiple episodes of pneumonia and otitis media from infancy. On examination, he appeared well-grown; however, tonsils were not visualized on throat examination. He had a significant family history with the death of elder brother due to severe pneumonia at the age of 5 years. Evaluation showed panhypogammaglobulinemia with absent B-cells.

- *Serum immunoglobulins:*
    - *IgG:* 218 mg/dL (345–1,236)
    - *IgA:* <23 mg/dL (14–159)
    - *IgM:* <21 mg/dL (43–207)
- *Lymphocyte subset analysis:*
    - *CD3:* 97% (4,627 cells/uL)
    - *CD19:* 0% (0 cells/uL)
    - *CD56:* 2.8% (134 cells/uL)

- *Genetic test:* Pathogenic mutation in *BTK* gene
- *Diagnosis:* X-linked agammaglobulinemia

Case 6

A 35-year-old gentleman was referred to the immunology services with a history of chronic diarrhea for the past 2 years and significant weight loss. In the past, he had a history of recurrent sinusitis from the age of 12 years.

- His serum immunoglobulins showed hypogammaglobulinemia [*IgG:* 272 mg/dL (639–1,349), *IgA:* 30 mg/dL (70–312), *IgM:* 35 mg/dL (56–352)].
- Lymphocyte subset analysis was normal [CD3: 72% (50–75), CD19: 15% (10–15) and CD56: 10% (5–10)].
- *Diagnosis:* Common variable immunodeficiency (CVID).

Case 7

A 7-year-old boy, second born of a second-degree consanguineous marriage, presented with a history of severe eczema from infancy, recurrent otitis media, and pneumonia. There was a history of sibling death due to a similar illness at 4 years of age. After extensive evaluation, he was referred to the immunology department.

- *Evaluation showed:*
  - *IgG:* 722 mg/dL (608–1,572)
  - *IgA:* 45 mg/dL (33–236)
  - *IgM:* 65 mg/dL (43–207)
  - *IgE:* 5,000 IU/L (<100)
- *Genetic studies:* Pathogenic mutation in the *DOCK8* gene
  - *Diagnosis*: DOCK8 deficiency (autosomal recessive, hyper-IgE syndrome)

Case 8

A 4-year-old boy presented with a history of recurrent episodes of pneumonia. He had been empirically treated with antitubercular therapy. He had been investigated elsewhere, and cystic fibrosis and congenital heart disease were excluded. He was now referred to the immunology department for further evaluation.

- *Immunoglobulin profile showed:*
  - *IgG:* <26 mg/dL (345–1,236)
  - *IgA:* <20 mg/dL (14–159)
  - *IgM:* >560 mg/dL (43–207)
- *Lymphocyte subset assay:* B- and T-cells normal
- *Genetic test:* Pathogenic mutation in *CD40L* gene
- *Diagnosis:* Hyper-IgM syndrome (X-linked)

Case 9

A 12-year-old girl, presented with a history of recurrent otitis media and pneumonia. She had had two episodes of severe pneumonia, requiring oxygen support. Having excluded lung and cardiac anomalies, she was referred to the immunology services.

- The immunoglobulin profile is as follows:
  - *IgG:* 1,650 mg/dL (608–1,572)
  - *IgA:* <20 mg/dL (33–236)
  - *IgM:* 112 mg/dL (52–242)
- The possibility of IgA deficiency was considered; however, given the severe phenotype, serum IgG subclasses were tested:
  - *IgG1:* 1,425 mg/dL (423–939)
  - *IgG2:* 15 mg/dL (33–236)
  - *IgG3:* 100 mg/dL (27–107)
  - *IgG4:* 27 mg/dL (8–32)
- *Diagnosis:* IgG2 subclass deficiency with IgA deficiency.

Immunoglobulins

Immunoglobulins are glycoproteins produced by plasma cells (activated B cells), which play an important role in immune response against

TABLE 33.3: Immunological profile and IEI.

Immunological profile	*Likely IEI*
Panhypogammaglobulinemia in a boy child	X-linked agammaglobulinemia
Low IgG, IgA, and/or IgM with normal B-cells	Common variable immunodeficiency (CVID)
High IgE levels	Hyper-IgE syndromes (AD/AR), Wiskott-Aldrich syndrome, Omenn syndrome
Low IgG, IgA, and high IgM	Hyper-IgM syndrome*
High IgG	Chronic granulomatous disease, HIV, and systemic lupus erythematosus

*50% of children with hyper-IgM syndrome have normal IgM levels.
(AD: autosomal dominant; AR: autosomal recessive; IEI: inborn errors of immunity; HIV: human immunodeficiency virus)

infections. These include IgG, IgM, IgA, IgE, and IgD. IgG antibodies are the most abundant isotype in the serum. The four subclasses of IgG include IgG1, IgG2, IgG3, and IgG4. IgG1 is around 65% of the total IgG. IgG2 forms an important host defense against bacteria that are encapsulated.

Children and adults with immunoglobulin defects present with recurrent infections, and they are said to have humoral immunodeficiencies. Initial screening is done by measuring serum levels of the major circulating immunoglobulin classes: IgG, IgA, IgM, and IgE. This is usually done using nephelometry (for IgG, IgA, and IgM), a method that uses light to measure the scattered light from protein-antibody complexes in the sample. Total IgE and allergen-specific IgE levels are measured using a solid-phase immunoassay.

When comparing antibody levels, it is important to use age-matched reference intervals, typically provided as 95% confidence intervals (CI). If immunoglobulin levels are low, it is important to also check the serum albumin level to rule out protein loss as the cause. Another useful test is measuring IgG subclass levels, particularly for those with selective IgA deficiency and recurrent sinopulmonary infections **(Table 33.3)**.

Case 10

A 2-year-old boy, a product of a nonconsanguineous marriage, presented with a history of cervical lymphadenitis and several episodes of pneumonia. Recently, he developed blood in stools and was evaluated by the gastroenterology team. Inflammatory bowel disease had been excluded.

- *Investigations:*
  - *CBC:* Hb 9.2 g/dL, TC 24,000/mm^3 ($N_{70\%}$ $L_{20\%}$ M_6 E_4), PC 500,000/mm^3
  - Erythrocyte sedimentation rate (ESR) 100 mm/h, C reactive protein (CRP) 68 mg/L (<6)
- *Immunoglobulins:*
  - *IgG:* 2,240 mg/dL (345–1,236)
  - *IgA:* 198 mg/dL (14–159)
  - *IgM:* 280 mg/dL (43–207)
- NBT and DHR showed impaired oxidative burst.
- *Diagnosis:* Chronic granulomatous disease (CGD)

Nitroblue Tetrazolium and Dihydrorhodamine

Nitroblue tetrazolium test is a simple and cost-effective test for the diagnosis of CGD; however, it is observer-dependent. Hence, DHR test is now the screening test of choice for CGD.

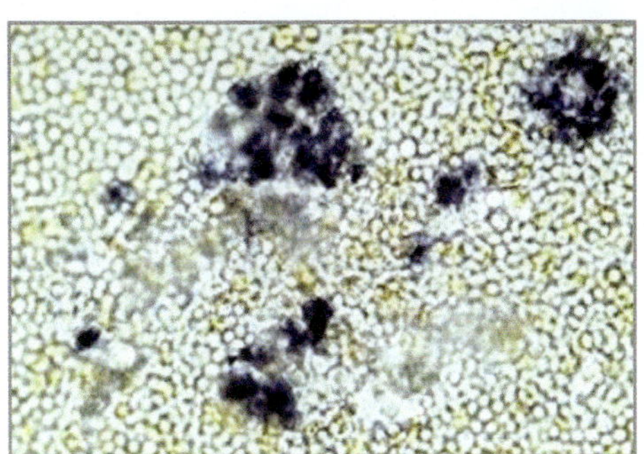

Fig. 33.1: *NBT test:* Blue-black formazan granules suggestive of normal oxidative burst.

- *Principle of NBT test:* NBT is a yellow dye that produces blue-black formazan granules when reduced. The formation of formazan granules indicates a normal oxidative burst **(Fig. 33.1)**.
- *Principle of DHR:* DHR is a flow cytometry-based test. Neutrophils are stimulated with phorbol myristate acetate (PMA) and DHR is oxidized to produce rhodamine, which is fluorescent. The degree of fluorescence defines the function of neutrophils.

Message: Recurrent suppurative infections/nonresolving pneumonia + High serum immunoglobulins = Evaluate for CGD

Case 11

A 3-month-old girl was hospitalized with severe pneumonia and oral thrush. She was noted to have failure to thrive. Her hemogram showed lymphopenia and was, therefore, further evaluated. Lymphocyte subset analysis showed markedly reduced T-cells.

- *CD3:* 2% (50–70%)
- *CD19:* 91% (10–15%)
- *CD56:* 3% (5–10%)

Diagnosis: SCID

Lymphocyte Subset Analysis

The lymphocyte subset includes T-cell, B-cell, and natural killer (NK) cell counts, which are performed by flow cytometry. The markers for different lymphocytes are as follows:

- *T-cells:* CD3
- *B-cells:* C19
- *NK cells:* CD56

CD3 count <300/mm^3 is a diagnostic indicator of SCID. In some cases, there may be a low CD3 count, but not <300/mm^3. This can make diagnosis challenging. When faced with such situations, testing for naïve T-cells and recent thymic emigrants is recommended, as these are expected to be low in individuals with SCID. The immunological phenotype can suggest the underlying genetic defect in SCID **(Table 33.4)**.

TABLE 33.4: Lymphocyte subset and associated types of severe combined immunodeficiency (SCID).

Lymphocyte subset	*Types of SCID*
T-B-NK–	ADA deficiency
T-B+NK–	IL2RG, JAK3
T-B-NK+	RAG1, RAG2, DCLRE1C, DNA ligase IV, Cernunnos
T-B+NK+	IL17Rα, Coronin 1a

(ADA: adenosine deaminase; DNA: deoxyribonucleic acid; IL2RG: interleukin-2 receptor gamma; IL17Rα: interleukin 17-alpha; JAK3: Janus kinase 3; T-B-NK: T-cell, B-cell, and natural killer)

Discussion on genetic evaluation is beyond the scope of this chapter and will not be discussed in detail. However, a few points on genetics and IEI **(Table 33.5)**:

- Majority of IEIs are monogenic.
- Exome sequencing would aid in arriving at a final diagnosis in the majority of IEI.
- Microdeletions are detected by array comparative genomic hybridization (CGH)/fluorescence in situ hybridization (FISH).
- Large deletions and complex mutations can be missed on next generation sequencing (NGS).

TABLE 33.5: Diagnostic tests, tubes, and methodology.

Tests	*Tubes*	*Methodology*
Immunoglobulins (IgG, IgA, and IgM)	Serum	Nephelometry/turbidimetry
IgE	Serum	ELISA
Lymphocyte subsets	EDTA	Flow cytometry
NBT	Sodium heparin/EDTA	Microscopy
DHR	Sodium heparin/EDTA	Flow cytometry
CD18, CD11	Sodium heparin/EDTA	Flow cytometry
Whole exome sequencing	EDTA	NGS

(DHR: dihydrorhodamine; EDTA: ethylenediaminetetraacetic acid; ELISA: enzyme-linked immunosorbent assay; NBT: nitroblue tetrazolium; NGS: next-generation sequencing)

Hence, choosing the right platform for genetic testing is very important in attaining an appropriate diagnosis. Lastly, as highlighted previously, a negative genetic test does not exclude IEI.

SUMMARY

Tests for IEI include basic screening such as complete blood counts, lymphocyte subsets, and immunoglobulin levels, followed by functional assays like neutrophil oxidative burst and lymphocyte proliferation assays. Advanced diagnostics involve flow cytometry-based protein expression, cytokine signaling studies, and next-generation sequencing for genetic confirmation. Interpretation requires integrating clinical features with laboratory and molecular findings to guide the diagnosis and management.

KEY POINTS

- The most important step in the diagnosis of IEI is clinical suspicion.
- The presence of cytopenia provides an important clue to the underlying IEI. A detailed review of the differential counts is thus warranted.
- NBT and DHR can be used as screening tests for CGD.
- Serum immunoglobulins must be looked at, in children and adults with suspected humoral and combined immunodeficiencies.
- Choosing an appropriate genetic test is crucial while arriving at a diagnosis of IEI.

SUGGESTED READING

1. Devonshire AL, Makhija M. Approach to primary immunodeficiency. Allergy Asthma Proc. 2019;40(6):465-9.
2. Patra PK, Priyanka P, Singh P, Reddy P, Sharma N, Yagavan P. Approach to primary immunodeficiency disorders. J Int Med Res. 2024;2(1):10-16.
3. Sullivan KE, Stiehm ER (Eds). In: Stiehm's Immune Deficiencies: Inborn Errors of Immunity, 2nd edition. New York: Academic Press (Elsevier); 2020.

34 CHAPTER

Anaphylaxis: Diagnosis and Management

Vikram Patra

INTRODUCTION

Anaphylaxis represents one of the most serious medical emergencies in allergic disease, characterized by a rapid-onset, systemic hypersensitivity reaction that can cause death within minutes of exposure to an allergen. With a global incidence escalating at 5.3% annually and affecting approximately 1–2% of the population worldwide, this condition has emerged as a significant public health concern requiring immediate recognition and intervention. Despite its potentially fatal nature, the mortality rate remains relatively stable at 0.5–1 per million population due to improved emergency protocols and widespread availability of epinephrine autoinjectors. The condition presents unique clinical challenges, including its biphasic nature with potential secondary reactions occurring hours after initial resolution, variable presentations that may lack typical skin manifestations, and the influence of cofactors such as exercise, medications, and comorbidities that can amplify reaction severity. Recent therapeutic advances, including the 2024 FDA approval of intranasal epinephrine and refined diagnostic criteria from the World Allergy Organization, continue to evolve the management landscape. This chapter provides comprehensive guidance on the diagnosis and management of anaphylaxis, integrating evidence-based protocols with emerging innovations to optimize outcomes for patients at risk of this life-threatening condition.

DEFINITION AND OVERVIEW

As per the World Allergy Organization (WAO) 2020 guidelines, anaphylaxis is a serious systemic hypersensitivity reaction that is usually rapid in onset and may cause death. Severe anaphylaxis is characterized by potentially life-threatening compromise in breathing and/or the circulation and may occur without typical skin features or circulatory shock being present. It occurs when the immune system overreacts to a trigger (such as food, insect stings, or medications) by releasing mediators such as histamine, leading to symptoms such as skin rashes, airway obstruction, and cardiovascular collapse. The hallmark of anaphylaxis is its *rapid onset*, often within minutes of exposure to an allergen, and it requires immediate medical attention to prevent fatalities.

CLINICAL RELEVANCE

Anaphylaxis is a major cause of emergency room visits and hospitalization due to allergic reactions. According to recent studies, the incidence of anaphylaxis has been increasing, driven in part by the rise in food allergies, insect venom sensitivity, and increased awareness and reporting.

Additionally, healthcare systems are more attuned to recognizing and responding to these reactions in both children and adults.

EPIDEMIOLOGY

While the exact prevalence of anaphylaxis is difficult to pinpoint, some studies estimate that anaphylaxis affects approximately 1–2% of the population globally. Notably, food allergies are responsible for the highest rates of anaphylaxis in children, while adults often experience reactions due to medications or insect stings.

PATHOPHYSIOLOGY OF ANAPHYLAXIS (FLOWCHART 34.1)

Immunologic Mechanisms

Anaphylaxis is primarily mediated by a *type I hypersensitivity reaction* in which the immune system produces immunoglobulin E (IgE) antibodies in response to an allergen. These IgE antibodies bind to *mast cells* and *basophils*. Upon re-exposure to the allergen, these immune cells release a variety of inflammatory mediators (histamine, prostaglandins, and leukotrienes), leading to vasodilation, increased vascular permeability, bronchoconstriction, and other symptoms. The *immune cascade* also involves the activation of T-cells and the release of cytokines, contributing to systemic inflammation and shock.

Nonimmunologic Mechanisms

Anaphylactoid reactions, which resemble anaphylaxis but are not IgE mediated, may occur in response to certain drugs, contrast agents, or physical triggers such as exercise. These reactions are often less understood but are similarly characterized by the release of mediators from mast cells and basophils, though without prior sensitization.

Systemic Impact

The *cardiovascular system* is typically affected first, with rapid onset of hypotension due to vasodilation and increased capillary permeability. *Airway compromise* often follows, with laryngeal edema or bronchospasm

Flowchart 34.1: Mechanism of anaphylaxis.

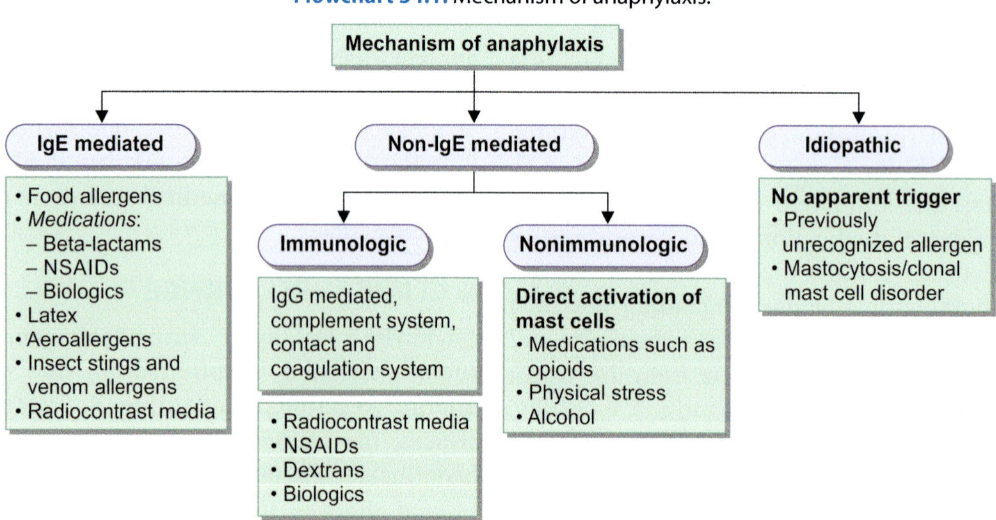

(IgG: immunoglobulin G; NSAIDs: nonsteroidal anti-inflammatory drugs)

leading to breathing difficulties. The *gastro-intestinal system* can also be involved, leading to nausea, vomiting, and abdominal cramping. *Skin symptoms* such as urticaria (hives) and angioedema (swelling of the skin) are common as well.

RECOGNIZING ANAPHYLAXIS: DIAGNOSIS

Clinical Features and Symptoms

Anaphylaxis typically begins within minutes to hours after exposure to a trigger. Common early symptoms include:

- *Skin manifestations:* Urticaria, angioedema, flushing, and pruritus
- *Respiratory symptoms:* Wheezing, shortness of breath, throat tightness, cough, and stridor (due to airway swelling)
- *Cardiovascular symptoms:* Dizziness, hypotension, tachycardia, and potential loss of consciousness (syncope)
- *Gastrointestinal symptoms:* Vomiting, diarrhea, and abdominal cramps

Diagnostic Criteria

The National Institute of Allergy and Infectious Diseases (NIAID) and Food Allergy and Anaphylaxis Network (FAAN) guidelines 2006 outlined the criteria for diagnosing anaphylaxis **(Table 34.1)**. These criteria have been widely adopted and were found to be 95% sensitive and 71% specific in a prospective validation study among emergency department (ED) patients. Knowledge deficits regarding anaphylaxis recognition and treatment continue to be revealed. In an effort to simplify anaphylaxis diagnostic criteria, in 2019 the WAO Anaphylaxis Committee proposed revisions to the definition for the clinical diagnostic criteria for anaphylaxis, which was subsequently largely adopted by the WAO 2020 guidelines **(Table 34.1)**.

Laboratory Investigations

Anaphylaxis diagnosis is clinical. Serum tryptase level may help to support the diagnosis. The European Academy of Allergy and Clinical Immunology (EAACI) task force suggests measuring serum tryptase *30 minutes to 2 hours after the start of the reaction* and *baseline tryptase* at least 24 hours after complete resolution of symptoms. A level of serum tryptase 30 minutes to 2 hours after the start of the reaction (1.2 × Baseline tryptase) + 2 μg/L supports a diagnosis of anaphylaxis **(Fig. 34.1)**. But, failing to find an elevated tryptase level does not rule out anaphylaxis, particularly in children and with food triggers overall. *Most important, collecting samples for serum tryptase should not delay initial treatment.*

Differential Diagnosis

Several conditions can mimic anaphylaxis, including:

- *Vasovagal syncope* (fainting due to low blood pressure)
- *Asthma exacerbations* with wheezing and respiratory distress
- *Cardiac events* (e.g., arrhythmias or myocardial infarction) presenting with chest pain and hypotension
- *Exercise-induced anaphylaxis*, which requires careful history taking

Anaphylaxis Triggers

- *Food:* Peanuts, tree nuts, shellfish, milk, egg, wheat, and soy are the most common triggers.
- *Insect stings:* Bees, wasps, and fire ants
- *Medications:* Antibiotics (penicillin), nonsteroidal anti-inflammatory drugs (NSAIDs), anesthetics, and contrast agents used in imaging studies
- *Idiopathic triggers:* In some cases, anaphylaxis occurs without an identifiable trigger.

TABLE 34.1: NIAID 2006 and WAO 2020 side-by-side comparison.

NIAID criteria (2006)	***WAO criteria (2020)***
Anaphylaxis is highly likely when any one of the following three criteria are fulfilled: 1. Acute onset of an illness (minutes to several hours) with involvement of the skin, mucosal tissue, or both (e.g., generalized hives, pruritus or flushing, swollen lips-tongue-uvula) and at least one of the following: a. Respiratory compromise (e.g., dyspnea, wheeze—bronchospasm, stridor, reduced PEF, and hypoxemia) b. Reduced blood pressure (BP) or associated symptoms of end-organ dysfunction [e.g., hypotonia (collapse), syncope, and incontinence] 2. Two or more of the following that occur rapidly after exposure to a likely allergen for that patient (minutes to several hours): a. Involvement of the skin mucosal tissue (e.g., generalized hives, itch-flush, and swollen lips-tongue-uvula) b. Respiratory compromise (e.g., dyspnea, wheeze—bronchospasm, stridor, reduced PEF, and hypoxemia) c. Reduced BP or associated symptoms of end-organ dysfunction [e.g., hypotonia (collapse), syncope, incontinence] d. Persistent gastrointestinal symptoms (e.g., crampy abdominal pain and vomiting) 3. Reduced BP after exposure to known allergen for that patient (minutes to several hours): a. *Infants and children:* Low systolic BP (age specific) or >30% decrease in systolic BP b. *Adults:* Systolic BP <90 mm Hg or >30% decrease from that person's baseline	Anaphylaxis is highly likely when any one of the following two criteria are fulfilled: 1. Acute onset of an illness (minutes to several hours) with involvement of the skin, mucosal tissue, or both (e.g., generalized hives, pruritus or flushing, swollen lips-tongue-uvula) and at least one of the following: a. Respiratory compromise (e.g., dyspnea, wheeze—bronchospasm, stridor, reduced PEF, and hypoxemia) b. Reduced BP or associated symptoms of end-organ dysfunction [e.g., hypotonia (collapse), syncope, incontinence] c. Severe gastrointestinal symptoms (e.g., severe crampy abdominal pain and repetitive vomiting), especially after exposure to nonfood allergens 2. Acute onset of hypotension or bronchospasm or laryngeal involvement after exposure to a known or highly probable allergen for that patient (minutes to several hours), even in the absence of typical skin involvement.

(NIAID: National Institute of Allergy and Infectious Diseases; PEF: peak expiratory flow; WAO: World Allergy Organization)

- *Exercise induced:* A rare form triggered by physical exertion, often in conjunction with food ingestion.

Cofactors

There are various factors, which increase severity and risk of anaphylaxis. These are mentioned in **Table 34.2**.

IMMEDIATE MANAGEMENT OF ANAPHYLAXIS

Initial Steps

- *Recognition:* Immediate recognition of the signs of anaphylaxis is crucial.
- *Call for help:* Activating emergency services (e.g., calling 911) ensures quick access to advanced care.

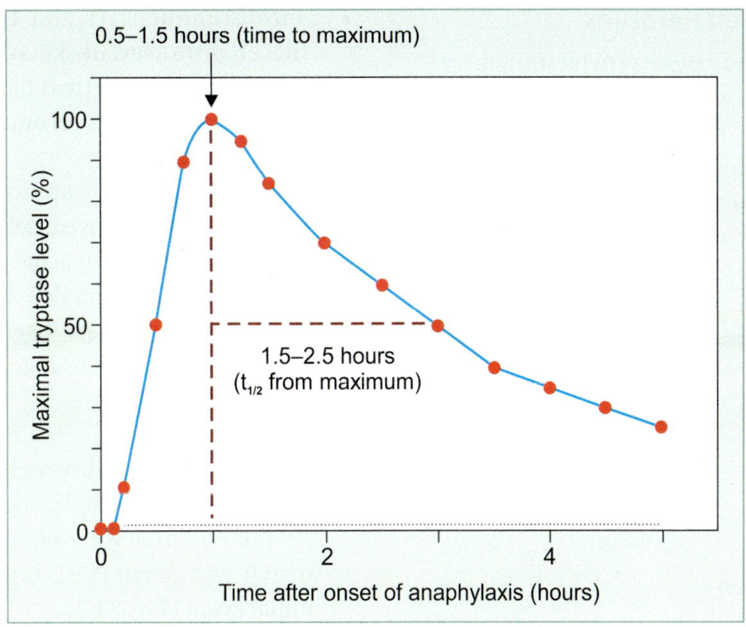

Fig. 34.1: Serum tryptase timeline.

TABLE 34.2: Factors increasing severity and risk of anaphylaxis.

Factors increasing severity	***Concomitant diseases increasing risk***
Physical and emotional stress	Asthma
Sleep deprivation and travel	Allergic rhinitis and atopic eczema
Acute ongoing infection	Cardiovascular diseases
Premenstrual state	Mastocytosis/clonal mast cell disorders
Concurrent use of medication (ACE inhibitors/beta-blockers/ NSAIDs), alcohol, or recreational drugs	Psychiatric diseases

(ACE: angiotensin-converting enzyme; NSAIDs: nonsteroidal anti-inflammatory drugs)

- *Airway management:* Ensuring the airway is open and supporting breathing with supplemental oxygen if necessary.
- *Circulatory support:* Fluid resuscitation to manage hypotension and support circulation

Epinephrine Administration

Epinephrine is the *first-line treatment* for anaphylaxis **(Table 34.3)**.

- *Dosage and administration:* In adults, 0.3 mg of epinephrine is typically administered intramuscularly (IM), whereas 0.01 mg/kg is used for children.
- *Mechanism of action:* Epinephrine reverses the effects of anaphylaxis by causing *vasoconstriction, bronchodilation,* and *reduction of edema.*
- *Timing:* Immediate administration is critical, and the injection should be repeated every 5–10 minutes if symptoms persist or worsen.
- *Intravenous epinephrine is typically reserved for severe cases or those requiring intensive care management.*

Adjunctive Therapies

- High-flow *oxygen* is to be started.
- *Intravenous crystalloid fluid* at 10 mL/kg (500 mL maximum) should be started simultaneously with first-dose adrenaline if there is circulatory collapse or if no response after second-dose adrenaline.

TABLE 34.3: Adrenaline dose as per age and weight range.

Age range	*Weight range*	*Dose of adrenaline*
<1 year	<7.5 kg	0.01 mL/kg
1–5 years	7.5 to 25–30 kg	0.15 mL
6–12 years	>25–30 kg	0.3 mL
Adolescents and adults	–	0.3 mL
Overweight adult or history of previous severe anaphylaxis in past	–	0.5 mL

- *Antihistamines* (H1 and H2 blockers): These help to alleviate skin symptoms such as hives but do not treat life-threatening symptoms such as bronchospasm or hypotension.
- *Corticosteroids:* They are used to reduce inflammation and prevent delayed reactions but are not effective in acute anaphylaxis.
- *Bronchodilators:* Inhaled beta-agonists such as *albuterol* are used to manage bronchospasm if wheezing is present.

Monitoring and Observation

- Patients should be observed for 4–6 hours after an anaphylactic episode to monitor for the potential for a *biphasic reaction*, which can occur 4–12 hours after the initial event **(Fig. 34.2)**.
- Close monitoring of vital signs, respiratory function, and mental status is essential.
- *Criteria for discharge*: Patients should not be discharged until they are symptom free and have demonstrated stable vital signs.

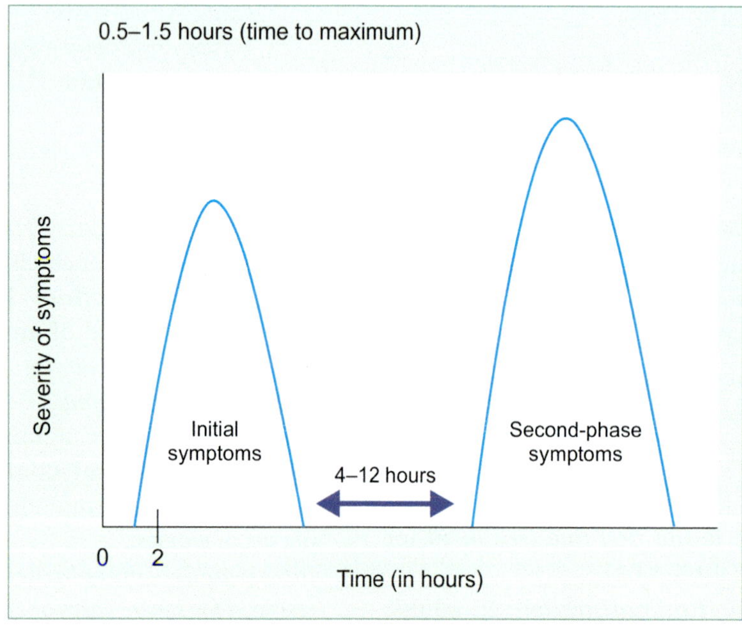

Fig. 34.2: Biphasic anaphylactic reaction.

PREVENTION AND LONG-TERM MANAGEMENT

Identifying and Avoiding Triggers

- *Detailed history:* A thorough patient history is critical to identify potential triggers.
- *Avoidance strategies:* Patient education on identifying allergens (e.g., reading food labels, avoiding known insect habitats)
- *Cross-contamination risks:* For food allergies, awareness of how allergens can spread in shared kitchens or restaurants is key.

Anaphylaxis Action Plans

- Creating a personalized emergency action plan is essential for at-risk individuals.
- The plan should include specific instructions on *when and how to use epinephrine*, along with clear guidance on when to seek emergency care.
- *Education:* Patients and caregivers must be educated on the *use of epinephrine autoinjectors*. This education is critical to ensure that the right dose is administered at the right time.

Desensitization and Immunotherapy

- *Oral immunotherapy (OIT):* An emerging treatment for food allergies, OIT involves the gradual administration of increasing amounts of the allergen under medical supervision. This approach has shown promise in reducing the severity of reactions over time.
- *Venom immunotherapy (VIT):* For insect sting allergies, VIT has proven highly effective in reducing the risk of anaphylaxis from future stings.
- *Safety considerations:* These therapies are still evolving, and safety protocols must be followed closely to prevent severe reactions during desensitization.

ADVANCES IN ANAPHYLAXIS RESEARCH AND EMERGING THERAPIES

Biologic and Targeted Therapies

Advances in immunology have led to the exploration of biologics (e.g., *omalizumab*) as adjunctive treatments. These drugs work by inhibiting IgE and mast cell activation, offering new hope for patients with severe or refractory anaphylaxis.

Epinephrine Delivery Devices

New methods for delivering adrenaline (epinephrine) for anaphylaxis aim to provide faster, more user-friendly options beyond traditional injections such as the EpiPen. The three significant developments are given as follows:

1. *Intranasal epinephrine spray (Neffy):* Approved by the Food and Drug Administration (FDA) in August 2024, Neffy is the first nasal spray for treating anaphylaxis. It provides a needle-free option for emergency use in adults and children weighing at least 30 kg (66 pounds). This delivery system addresses common barriers such as fear of injections, particularly in children. Studies have shown that Neffy delivers epinephrine with comparable efficacy to injected options, achieving similar blood concentration levels and therapeutic effects such as increased blood pressure. However, it comes with warnings about use in individuals with certain nasal conditions (e.g., nasal polyps).
2. *Wearable devices and patch technology:* Researchers are exploring wearable patches that administer epinephrine via the skin in emergencies. These devices aim to simplify adrenaline delivery by providing a less invasive and potentially more accessible solution, though most are still in development or trial phases.

3. *Autoinjector technologies:* New autoinjector technologies have made epinephrine more accessible, especially for children and those with physical limitations. Devices that include *autodosing features* or *clear instructions* improve user confidence and compliance.

Precision Medicine

New research focuses on *genetic and immunological biomarkers* to predict an individual's risk of anaphylaxis, leading to more tailored prevention strategies.

SUMMARY

Anaphylaxis remains a potentially fatal medical emergency that requires immediate recognition, prompt treatment, and long-term preventive strategies. As research continues, new therapies and diagnostic tools are improving outcomes, while greater public awareness and better patient education are key to reducing morbidity and mortality.

KEY POINTS

- Anaphylaxis is a severe, systemic hypersensitivity reaction that can rapidly become life-threatening, even in the absence of skin symptoms.
- The most common triggers include foods, medications, and insect stings, though idiopathic and exercise-induced cases also occur.
- Diagnosis is clinical (NIAID/WAO criteria); do not delay treatment to wait for labs.
- Epinephrine is the first-line treatment and must be administered intramuscularly without delay; adjunctive therapies are secondary.
- Observation is essential after an acute episode due to the risk of biphasic reactions, which may occur several hours later.
- Long-term management focuses on trigger avoidance, patient education, and provision of personalized anaphylaxis action plans with autoinjectors.
- Emerging therapies such as biologics, oral immunotherapy, and novel epinephrine delivery systems hold promise for improving patient outcomes

SUGGESTED READING

1. Cardona V, Ansotegui IJ, Ebisawa M, El-Gamal Y, Rivas MF, Fineman S, et al. World Allergy Organization Anaphylaxis Guidance 2020. World Allergy Organ J. 2020;13(10): 100472.
2. Golden DBK, Wang J, Waserman S, Akin C, Campbell RL, Ellis AK, et al. Anaphylaxis: A 2023 Practice Parameter Update. Ann Allergy Asthma Immunol. 2024;132(2):124-76.
3. Muraro A, Worm M, Alviani C, Cardona V, Galvin AD, Garvey LH, et al. EAACI guidelines: anaphylaxis (2021 update). Allergy. 2022;77(2):357-77.
4. Shaker MS, Wallace DV, Golden DBK, Oppenheimer J, Bernstein JA, Campbell RL, et al. Anaphylaxis—a 2020 practice parameter update, systematic review, and Grading of Recommendations, Assessment, Development and Evaluation (GRADE) analysis. J Allergy Clin Immunol. 2020;145(4):1082-123.
5. U.S. Food and Drug Administration. (2024). FDA Approves First Nasal Spray for Treatment of Anaphylaxis. [online] Available from https://www.fda.gov/news-events/press-announcements/fda-approves-first-nasal-spray-treatment-anaphylaxis. [Last accessed April, 2025].

35 CHAPTER

Allergic Conjunctivitis

Arjun V, Vivek Oommen Varghese

INTRODUCTION

Allergic conjunctivitis, which includes seasonal and perennial forms, is a common condition that affects sensitized individuals, particularly children and young adults. The prevalence rates can reach up to 40% in certain populations. A significant number of people with allergic conjunctivitis also have allergic rhinitis (60%), and there are additional associations with asthma, atopy, and dermatitis. Environmental factors such as passive smoke, pollution, and irritants can contribute to the development of allergic conjunctivitis. Seasonal allergic conjunctivitis is primarily caused by outdoor allergens, with peak exposure during pollen seasons, while perennial allergic conjunctivitis is associated with indoor allergens such as dust, dust mites, pets, and mold. Avoiding exposure to these allergens can reduce symptoms. Vernal keratoconjunctivitis (VKC), a more chronic form of allergic conjunctivitis, is more prevalent in younger males and is commonly seen in warmer climates, especially closer to the equator. It typically begins before the age of 10 years and often resolves by puberty, with a higher occurrence during spring and summer.

EPIDEMIOLOGY

The global prevalence of allergic conjunctivitis varies significantly based on geographic location, with incidence rates decreasing as distance from the equator increases. For example, India reports a prevalence of approximately 5%, while countries closer to the equator, such as Ethiopia and Egypt, have higher rates of 5–7 and 3%, respectively. In temperate climates, prevalence is significantly lower, with Italy reporting 0.27%, Sweden 0.087%, and Finland 0.03%.

PATHOPHYSIOLOGY

The conjunctival epithelium is primarily composed of epithelial cells with minimal cellular infiltration. In allergic conjunctivitis, mast cells and eosinophils migrate from the underlying stroma into the epithelium. Mast cells release preformed mediators such as tryptases and histamines, as well as newly synthesized mediators derived from arachidonic acid upon encountering allergens. VKC involves cytokine-induced cells, primarily interleukin-4 (IL-4)-producing CD4 T cells.

The ocular surface damage is caused by eosinophils, reaching the epithelium and releasing destructive proteins such as eosinophilic major basic proteins and cationic proteins. This cycle repeats, resulting in the production of giant papillae with fibroblastic and mucoid deposits on the surface. The destruction of the corneal epithelium is caused by the action of elastase. Following the destruction of the corneal epithelium, fibrin, which entangles the mucoid discharge, leads to the production of plaque. Further erosion of the epithelium, along with the deposition of fibroblasts and mucus, leads to the formation of shield ulcers. These ulcers are primarily an immune phenomenon, and they are responsive to steroids.

SIGNS AND SYMPTOMS

Allergic conjunctivitis typically presents with tearing, itching, and redness, often accompanied by edema. The nature of the discharge varies depending on the type of allergic conjunctivitis, with watery discharge common in seasonal and perennial cases and mucoid or ropy discharge characteristic of VKC. Itching is a predominant symptom in most cases, while conjunctival hyperemia and eyelid edema are often associated with redness. Chronic allergic conjunctivitis can lead to additional symptoms such as photophobia, ocular pain, vision impairment, and discharge. Persistent itching and pain may result in periorbital skin changes and lid drooping, and chronic edema can lead to conjunctival pigmentation, particularly in children. Tearing and photophobia are frequently associated with other vasomotor symptoms such as rhinitis and nasal secretions. Photophobia is a significant indicator of corneal epithelial involvement and severe disease activity, posing a risk of blinding complications and permanent vision damage. Conjunctival hyperemia, chemosis, papillae, and mucoid discharge are common clinical examination findings in allergic conjunctivitis. Chronic conjunctivitis may lead to perilimbal pigmentation, conjunctival scarring, and subconjunctival fibrosis. Corneal involvement in allergic conjunctivitis may start with epithelial stippling or erosions, progressing to macroerosions and shield ulcers if the condition worsens.

COMPLICATIONS

Vernal keratoconjunctivitis can lead to complications such as keratoconus, often caused by chronic eye rubbing. The indiscriminate use of corticosteroids, especially in individuals who are responsive to steroids, can raise the risk of steroid-induced glaucoma. In severe instances, VKC can lead to blinding complications, affecting 5–30% of patients.

Shield Ulcer

Untreated allergic conjunctivitis can lead to shield ulcers, which are classified using Cameron's grading system from grades 1 to 3. Grade 1 ulcers initially show a clear, eroded epithelial surface and severe photophobia. As the condition progresses, the ulcer base may become translucent or yellow, and in grade 3, an elevated plaque with underlying vascularization can develop. Grade 3 ulcers, a serious complication, often need both medical and surgical management, such as plaque removal and amniotic membrane transplantation.

Atopic Keratoconjunctivitis

Atopic conjunctivitis is a chronic and severe condition that affects both eyes and typically starts between the ages of 20 and 50 years. It is often linked to atopic dermatitis, occurring in about 25–42% of cases, and is more common in males than females. A personal or family history of atopic dermatitis is frequently seen in individuals with atopic conjunctivitis, and it is often triggered by a type 4 hypersensitivity reaction. In contrast to vernal or allergic conjunctivitis, atopic conjunctivitis, tends to occur during cold season.

MANAGEMENT

The management of allergic conjunctivitis is summarized using the ALAMS acronym:

Avoidance, lubricants, antihistamines, mast cell stabilizers, steroids, surgery, or supportive therapy.

Avoidance

Avoidance is crucial and involves minimizing exposure to allergens; washing the face, hands, and hair frequently; and wearing goggles to reduce allergen load. Patients should be advised to avoid eye rubbing, as it can worsen inflammation through mast cell degranulation and lead to complications such as keratoconus. Supportive measures include using preservative-free, refrigerated lubricants to flush out allergens and reduce inflammation, along with cold compresses to reduce vascularity and induce vasoconstriction. When using lubricants in allergic conjunctivitis, it is important to use preservative-free lubricants to prevent further damage to the ocular surface.

Alpha agonists can cause rebound redness and should be avoided in cases of chronic allergic conjunctivitis. Nonsteroidal anti-inflammatory drugs (NSAIDs) may worsen ocular surface damage, especially in cases with corneal involvement.

Medical Management

Antihistamines and Dual-action Agents

The primary pharmacological approaches to managing allergic conjunctivitis include antihistamines, mast cell stabilizers, and dual-acting agents.

Antihistamines competitively inhibit H1 receptors, inhibiting the release of histamine and other inflammatory mediators, leading to reduced vasodilation, edema, and itching. High-affinity H1 receptor antagonists provide rapid symptom relief but may take several weeks to achieve optimal efficacy. Mast cell stabilizers, such as cromolyn sodium, prevent mast cell degranulation and the subsequent release of inflammatory mediators, making them useful for preventing allergic reactions in individuals with known triggers. Dual-acting agents, combining antihistamine and mast cell-stabilizing properties, offer a convenient and effective approach to managing allergic conjunctivitis by providing immediate symptom relief and long-term protection. Topical medications such as alcaftadine, bepotastine, and olopatadine are commonly used, with the choice of medication and dosage depending on the severity of symptoms. While dual-acting agents and antihistamines often provide adequate relief, cromolyn sodium may be more suitable for individuals with perennial allergies.

Steroids

Topical corticosteroids are a valuable therapeutic option for allergic conjunctivitis as they inhibit phospholipase A2, suppressing the production of inflammatory mediators such as prostaglandins and cytokines. In addition, they directly affect mast cells and eosinophils, reducing their migration and differentiation. The choice of corticosteroid and dosage depends on the severity of inflammation and the presence of underlying ocular surface disease. For mild-to-moderate cases, surface corticosteroids such as fluorometholone or loteprednol may suffice. However, severe or refractory inflammation may require more potent corticosteroids such as prednisolone or dexamethasone. To minimize potential side effects, corticosteroids should be used judiciously and monitored closely to manage elevated intraocular pressure and posterior subcapsular cataracts. In cases requiring long-term corticosteroid therapy, lower dosages and intermittent dosing schedules are preferred. Steroid-sparing agents, such as antihistamines or mast cell stabilizers, can be used in conjunction with corticosteroids to reduce the overall steroid dosage and minimize potential side effects. By combining these approaches, clinicians can effectively manage allergic conjunctivitis while minimizing the risk of complications.

Supratarsal Steroids

In severe or refractory cases of VKC, supratarsal corticosteroids are used temporarily to suppress inflammation. The procedure involves eversion of the superior tarsus under aseptic conditions and appropriate anesthesia, followed by the creation of a subconjunctival bleb through injection of a local anesthetic. A parenteral corticosteroid, such as triamcinolone or dexamethasone, is then injected into the bleb. Supratarsal injections can significantly reduce inflammation, promote regression of tarsal papillae, and prevent further damage to the ocular surface. Patients need close monitoring for potential complications, including elevated intraocular pressure, eyelid necrosis, and subcutaneous fat atrophy. Since supratarsal corticosteroids offer temporary relief, long-term maintenance therapy with steroid-sparing agents is essential.

Immunomodulators

Immunomodulatory agents such as cyclosporine A and tacrolimus are commonly used instead of steroids for severe or refractory allergic conjunctivitis. These agents work by inhibiting lymphocyte activation and suppressing the release of inflammatory mediators. Cyclosporine, available in concentrations from 0.05 to 2%, is often used to treat allergic conjunctivitis, especially VKC. Long-term therapy is usually necessary to effectively control inflammation, and studies such as VEKTIS have shown that cyclosporine reduces symptoms, signs, and the need for rescue corticosteroids. Tacrolimus, another immunomodulatory agent, is a calcineurin inhibitor that has demonstrated effectiveness in managing refractory VKC. It is typically applied as an ointment once or twice daily and has been observed to reduce the size of conjunctival papillae. Tacrolimus may be considered when cyclosporine is ineffective or not well tolerated. Both cyclosporine and tacrolimus may cause local discomfort, such as stinging or burning sensations, upon application.

Immunotherapy

Immunotherapy and biological agents are alternative treatments for severe or refractory allergic conjunctivitis, particularly VKC. Immunotherapy involves administering allergen extracts to desensitize the immune system, and it is recommended for cases with a well-defined systemic allergic response. Both subcutaneous and sublingual immunotherapy have been proven to improve ocular surface conditions and reduce the need for rescue medications. While no significant side effects have been reported, the optimal method may vary based on individual patient factors.

Biologicals

Biological agents, such as monoclonal antibodies, offer targeted therapy for severe VKC. Omalizumab, an immunoglobulin E (IgE) inhibitor, has been effective in reducing signs and symptoms of VKC, especially in refractory cases. Dupilumab, an interleukin-4 receptor alpha inhibitor, has shown promising results in resolving shield ulcers, promoting corneal re-epithelialization and reducing giant papillae in atopic keratoconjunctivitis. It is important to note that the use of biological agents for allergic conjunctivitis is often off-label and should be considered in consultation with an allergist.

Surgery

Surgical intervention may be necessary for VKC or allergic keratoconjunctivitis, especially when giant papillae or shield ulcers are present. Giant papillae can be treated by excision with mitomycin C application or through ocular surface reconstruction using methods such as amniotic membrane, autologous conjunctival graft, or buccal mucosal graft in severe cases. Other techniques for reducing papillae include cryotherapy or carbon dioxide laser ablation. Shield ulcer management involves debridement of the ulcer and plaque removal, followed by amniotic membrane application to aid re-epithelialization. This process effectively removes thick mucoid discharge and promotes wound healing through the protective and proepithelializing properties of the amniotic membrane. In some cases, supratarsal corticosteroids may be used in combination with the procedure to reduce inflammation.

STEPLADDER APPROACH

Vernal keratoconjunctivitis can be graded from mild to severe, providing important information about the disease's severity and informing treatment decisions. Mild cases, which show symptoms, and mild papillae may need antihistamines as necessary. Moderate cases, characterized by corneal epithelial erosions, limbal papillae, inflammation, and Horner–Trantas dots, typically require topical corticosteroids to address the inflammation. Chronic moderate cases, with cobblestone papillae and ocular surface damage, often require long-term therapy with stronger corticosteroids or steroid-sparing agents. Severe cases, marked by macroerosions, conjunctival granulomas, and pannus formation, may need aggressive management. In severe cases, there is a risk of blinding complications such as shield ulcers, corneal scarring, and limbal stem cell deficiency. Recent recommendations a paradigm shift in protocol have led to the use of topical calcineurin inhibitors such as cyclosporine and tacrolimus as a primary treatment for chronic, intermittent, and severe keratoconjunctivitis. These agents offer potential benefits, including a favorable side effect profile and good tolerability, making them appealing alternatives to corticosteroids.

SUMMARY

Allergic conjunctivitis encompasses a spectrum of condition from benign, self-limiting seasonal illnesses to chronic, resistant conditions that might potentially be blinding, such as VKC. Treatment strategies vary based on disease severity, with a progressive approach starting from avoidance, medical therapy, and to surgical intervention.

KEY POINTS

- Allergic conjunctivitis is common in children and young adults and is often associated with rhinitis, asthma, and atopic dermatitis.
- It includes seasonal, perennial, vernal, and atopic types with symptoms such as itching, tearing, redness, and ropy discharge.
- Allergens activate mast cells and eosinophils, leading to inflammation and damage to the ocular surface.
- Severe cases can cause shield ulcers and even vision loss.
- Management involves avoidance of allergens, lubricants, antihistamines, mast cell stabilizers, steroids, and surgery if needed.
- Calcineurin inhibitors and biologicals are useful in chronic or severe cases, and surgery may be required in case of shield ulcers and giant papillae.

SUGGESTED READING

1. Aït-Khaled N, Pearce N, Anderson HR, Ellwood P, Montefort S, Shah J, et al. Global map of the prevalence of symptoms of rhinoconjunctivitis in children: the International Study of Asthma and Allergies in Childhood (ISAAC) phase three. Allergy. 2009;64(1):123-48.
2. Leonardi A, Silva D, Perez Formigo D, Bozkurt B, Sharma V, Allegri P, et al. Management of ocular allergy. Allergy. 2019;74(9):1611-30.
3. Mehta JS, Chen WL, Cheng ACK, Cung LX, Dualan IJ, Kekunnaya R, et al. Diagnosis, management, and treatment of vernal keratoconjunctivitis in Asia: recommendations from the management of vernal keratoconjunctivitis in Asia Expert Working Group. Front Med. 2022;9: 882240.
4. Villegas BV, Benitez-del-Castillo JM. Current knowledge in allergic conjunctivitis. Turk J Ophthalmol. 2021;51(1):45-54.

CHAPTER 36

Allergen Avoidance Measures

Soundarya M

INTRODUCTION

One of the important tenets in the management of allergies is the avoidance of the inciting allergen. This holds true more so for food and venom allergies than aeroallergens, as the risk of anaphylaxis is much higher even with small accidental exposures in food/venom allergies than exposure to aeroallergens. This chapter focuses on the main avoidance measures and steps that can be taken to minimize exposure to allergens.

AEROALLERGENS

Advantages of Aeroallergen Control

- To maintain the effectiveness of the treatment measures
- To help taper the medications
- To improve quality of life in children with respiratory allergies
- To prevent complications in childhood asthma
- To prevent development of allergies in future generation, i.e., control atopic march

This is also one of the most frequently asked questions by parents as to whether anything can be done from apart from medication.

Evidence states that sensitization to inhaled allergens in a 4-year-old child (19.2%) is much more common than sensitization to food allergens (3.5%). The recent ARIA guidelines 2020 show that the counseling regarding avoidance of the inciting allergen should be the first step in the management.

Allergen Control Measures

- *House dust mite (HDM):* Here, the fecal particles are the allergenic component.
  - *Control measures in bedroom*:
    - *Remove carpets and avoid velvet cushion/sofa covers:* These act as reservoirs for the HDM allergen, as the allergen is heavy and does not stay airborne for long.
    - Remove stuffed toys from bedroom
    - *Washing all bed/cushion linen in hot water weekly (140°F/65°C):* The hot water kills the mites and dislodges the mite allergen.
    - *Sun drying of bed mattresses:* The mites survive in the relative humidity of 35–40% and by sun drying, the mites die as the humidity is not amenable to its survival.
    - *Mite-proof covers:* A thread count of >246 per square inch implies a very tight weave through which mite allergens cannot come out and become airborne.
    - Use of feather pillows, rather than synthetic pillows, as the covers of feather pillows are more tightly woven.

- *Measures in whole house*:
  - *Vacuum cleaning:* This reduces dust disturbances. It is better done when the child is out of the house. A vacuum cleaner that is fitted with high-efficiency particulate air (HEPA) filter is better, so that the allergen does not get airborne.
  - *HEPA filters:* High-frequency particulate absorbers absorb 99.7% of particles, which are of 0.3 μm.
  - *Humidity control:* To be kept at 45% or less for 22 hours a day in air conditioning control or by using dehumidifiers
  - Wet mopping rather than dusting prevents the allergen from becoming airborne.
  - Remove/avoid upholstered furniture/curtains, and use vinyl/rexin covers/blinds
  - *Acaricides:* These have been described to be of use; however, they do not have any long-term use in the management of HDM.
  - *Air purifiers:* These are also described in the control measures; however, they are of limited use due to its short airborne period.

  Numerous studies have described the multitude of the measures given above in isolation and combination. Collating the evidence, multifaceted, individualized, home-based, comprehensive avoidance measures have consistently demonstrated a significant reduction of HDM allergens. However, maintaining this practice over time is of great importance in achieving success.

  Physicians should adopt a pragmatic approach to mite allergen avoidance and advise sensitized patients to implement a multifaceted set of measures to achieve as great a reduction in exposure as possible, in conjunction with adequate treatment.

- *Cockroach allergen:* The cockroach frass is the main allergenic component present in kitchens and areas of food storage.

Measures: Blocking entry of the cockroach, withholding sources of food/shelter of the pest along with extermination of the existent pest. The three main approaches for this are given as follows:

1. *To control sources of attraction for cockroaches:*
   a. Food sources in kitchen and in other rooms and cupboards must be kept clean and covered.
   b. Seal drains and points of entry such as cracks and garbage collections.
   c. Avoid piling of used utensils in sinks as these attract cockroaches.
2. *To exterminate the existent cockroaches*:
   a. Integrated pest management using gel baits that are impregnated with pesticides such as fipronil or indoxacarb.
   b. Use of sticky traps and baits
   c. Remove excess vegetation to prevent breeding of cockroaches
   d. Seal garbage collection areas
3. *To remove the cockroach antigen*:
   a. Vacuum cleaning with HEPA filters to remove the suspended airborne allergen.
   b. Removal of carpets and mattresses where cockroaches were found.
   c. Use of sticky baits traps for monitoring, so that the integrated measures can be redone at regular intervals.

Collating all the evidence after analyzing all the above measures in isolation or combination, evidence states that integrated pest control management, including baits in households, helps in the reduction of cockroach allergen; however, this has to be sustained as well as accompanied by adequate management of the asthma to have any significant benefit.

- *Pollens:* These are larger allergens having 2–20 μm in size and mainly cause allergic rhinitis.
    - Measures to control pollen exposure:
        - *Use of masks:* Mouth and nose masks (N95—95% of PM 2.5) help to protect against entry of the large pollen particles; however, very small pollens may still enter.
        - Nasal irrigation done regularly using normal saline/hypertonic saline helps to flush the adherent pollen particles from the nasal mucosa.
        - Bathing after coming from outside helps to remove pollens from skin and scalp.
        - Following pollen forecasts:
            - Staying indoors on high pollen count days
            - Staying indoors during thunderstorms, as the thunder and lightning tend to break the pollen grains suspended in the air into smaller, charged particles, which can precipitate asthma (thunderstorm asthma).
        - Reduction in pollution exposure, especially diesel exhaust particles (DEPs), helps to reduce the effect of pollen allergy, as the DEP acts as a carrier for the charged pollen grains. Using better transport facilities to avoid pollution or choosing work options that reduce the exposure to pollution.
- *Pet dander:* The main allergens are Can f 1 (dog), which is the heavier antigen but can be airborne, settles in house and on carpets and Fel d 1 (cat), which is a light antigen; however, it has a sticky nature, can remain airborne for days, carried around with wind, and attaches to carpets and upholstered furniture.
    - Control measures:
        - Remove carpeting and upholstered furniture, as these are reservoirs of the antigen.
        - Vacuum cleaning with HEPA filters
        - Removing the pet, if possible; though this is difficult, as most children do not want to give up their pet.
        - Regularly washing the pet helps to some extent; however, this is not useful as the only measure.
        - Air purifiers may help but are ineffective if pet is at home, and in case of Fel d 1, this proves even more ineffective as it is a sticky allergen.
        - No hypoallergenic breeds exist; hence, they must not be advised.
        - Neutering or spaying of pets has been attempted, as male cats produce more Fel d 1; however, there has not been much evidence of this being helpful.

        Upon collating all the studies on control measures of pet dander and their effectiveness, consensus is that a multifaceted approach, including frequent washing, cleaning the house, and using bed covers along with appropriate control of allergies, is more helpful than isolated measures.
- *Molds:* Mold spores are released in large numbers. *Mucor, Penicillium, Aspergillus, Rhizopus, Alternaria,* and *Cladosporium* are indoor fungi that thrive in dampness, darkness, and poor ventilation.

- Measures of control:
  - Avoid dampness and seal leaks: Humidity is one of the main harbingers for molds to grow and produce spores.
  - Dehumidifiers can help if ambient humidity is more as dryness reduces mold and spore concentration.
  - Improving ventilation and light in basements
  - Avoiding the use of saunas and pools till allergy is controlled and mold source is treated.
  - Treatment of the mold source with removal of the damp material, cleaning of the area, proofing with damp-proof materials, and use of HEPA filters in exhaust
  - Reduce plants and soil in the house as soil is one of the main sources of mold.

  Scientific evidence when collated states that good mold control has multiple benefits and reduces the asthma symptoms, ER visits, and medication scores, thereby improving quality of life. When this is combined with a multifaceted approach by controlling environmental tobacco smoke, HDM, and cockroach allergens, it significantly reduced asthma morbidity in children.

- *Rodent:* Typically, the mouse is the main rodent infestation. While coexisting with cockroach, evidence suggests that mouse allergen is the major allergen in urban cities with the main allergenic component being the mouse urinary antigen.

  Control measures: Integrated pest management is the main stay, which caters to multiple pest infestations. The main prongs are given as follows:
  - Removal of factors, such as food, that lead to rodent infestation
  - Thorough cleaning of areas of food cooking, consumption, and storage
  - Blocking pathways of rodent entry
  - Removal of rodents using traps and rodenticides

    When all scientific evidence is collated, it states that control of the mouse allergen is conflicting and difficult as various areas of exposures, in schools and homes, etc., are to be considered. Composite control measures that work include control of cockroach, mold, and mouse allergens in various environments is needed for better clinical benefit.

  Control of environmental pollution also goes a long way in reducing the allergenicity of pollens and in control of asthma, as pollutants themselves are irritants to airways and stimulate inflammation. The GINA guidelines 2023 state that:

- *Level A evidence:* Encouraging cessation of smoking among family members and to provide resources and help for achieving the same.
- *Level B evidence:* Encouraging people to use nonpolluting heating and cooking sources and for venting out sources of indoor pollution.

Other Allergens

In conditions such as allergies to occupational allergens, adequate barrier precautions must be used to avoid exposure, and measures to remove the allergen such as HEPA filters must be used.

Food and Venom Allergens

Food allergies can be life-threatening and cause anaphylaxis and despite the initial episodes being seemingly mild, any next exposure can result in severe anaphylaxis.

Hence, in food and venom exposures, the risk assessment is very important. In situations, where there is a high risk of accidental exposure, evaluation and desensitization are the best options. In situations where the risk of accidental exposure is low, avoidance of the allergen is the best option. It is also important to understand the cross-reactive antigens in these allergens and minimize their exposure as well to avoid the risk of anaphylaxis.

SUMMARY

Avoidance measures are a very important and integral part of control in childhood allergies along with the pharmacotherapy. The main control measures advised in the environment are for aeroallergens as other allergens are avoided at source, like food, drugs and venom. The most common aeroallergen is the house dust mite and this is mainly controlled by avoiding warm and humid environment in the house and removing the fecal mite particles by hot washing and using covers. Control of source of food and maintaining cleanliness near food spaces helps control the cockroach allergen. Good waterproofing, ventilation and removal of molds have proven to be the best evidence in asthma control due to mold. Similarly, controlling pollen exposure and pet dander contributes to optimum control in specific childhood respiratory allergies.

KEY POINTS

- Allergen avoidance measures help to control the inciting agent, and enhances the effect of the treatment measures and achieves optimum control.
- House dust mite allergen is very difficult to control and the concentration can be reduced by maintaining a dry and cool environment, using mite covers and removal of mite concentrating areas like carpets and upholstery.
- Cockroach antigen is controlled by keeping the kitchen and garbage collection clean and dry without food spillage and soiling. Use of sticky baits and integrated pest control helps in managing the cockroach allergies.
- Mold control by using damp-proofing, removal of the seepage source and keeping areas dry is well proven in controlling asthma.
- Control of outdoor allergens, such as pollen, is more difficult and using masks, staying indoors on high-pollen-count days may help.

SUGGESTED READING

1. Aggarwal P, Senthilkumaran S. Dust Mite Allergy. [Updated 2022 Aug 8]. In: StatPearls [Internet]. Treasure Island (FL): StatPearls Publishing; 2023. [online] Available from https://www.ncbi.nlm.nih.gov/books/NBK560718/. [Last accessed September, 2025]
2. Ahrens B, Posa D. Prevention of allergies in childhood - where are we now?. Allergol Select. 2017;1(2):200-13. Published 2017 Aug 4. doi:10.5414/ALX01807E.
3. Cipriani F, Calamelli E, Ricci G. Allergen Avoidance in Allergic Asthma. Front Pediatr. 2017;5:103. doi:10.3389/fped.2017.00103
4. De Lucca SD, Taylor DJ, O'Meara TJ, Jones AS, Tovey ER. Measurement and characterization of cockroach allergens detected during normal domestic activity. J Allergy Clin Immunol. 1999;104(3 Pt 1):672-80. doi: 10.1016/s0091-6749(99)70341-6. PMID: 10482845.
5. GINA Main report 2024.
6. Institute of Medicine (US) Committee on Damp Indoor Spaces and Health. Damp Indoor Spaces and Health. Washington (DC): National Academies Press (US); 2004.
7. Wilson JM, Platts-Mills TAE. Home Environmental Interventions for House Dust Mite. J Allergy Clin Immunol Pract. 2018;6(1):1-7. doi:10.1016/j.jaip.2017.10.003
8. Zuiani C, Custovic A. Update on House Dust Mite Allergen Avoidance Measures for Asthma. Curr Allergy Asthma Rep. 2020;20(9):50. doi:10.1007/s11882-020-00948-y

CHAPTER 37

Rational Use of Antiallergy Medications

Shambo S Samajdar

INTRODUCTION

The management of allergic disorders such as allergic rhinitis, asthma, urticaria, and conjunctivitis involves a wide variety of pharmacological agents. These medications range from first-line treatments such as antihistamines and corticosteroids to more specialized therapies such as biologics and immunotherapy. With the growing prevalence of allergic conditions globally, healthcare professionals must adopt a rational approach to the use of antiallergy medications. Rational drug use ensures that medications are used appropriately based on the patient's specific condition, at the correct dose, for the correct duration, and with careful consideration of adverse effects and interactions.

This chapter provides an overview of various drug classes used in allergy treatment, emphasizing appropriate prescribing practices for allergy specialists.

WORLD HEALTH ORGANIZATION PRINCIPLES OF RATIONAL MEDICATION USE

The World Health Organization (WHO) has outlined the core principles that ensure the rational use of medications given as follows:

- Right patient
- Right drug
- Right dose
- Right route
- Right time

These principles ensure that each patient receives treatment tailored to their specific conditions and needs while minimizing the risk of adverse drug reactions (ADRs) and preventing unnecessary drug use. Rational drug use is especially critical for allergy medications, where polypharmacy and inappropriate prescribing can lead to significant complications.

CLASSES OF ANTIALLERGY MEDICATIONS

Antihistamines

Antihistamines are the most commonly used class of medications for allergic conditions. They block histamine receptors (H1 receptors), reducing the effects of histamine, which is a major mediator in allergic reactions.

First-generation Antihistamines

First-generation antihistamines, such as diphenhydramine, hydroxyzine, and chlorpheniramine, are effective for short-term relief but have significant side effects due to their ability to cross the blood–brain barrier. These include sedation, cognitive impairment, and anticholinergic effects such as dry mouth and urinary retention.

Clinical use: These agents are mainly used in acute allergic reactions, such as urticaria and allergic rhinitis. However, due to their sedative properties, their use is generally limited to short-term applications.

Key considerations:

- *Elderly patients:* They should generally avoid first-generation antihistamines due to the increased risk of falls and confusion.
- *Pediatric use:* Promethazine is contraindicated in children under 2 years due to the risk of severe respiratory depression and other adverse effects.

Second-generation Antihistamines

Second-generation antihistamines, including cetirizine, loratadine, fexofenadine, and desloratadine, are preferred for long-term management due to their reduced sedative effects. These drugs selectively target peripheral H1 receptors and have a more favorable safety profile compared to first-generation agents.

Clinical use: Effective in managing chronic allergic rhinitis, chronic urticaria, and allergic conjunctivitis.

Table 37.1 includes data on routes of excretion, use in renal impairment, liver metabolism, potential drug interactions, and pregnancy safety categories.

Key considerations:

- *Renal impairment:*
    - *Levocetirizine:* It requires dose adjustment in patients with impaired kidney function; contraindicated in severe renal impairment.
    - *Bilastine, fexofenadine, and ebastine:* No significant adjustment needed in renal impairment
- *Liver impairment:*
    - *Desloratadine and fexofenadine:* Generally safe for use in patients with hepatic impairment
    - *Mizolastine and rupatadine:* Not recommended or contraindicated in patients with significant liver disease due to extensive hepatic metabolism.
- *Pregnancy:*
    - *Bilastine and fexofenadine:* Category B, considered relatively safe in pregnancy
    - *Loratadine:* Although classified as category B, some studies suggest an increased risk of hypospadias with maternal use.
- *Cardiovascular concerns:*
    - *Ebastine, mizolastine, and rupatadine:* Should be used with caution in patients with preexisting cardiovascular conditions, particularly those prone to QT prolongation or electrolyte imbalances.

Cysteinyl Leukotriene Receptor Antagonists

Leukotriene receptor antagonists, such as montelukast, block the action of leukotrienes, which are inflammatory mediators that contribute to asthma, allergic rhinitis, and other allergic conditions. Montelukast is particularly useful in patients who have both asthma and allergic rhinitis.

Clinical Use

Montelukast is approved for the treatment of asthma, allergic rhinitis, and exercise-induced bronchoconstriction. It is also indicated in patients with aspirin-exacerbated respiratory disease (AERD).

Key Considerations

- *Neuropsychiatric effects:* Montelukast has been associated with neuropsychiatric side effects such as mood changes, anxiety, and suicidal thoughts, particularly in children.

TABLE 37.1: Comprehensive prescribing considerations for second-generation antihistamines.

Drugs	*Fecal excretion*	*Renal excretion*	*Liver metabolism*	*Use in renal impairment*	*Use in hepatic impairment*	*Pregnancy category*	*Cardiovascular considerations*
Bilastine	67%	33%	No	Not necessary	No dose adjustment needed	B	None in particular
Desloratadine	47%	45%	Extensive (3-hydroxydesloratadine)	Use with caution in serious kidney failure	Not necessary	C	None in particular
Ebastine	66%	None	Extensive (CYP3A4, CYP2J, CYP4F)	No dose adjustment needed	Not necessary for mild/moderate impairment; do not exceed 10 mg in severe impairment	C	Use with caution in patients with prolonged QT interval or hypokalemia
Fexofenadine	80%	11%	Minimal (5%)	No dose adjustment needed	Not necessary	B	None in particular
Levocetirizine	13%	85%	Minimal (14%)	Adjust dose according to creatinine clearance; contraindicated if <10 mL/min	No dose adjustment necessary	B	None in particular
Mizolastine	84–95%	8–15%	Extensive (>65%, UGT, CYP3A4)	No specific guidance	Contraindicated in serious hepatic impairment	B	Contraindicated in patients with significant cardiac illness or arrhythmias
Rupatadine	61%	35%	Extensive (CYP3A4, biliary elimination)	Use with caution due to lack of experience	Not recommended in serious hepatic impairment	C	Use with caution in patients with prolonged QT interval, hypokalemia, or arrhythmias

- *Efficacy:* While montelukast is beneficial in managing mild-to-moderate asthma, it is not as effective as inhaled corticosteroids (ICSs) and is typically used as an adjunct therapy.

Corticosteroids

Corticosteroids are potent anti-inflammatory agents that play a critical role in the management of severe allergic reactions, asthma, and chronic allergic conditions. They inhibit inflammatory cytokines and mediators, thereby reducing inflammation and immune responses.

Inhaled Corticosteroids

Inhaled corticosteroids, such as fluticasone and budesonide, are the cornerstone of long-term asthma management. They target airway inflammation and are highly effective in controlling symptoms and preventing exacerbations.

Clinical use: ICSs are indicated for patients with persistent asthma and allergic rhinitis. They are often combined with long-acting beta-agonists (LABAs) for better symptom control in moderate-to-severe asthma.

Key considerations:

- *Adverse effects:* Long-term use of ICS can cause oral candidiasis (thrush) and, at high doses, may lead to systemic side effects such as adrenal suppression and osteoporosis.
- *Patient education:* Proper inhaler technique, including the use of spacers, is essential to minimize local side effects such as throat irritation and hoarseness.

Systemic Corticosteroids

Systemic corticosteroids, such as prednisone and methylprednisolone, are reserved for the management of severe allergic reactions or acute asthma exacerbations.

Clinical use: Short courses of systemic corticosteroids are used in acute exacerbations of asthma or severe allergic conditions such as angioedema and anaphylaxis.

Key considerations:

- *Short-term use:* Systemic corticosteroids should only be used for short periods to avoid serious side effects such as adrenal suppression, hyperglycemia, and hypertension.
- *Tapering:* Gradual dose reduction is necessary when discontinuing long-term corticosteroid therapy to prevent adrenal insufficiency.

Immunotherapy

Allergen immunotherapy (AIT) involves gradually exposing patients to increasing doses of allergens to desensitize their immune system and reduce allergic reactions over time. AIT is the only disease-modifying treatment for allergic conditions such as allergic rhinitis and allergic asthma.

Subcutaneous Immunotherapy

Administered via injections, subcutaneous immunotherapy (SCIT) is highly effective but carries a risk of systemic allergic reactions, including anaphylaxis.

Sublingual Immunotherapy

It involves placing allergen tablets or drops under the tongue. Sublingual immunotherapy (SLIT) has a better safety profile compared to SCIT, though it requires longer treatment durations and daily administration.

Key Considerations

- *Patient selection:* AIT is typically reserved for patients with moderate-to-severe allergic rhinitis or asthma who are not adequately controlled with pharmacotherapy.

- *Risk of anaphylaxis:* SCIT should be administered in a controlled setting where immediate medical intervention is available in case of systemic reactions.

Biologic Therapies

Biologics represent a more targeted approach to managing severe allergic diseases by modulating specific immune pathways involved in the allergic response.

Omalizumab (Anti-immunoglobulin E)

Omalizumab is a monoclonal antibody that binds to immunoglobulin E (IgE), preventing it from activating mast cells and basophils. It is indicated for patients with severe persistent asthma and chronic idiopathic urticaria that are not well controlled with standard therapies.

Clinical use: Omalizumab is used in patients with elevated IgE levels who experience frequent exacerbations despite high-dose inhaled corticosteroids.

Key considerations:
- *Administration:* Omalizumab is administered subcutaneously every 2–4 weeks depending on the patient's weight and IgE levels.
- *Adverse effects:* There is a small risk of anaphylaxis, so administration should occur in a setting equipped to manage allergic reactions.

Mepolizumab and Benralizumab (Anti-interleukin-5)

Mepolizumab and benralizumab are monoclonal antibodies that target interleukin-5 (IL-5), a cytokine responsible for eosinophilic inflammation in asthma.

Clinical use: These biologics are indicated for patients with severe eosinophilic asthma, particularly those who continue to have exacerbations despite standard therapy.

Key considerations:
- *Eosinophil monitoring:* Eosinophil levels should be monitored to evaluate treatment response.
- *Administration:* Both drugs are administered subcutaneously; benralizumab requires an initial loading phase followed by less frequent maintenance dosing.

Additional considerations:
- *Blood eosinophil count:* Mepolizumab and benralizumab are particularly indicated in patients with elevated eosinophil counts (≥150 cells/μL).
- *Coexisting conditions:*
  - *Omalizumab:* Suitable for patients with chronic urticaria, allergic rhinitis, or chronic rhinosinusitis (CRS)
  - *Dupilumab:* Effective for patients with CRS and nasal polyposis, particularly those with atopic dermatitis

Dosing and frequency:
- *Benralizumab:* After an initial three-dose loading phase (every 4 weeks), the dosing frequency is reduced to every 8 weeks for long-term maintenance.
- *Omalizumab:* Dosing is highly individualized based on body weight and IgE levels, with administration occurring every 2–4 weeks.

Mechanism of action: Omalizumab works by blocking IgE from binding to its receptors on mast cells, preventing allergic inflammation.
- Mepolizumab and benralizumab target IL-5 or its receptor, directly affecting eosinophils involved in the inflammatory response.
- Dupilumab inhibits both IL-4 and IL-13, blocking type 2 inflammatory pathway, which is key in conditions such as atopic dermatitis.

Table 37.2 consolidates all the important information regarding biologics used

TABLE 37.2: Comprehensive overview of biologics for asthma and allergic disorders: Indications, dosing, and key considerations.

Biologics	*Indication*	*Age group*	*Onset*	*Allergy prerequisite*	*Dominant biomarker*	*Coexisting conditions*	*Dose*	*Frequency*
Omalizumab (Anti-IgE)	Severe allergic asthma	Children, adolescents, and young adults	Childhood	IgE sensitization to perennial allergens	Serum total IgE (for dosing)	Allergic rhinitis, chronic rhinosinusitis (CRS) with nasal polyps and chronic urticaria	75–375 mg SC (dose depends on weight and IgE levels)	Every 2 or 4 weeks
Mepolizumab (Anti-IL-5)	Severe eosinophilic asthma	Adults	Adulthood	Irrespective of allergy	Increased blood eosinophil count	CRS with nasal polyps	100 mg SC (pen autoinjector)	Every 4 weeks
Benralizumab (Anti-IL-5R)	Severe eosinophilic asthma	Adults	Adulthood	Irrespective of allergy	Increased blood eosinophil count (>150 cells/μL)	CRS with nasal polyps	30 mg SC	First three doses every 4 weeks and then every 8 weeks
Dupilumab (anti-IL-4/IL-13)	Type 2 inflammation in asthma and dermatitis	Adults	Adulthood	Irrespective of allergy	Type 2 inflammation markers	CRS with nasal polyps, atopic dermatitis, and chronic urticaria	Varies based on clinical trial	Varies based on clinical trial

(IgE: immunoglobulin E; IL-5: interleukin-5)

for managing severe asthma and related conditions, highlighting key prescribing considerations for allergy specialists.

Mast Cell Stabilizers

Mast cell stabilizers, such as cromolyn sodium and nedocromil, prevent the release of histamine and other mediators from mast cells. These agents are primarily used for the prophylactic treatment of asthma and allergic rhinitis.

Clinical Use

Cromolyn is especially effective in preventing exercise-induced bronchoconstriction and managing allergic rhinitis in pediatric populations.

Key Considerations

- *Prophylactic use:* Mast cell stabilizers are not suitable for acute relief of symptoms and must be used preventively.
- *Safety profile:* These drugs have a favorable safety profile and are well tolerated, making them ideal for use in children and pregnant women.

Decongestants

Decongestants, such as pseudoephedrine and phenylephrine, provide short-term relief from nasal congestion by constricting nasal blood vessels. However, they are associated with significant side effects, particularly cardiovascular complications.

Clinical Use

Decongestants are often used for acute relief of nasal congestion in allergic rhinitis, but prolonged use is discouraged due to the risk of rebound congestion (rhinitis medicamentosa).

Key Considerations

- *Short-term use:* Decongestants should not be used for >5–7 days to avoid rebound effects.
- *Cardiovascular risks:* Patients with hypertension, arrhythmias, or other cardiovascular conditions should avoid decongestants due to their sympathomimetic effects.

Others (Vitamin D and Crisaborole)

Emerging evidence suggests that vitamin D may play a role in modulating immune response in allergic conditions. Vitamin D supplementation has shown promise in improving asthma control and reducing the severity of allergic rhinitis.

Crisaborole, a phosphodiesterase-4 (PDE-4) inhibitor, is used primarily in the management of atopic dermatitis. It helps reduce inflammation and pruritus in mild-to-moderate cases.

CONCLUSION

The rational use of antiallergy medications is essential for optimizing therapeutic outcomes and ensuring patient safety. Allergy specialists must tailor treatments to individual patient needs, taking into account the severity of the allergic condition, comorbidities, and potential adverse effects. The introduction of biologics and immunotherapy has expanded the therapeutic landscape for patients with severe allergic diseases, offering new avenues for disease control. By adhering to the principles of rational medication use, healthcare providers can effectively manage allergic disorders while minimizing the risks of adverse effects and drug interactions.

KEY POINTS

- This chapter covers the rational use of various pharmacological treatments for allergic disorders, including antihistamines, corticosteroids, leukotriene receptor antagonists, biologics, and immunotherapy.
- The WHO's principles of correct dosing, patient selection, and minimizing adverse reactions guide rational drug use for optimal therapeutic outcomes.
- First-generation antihistamines are effective but have sedative effects, while second-generation antihistamines are safer for long-term use.
- Biologics and immunotherapy have advanced as effective treatments for severe allergies, particularly in asthma and CRS patients.
- Special consideration is required for patients with renal or hepatic impairment to avoid drug interactions and adverse effects.

SUGGESTED READING

1. Barnes PJ. Pulmonary pharmacology. In: Brunton LL, Knollmann BC (Eds). Goodman & Gilman's: The Pharmacological Basis of Therapeutics, 14th edition. New York: McGraw-Hill Education; 2023.
2. Morita H, Matsumoto K, Saito H. Biologics for allergic and immunologic diseases. J Allergy Clin Immunol. 2022;150(4):766-77.
3. Randall KL, Hawkins CA. Antihistamines and allergy. Aust Prescr. 2018;41(2):41-5.
4. Samajdar SS, Moitra S, Sarkar S, Tripathi SK. Efficacy and safety of subcutaneous vs. sublingual immunotherapy in allergic rhinitis: a systematic review and meta-analysis. Clin Exp Allergy. 2025;55:199-201.
5. Samajdar SS, Moitra S. Advancing allergy practice in India for respiratory physician. J Assoc Chest Physicians. 2024;12(2):51-61.

CHAPTER 38

Sublingual Immunotherapy

Shilpa Nayak

INTRODUCTION AND HISTORICAL BACKGROUND

Allergen immunotherapy (AIT) is increasingly recognized as a crucial approach to managing allergy-related disorders, which currently affect approximately one third of the global population. While conventional antiallergic medications primarily focus on symptom control, they do not provide a cure or prevent the allergic march. In contrast, AIT is the only disease-modifying treatment for individuals with established immunoglobulin E (IgE)-mediated hypersensitivity to common allergens, such as pollens, house dust mites, and insect venom.

The evolution of AIT can be traced through several key milestones.

Early Foundations (Late 19th Century)

The scientific foundations for AIT were laid in the late 19th century when Charles Blackley (1873) demonstrated that pollen was a primary cause of hay fever. He developed skin and provocation tests to measure sensitization.

H Holbrook Curtis (1899) published an article on "The immunizing Cure of hay Fever," where he used subcutaneous injections of pollen extracts to treat patients. This early attempt at immunotherapy highlighted the potential of using allergens to modify immune responses.

Birth of Modern Immunotherapy (Early 20th Century)

A pivotal moment in AIT history occurred in 1911 when Leonard Noon published findings demonstrating that repeated subcutaneous injections of grass pollen extract could reduce sensitivity in individuals with hay fever. This study is often regarded as the formal introduction of AIT as a treatment modality.

Following Noon, Freeman conducted further studies in Europe, confirming that AIT could alleviate symptoms of allergic rhinitis and asthma during pollen seasons, thus establishing its clinical relevance.

Development and Standardization (Mid-20th Century)

Frankland performed the first double-blind placebo-controlled trials, establishing evidence-based practices for AIT.

SUBLINGUAL IMMUNOTHERAPY

In recent years, sublingual immunotherapy (SLIT) has emerged as a safe and effective alternative to traditional subcutaneous methods. This route offers greater convenience for patients while maintaining efficacy in desensitizing against allergens.

Instead of delivering the medication through injections under the skin (subcutaneously), it is placed under the tongue (sublingually). The dosage is gradually increased, allowing the body to build a tolerance to the allergen over time. This approach can effectively decrease sensitivity, leading to a reduction in the severity of symptoms and the frequency of allergy attacks.

Sublingual immunotherapy is a prominent form of AIT that has been extensively studied and shown to significantly reduce allergy symptoms compared to placebo. Research indicates that SLIT not only alleviates symptoms during the treatment period but may also provide lasting relief even after the treatment has ended. This characteristic positions immunotherapy as the only disease-modifying treatment available for allergies, underscoring its vital role in managing allergic conditions.

Indications

Aeroallergen immunotherapy should be considered for patients experiencing symptoms of *allergic rhinitis, rhinoconjunctivitis, and/or asthma* following natural exposure to allergens, particularly if they demonstrate specific IgE antibodies to relevant allergens. The decision to initiate immunotherapy should take into account the severity of the disease, the risk-benefit ratio, and the physician's ability to correlate clinical symptoms with appropriate allergy testing results. Initiating AIT early in the course of allergic disease may enhance its preventive benefits.

Potential Indications

- Atopic dermatitis
- Food allergy
- Oral allergy syndrome

Allergen immunotherapy is *not indicated* for conditions such as:

- Urticaria
- Angioedema

Key Factors in Patient Selection for Allergen Immunotherapy

The decision to initiate AIT is influenced by several critical factors, primarily related to patient selection. Proper identification of suitable candidates is essential for maximizing treatment efficacy and minimizing risks.

Allergic History and Diagnosis

Candidates should have a well-documented history of allergic conditions, ideally confirmed through current international diagnostic guidelines. A history of IgE-mediated allergies, such as allergic rhinitis or asthma, should typically span at least 2 consecutive years for seasonal allergies or 1 year for perennial allergies.

Allergen Sensitization

Patients often exhibit sensitization to multiple allergens, making it crucial to target specific allergens relevant to their symptoms. A detailed allergy profile, including skin testing and serum IgE levels, is necessary to confirm the causal role of identified allergens.

Severity and Persistence of Symptoms

The patient must demonstrate significant symptoms related to their allergies before starting AIT. This requirement ensures that therapy addresses substantial clinical issues rather than being initiated based on transient or mild symptoms.

Previous Treatments

Patients who have undergone AIT for the same or cross-reacting allergens within the past 5 years are generally excluded from new immunotherapy programs. This exclusion helps avoid potential adverse reactions and ensures the effectiveness of the therapy.

Comorbid Conditions

The presence of other medical conditions can affect both the safety and efficacy of AIT. For instance, patients with mastocytosis may be at higher risk for severe reactions during insect venom immunotherapy and require careful evaluation before enrollment.

Patient Preferences and Expectations

Understanding patient expectations regarding treatment outcomes is vital. Factors such as sociodemographic data, previous treatment experiences, and perceived benefits significantly influence the decision-making process for both patients and healthcare providers.

Environmental Considerations

Geographical location and environmental factors influencing allergen exposure must be considered when selecting allergens for immunotherapy. This includes seasonal variations in pollen levels and other local allergenic sources. In summary, a comprehensive evaluation encompassing allergic history, sensitization patterns, symptom severity, prior treatments, comorbidities, patient preferences, and environmental factors is crucial for selecting appropriate candidates for AIT.

Mechanism of Sublingual Immunotherapy (Figs. 38.1A and B)

- SLIT is associated with the retention of allergens in sublingual mucosa for several hours.
- Early increase in antigen-specific IgE and blunting of seasonal IgE.
- Persistent increase in antigen-specific IgG4- and IgE-blocking activity that parallel long-term clinical benefits of both subcutaneous immunotherapy (SCIT) and SLIT.
- Inhibition of eosinophils and reduction of adhesion molecules in target organs.
- An early (at 4–12 weeks) increase in peripheral phenotypic Tregs and delayed (at 12 months) immune deviation in favor of Th1 responses.
- Tregs are a specialized subset of CD4+ T cells recognized for their suppressive functions, primarily mediated through the secretion of anti-inflammatory cytokines such as *interleukin-10 (IL-10)* and *transforming growth factor-β (TGF-β)* and through inhibitory surface molecules such as *cytotoxic T-lymphocyte-associated antigen 4* (*CTLA-4)* and *programmed death 1* (*PD-1)*.
- Detection of CD25 + FOXP + phenotypic Treg cells in the sublingual mucosa
- Alterations in dendritic cell markers (e.g., increase in expression of complement component C1Q) that correlate with clinical response to treatment and merit further study.
- Clinical efficacy of SLIT biomarkers that are predictive of or surrogates for the clinical response to immunotherapy is not currently available for routine use.
- *Clinical outcomes post-AIT:* Following a successful course of AIT, there is often a correction of previously dysregulated Treg responses, which correlate with improved clinical outcomes for patients. This restoration of Treg function is vital for achieving long-term tolerance to allergens and may prevent new sensitizations, features consistent with the induction of tolerance.

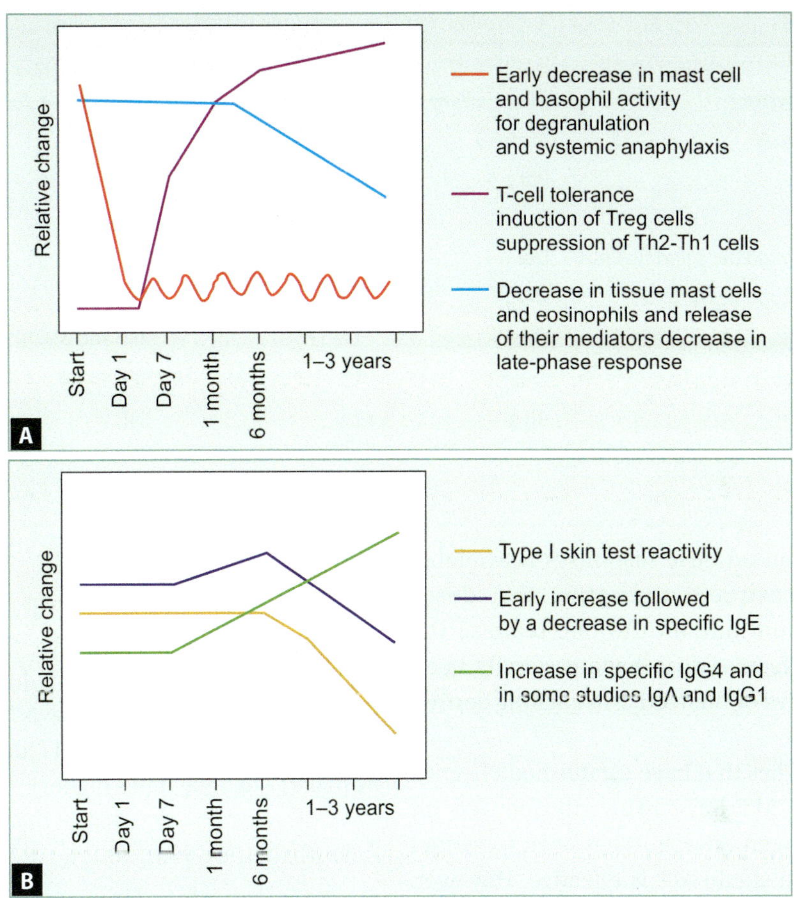

Figs. 38.1A and B: Steps in allergen-specific immunotherapy and their underlying mechanisms. (IgA: immunoglobulin A; IgE: immunoglobulin E; IgG1: immunoglobulin G1; IgG4: immunoglobulin G4)

Optimum/Effective Dose

Effective Dose of Individual Allergens for Subcutaneous Immunotherapy (Table 38.1)

A significant challenge in discussing doses for AIT is the variability in how allergen extract strength is expressed. Some expressions, such as weight by volume and protein nitrogen units, do not correlate with allergenic potency, which is defined as the quantity of allergenic proteins per unit volume of extract. Even when relevant measures are employed—such as skin testing reactions or in vitro inhibition assays—the units used can vary by company or regulatory agency, making them noninterconvertible. Additionally, measures of total allergenic potency often fail to identify differences in the relative amounts of major allergens within the extract. Despite these limitations, effective doses can be expressed as the quantity of the major allergen delivered as a maintenance dose. This method typically reveals a relatively narrow range of effective doses (3-20 μg of major allergen), with notable exceptions such as *Alternaria*, where significant improvement was achieved with only 1.6 μg of the major allergen Alt a 1.

TABLE 38.1: The effective dose of individual allergens for SCIT.			
Allergen extract	***Major allergen***	***Effective dosing (µg)***	***Less effective or ineffective dosing (µg)***
Short ragweed	Amb a 1	6–24	0.6 and 2
Timothy	Phl p 5	15 and 20	2[8]
Birch	Bet v 1	3.28 and 12	ND
Dermatophagoides pteronyssinus	Der p 1	7 and 12	0.7
Dermatophagoides farinae	Der f 1	10	ND
Cat dander	Fel d 1	11–17	0.6 and 3
Dog dander	Can f 1	15	0.6 and 3
Alternaria	Alt a 1	1.6	ND

(SCIT: subcutaneous immunotherapy)

Information on dose responses is available for most extracts, indicating that doses ranging from one fifth to one tenth of the proven effective dose have generally been less effective or ineffective in eliciting desired responses.

All studies that have established effective doses for AIT have primarily focused on single allergen extracts. It has been suggested that only a single AIT is effective. However, research conducted by Lowell and Franklin, as well as Franklin and Lowell, demonstrated the effectiveness of immunotherapy by manipulating the dose of ragweed in patients receiving extracts that included ragweed along with multiple other allergens. Additionally, the classic study by Johnstone and Crump showed that higher doses of multiple allergens were effective in treating childhood asthma, while lower doses were either less effective or provided no benefit.

At present, there is no universally accepted dosing schedule for SLIT, but it is recognized that SLIT doses are generally higher than those used in SCIT. The key comparisons between SLIT and SCIT dosing are given below.

Dosing Characteristics of Sublingual Immunotherapy

Individual SLIT doses can range from *0.0006 to 21 times* an individual SCIT dose, but the median monthly SLIT dose is ~49 times higher than the median SCIT dose (range from 0.017 to >500 times higher).

Administration Frequency

- *SLIT:* Typically administered daily after an initial dose given in a clinical setting
- *SCIT:* Administered monthly, requiring regular visits to a healthcare provider for injections.

Efficacy and Safety

Sublingual immunotherapy has emerged as a significant treatment modality for allergic rhinitis and asthma, demonstrating substantial efficacy in clinical trials.

Clinical Evidence Supporting Sublingual Immunotherapy

Efficacy in Allergic Rhinitis and Asthma

Numerous randomized controlled trials (RCTs) have established that SLIT significantly improves symptoms and reduces medication use in patients suffering from allergic rhinitis and asthma. A meta-analysis indicated that SLIT effectively decreases asthma symptom scores and reliance on rescue medications.

A systematic review highlighted that SLIT can prevent new sensitizations and the onset of asthma in patients with allergic rhinitis, particularly when treated with grass pollen extracts.

Long-term Benefits

Randomized controlled clinical trials with dust mite and pollen SLIT have demonstrated significant improvement in symptoms and medication use in patients with allergic rhinitis and asthma.

Effectiveness Across Age Groups

Meta-analyses confirm that SLIT is effective for both adults and children with allergic rhinitis and asthma. The therapy has shown comparable efficacy to traditional SCIT, albeit with a better safety profile.

Sublingual immunotherapy is increasingly favored for its safety profile compared to SCIT. SLIT must be administered by physicians with specialized training in allergy treatment. Patients must be well-informed about managing potential adverse reactions, handling unexpected treatment interruptions, and recognizing when to pause therapy.

Adverse Reactions

Local Reactions

The majority of adverse events associated with SLIT are localized and typically mild. Common local reactions include:

- *Oral symptoms:* Oromucosal pruritus, dysgeusia (altered taste), glossodynia (tongue pain), swollen tongue, mucosal edema, pharyngeal irritation, ear pruritus, lip swelling, mouth ulceration, and throat irritation
- *Gastrointestinal symptoms:* Nausea, vomiting, upper abdominal pain, lower abdominal pain, and diarrhea.

These local reactions often occur at the beginning of treatment and usually resolve within a few days or weeks without the need for medical intervention.

Systemic Reactions

While systemic side effects are rare, there have been isolated reports of anaphylaxis associated with SLIT. These cases have not resulted in fatalities. The risk factors for severe adverse events during SLIT remain largely undefined; however, patients with a history of systemic reactions to SCIT may be at an increased risk for similar responses during SLIT.

Severity of Reactions

In a study involving children receiving SLIT for multiple allergens, 92.5% of reported side effects were mild and self-resolving. Only a small fraction required medical advice due to moderate severity.

The overall incidence of serious adverse events (SAEs) during SLIT is low; estimates suggest that no more than 1 in 100 individuals will experience an SAE.

Need for Standardized Reporting of Side Effects

There is a pressing need for a standardized system to report adverse reactions related to AIT in both clinical and research settings. To address this, a classification system has been developed to grade local reactions from SLIT, aimed at standardizing reporting practices and helping the clinician to make informed decisions **(Table 38.2)**.

TABLE 38.2: WAO grading system for SLIT local adverse events.

Symptom/sign	*Grade 1—mild*	*Grade 2—moderate*	*Grade 3—severe*	*Unknown severity*
• Pruritus/swelling of mouth, tongue, or lip • Throat irritation • Nausea • Abdominal pain • Vomiting • Diarrhea • Heartburn • Uvular edema	• Not troublesome *And* • No symptomatic treatment required *And* • No discontinuation of SLIT because of local side effects	• Troublesome *Or* • *Requires symptomatic treatment* *And* • No discontinuation of SLIT because of local side effects	• Grade 2 *And* • *SLIT discontinued because of local side effects*	The treatment is discontinued, but there is no subjective and/or objective description of the severity from the patient/physician

Each local adverse event can be early (<30 minutes) or delayed

(SLIT: sublingual immunotherapy; WAO: World Allergy Organization)

Unmet Needs in Sublingual Immunotherapy

- Current optimal maintenance regimens are established only for specific allergens, namely grass, dust mites, and ragweed
- Lack of standardized regimens for seasonal allergies
- Insufficient research on mixed SLIT
- Need for allergen extract standardization
- Undefined duration for long-term effects.

SUMMARY

- Allergen immunotherapy (AIT) is the only disease-modifying treatment for IgE-mediated allergic conditions. Unlike conventional medications, AIT not only controls symptoms but also alters the natural course of allergic disease and provides long-term benefits even after treatment ends.
- AIT is recommended for patients with *allergic rhinitis, rhinoconjunctivitis, or asthma* with confirmed IgE sensitization to relevant allergens. Early initiation can improve preventive outcomes. Careful assessment of allergic history, allergen sensitization, symptom severity, comorbidities, previous treatments, and environmental exposure is crucial for selecting suitable candidates. AIT is not indicated for conditions like *urticaria.*
- SLIT promotes immune tolerance by increasing allergen-specific IgG4 and regulatory T cells, reducing eosinophil activity, and shifting immune responses toward Th1 pathways. These immunologic changes correlate with *long-term symptom control* and prevention of new sensitizations.
- SCIT (injections) delivers allergens monthly at lower doses, while SLIT requires *daily administration* at comparatively higher doses. Both methods show proven efficacy, though SLIT offers better safety and patient convenience.
- Randomized controlled trials and meta-analyses confirm SLIT's effectiveness in reducing symptoms, medication use, and risk of new sensitizations in adults and children. Most side effects are mild and local (oral or gastrointestinal); systemic reactions are rare but require physician oversight. A standardized grading system for adverse events has been developed to improve reporting.
- Key gaps remain in the standardization of allergen extracts, optimal dosing

schedules for mixed allergens, and duration of maintenance therapy. Further research is needed to refine these aspects and maximize AIT's potential.

KEY POINTS

- *Disease-modifying role:* Allergen immunotherapy (AIT) is the only treatment that alters the natural course of IgE-mediated allergic diseases, unlike symptomatic drugs, and provides long-term benefits even after discontinuation.
- *Patient selection:* AIT is indicated for allergic rhinitis, rhinoconjunctivitis, and asthma with confirmed IgE sensitization. Careful assessment of allergy history, severity, comorbidities, and environmental exposures is essential for identifying suitable candidates.
- *Mechanism of SLIT:* Sublingual immunotherapy (SLIT) induces tolerance by enhancing IgG4 and Treg activity, reducing eosinophilic inflammation, and shifting immune responses toward Th1, leading to sustained clinical improvement and prevention of new sensitizations.
- *Dosing and administration:* SCIT involves monthly injections at lower doses, whereas SLIT requires daily sublingual dosing at comparatively higher cumulative doses, offering greater safety and convenience.
- *Efficacy and safety:* Multiple RCTs and meta-analyses confirm SLIT's effectiveness in adults and children for reducing symptoms, medication use, and preventing asthma onset. Most side effects are mild and local; systemic reactions are rare but require monitoring.
- *Unmet needs:* Standardization of allergen extracts, optimized dosing for mixed allergens, and defining long-term maintenance regimens remain gaps, highlighting the need for further research to maximize AIT's potential.

SUGGESTED READING

1. Akdis M, Akdis CA. Mechanisms of allergen-specific immunotherapy. J Allergy Clin Immunol. 2007;119(4):780-9.
2. Blackley CH. Experimental Researches on the Causes and Nature of Catarrhus aestivus (HAy-Fever or Hay-Asthma). London: Bailliere, Tindeall and Cox; 1873. p. 73.
3. Burks AW, Calderon MA, Casale T, Cox L, Demoly P, Jutel M, et al. Update on allergy immunotherapy: American Academy of Allergy, Asthma & Immunology/ European Academy of Allergy and Clinical Immunology/PRACTALL consensus report. J Allergy Clin Immunol. 2013;131(5):1288-96.
4. Calderon MA, Simons FE, Malling HJ, Lockey RF, Moingeon P, Demoly P. Sublingual allergen immunotherapy: mode of action and its relationship with the safety profile. Allergy. 2012;67(3):302-11.
5. Cox LS, Linnemann DL, Nolte H, Weldon D, Finegold I, Nelson HS. Sublingual immunotherapy: a comprehensive review. J Allergy Clin Immunol. 2006;117(5):1021-35.
6. Curtis HH. The immunizing cure of hay fever. NY Med J. 1900;77:16-8.
7. Dávila I, Navarro A, Domínguez-Ortega J, Alonso A, Antolín-Amérigo D, Diéguez MC, et al. SLIT: indications, follow-up, and management. J Investig Allergol Clin Immunol. 2014;24(Suppl 1):1-35.
8. Frankland AW, Augustin R. Prophylaxis of summer hay-fever and asthma: a controlled trial comparing crude grass-pollen extracts with the isolated main protein component. Lancet. 1954;266:1055-7.
9. Freeman J. Further observations on the treatment of hay fever by hypodermic inoculations of pollen vaccine. Lancet. 1911;178:814-7.
10. Lee HY, Lee SM, Kang SY, Kim K, Kim JH, Ryu G, et al. KAAACI guidelines for allergen immunotherapy. Allergy Asthma Immunol Res. 2023;15(6):725.
11. Noon L, Cantar B. Prophylactic inoculation against hay fever. Lancet. 1911;177:1572-3.
12. Passalacqua G, Canonica GW. Allergen immunotherapy: history and future developments. Immunol Allergy Clin North Am. 2016;36(1):1-12.
13. Passalacqua G, Compalati E, Canonica GW. Sublingual immunotherapy: clinical indications in the WAO-SLIT position paper. World Allergy Org J. 2010;3:216-9.
14. Wise SK, Schlosser RJ. Subcutaneous and sublingual immunotherapy for allergic rhinitis: what is the evidence? Am J Rhinol Allergy. 2012;26(1):18-22.

CHAPTER 39

Immunotherapy in Food Allergy

Sowmya Arudi Nagarajan, Mosam Kamlesh Maroo

INTRODUCTION

Food allergy is an increasingly prevalent and important health issue in pediatric practice, affecting approximately 6–8% of children worldwide. It refers to an immune-mediated adverse reaction to food proteins that can lead to a broad spectrum of clinical manifestations, ranging from mild skin rashes to life-threatening anaphylaxis. In children, food allergies not only affect health but can also impact the quality of life, nutrition, growth, and psychological well-being of both the child and their family.

The diagnosis and management of food allergy in children require a careful clinical approach, including a detailed history, physical examination, appropriate use of diagnostic tests (such as skin prick tests, serum-specific IgE, and oral food challenges), and the implementation of dietary interventions. Increasing awareness of the distinction between food allergy and nonallergic food intolerance is crucial for preventing unnecessary dietary restrictions.

This chapter provides an overview of the pathophysiology, clinical presentation, diagnostic approach, and management strategies for food allergy in pediatric populations, emphasizing the importance of individualized care and the prevention of potentially severe complications.

WHAT IS FOOD ALLERGY?

Food allergy (FA) is an immune-mediated disorder that occurs reproducibly on exposure to a given food, with significant medical, psychosocial, and economic impacts on affected individuals and families.

IS FOOD ALLERGY OUR PROBLEM?

The Food Allergy Research & Education (FARE) states that 1 in 10 adults and 1 in 13 children suffer from FA, and over 40% of these are severe in nature. It describes FA as an epidemic in the United States. Even though precise numbers are not available in India, it is known that FA incidence is rising. FA impacts quality of life (QoL). Patients with FA suffer from anxiety, depression, bullying, and school absenteeism. Most of them are unable to visit restaurants or travel, fearing serious allergic reactions due to accidental allergen exposures.

Allergic reactions are triggered by ingestion, skin contact, and inhalation of food allergens. However, ingestion of an allergen remains the main concern for severe reactions.

WHAT ARE THE COMMON FOOD ALLERGENS?

The eight major food allergens are: (1) Milk, (2) egg, (3) peanut, (4) tree nuts, (5) wheat, (6) soy, (7) fish, and (8) crustacean shellfish. Even trace amounts of a food allergen can cause an allergic reaction. Although allergies to milk, egg, wheat, and soy often resolve in childhood, allergies to peanuts, tree nuts, and shellfish are generally lifelong.

Strict avoidance of relevant food allergens and early recognition and management of allergic reactions to food are important measures to prevent serious health consequences in individuals with food allergies. In 2021, the United States added sesame as the ninth major food allergen.

CAN FOOD ALLERGIES BE PREVENTED?

Delaying the introduction of allergenic foods does not provide protection against FA.

The Learning Early About Peanut Allergy (LEAP) study provided evidence that the age at which a child first eats peanuts and the frequency of peanuts in the diet can influence whether the child develops an allergy to peanuts. The LEAP findings demonstrate that early, sustained consumption of peanut products is associated with a substantial and significant decrease in the likelihood of developing peanut allergy.

In 2017, findings from the LEAP and related studies led to the release of new guidelines for the introduction of peanuts. These guidelines were developed by the National Institute of Allergy and Infectious Diseases (NIAIDs), a division of the National Institutes of Health (NIH). They call for the introduction of infant-safe peanut-containing foods as early as 4–6 months to help prevent a peanut allergy later in life.

A follow-up to the LEAP trial, Persistence of Oral Tolerance to Peanut (LEAP-On), showed that children who consumed peanuts from infancy through age 5 years, followed by 1 year of peanut avoidance, were 74% less likely to have peanut allergy than children who avoided peanuts up until age 6 years. This suggests that the tolerance to peanuts induced by the early introduction can persist even without repeated exposures.

CAN FOOD ALLERGIES BE TREATED?

The standard of care for FA is strict dietary avoidance of the implicated allergen(s) with ready access to injectable epinephrine and an emergency action plan in case of accidental ingestion.

In February 2024, the US Food and Drug Administration (FDA) approved the injectable biologic medication Xolair® (omalizumab) to treat FA in certain adults and children 1 year or older to reduce type I allergic reactions, including reducing the risk of anaphylaxis. The study participants were allergic to peanuts and at least two other foods, and they received Xolair treatment for 16 weeks. Two thirds of the treatment group were able to ingest a significant amount of peanuts compared to only 7% in the placebo group. This biological therapy was effective in increasing the allergic reaction threshold for peanuts and other common food allergens. Finally, patients who take Xolair must continue to avoid the foods to which they are allergic and carry epinephrine autoinjectors.

An oral peanut-based immunotherapy treatment for peanut allergy, Palforzia®, was approved in January 2020 by the US FDA, but this treatment is not appropriate for every peanut-allergic patient and is approved only for patients from age 4 to 17 years.

WHAT IS IMMUNOTHERAPY?

Immunotherapy involves intentional exposure to the food allergen, starting with very small amounts and increasing more or less gradually depending on the approach

TABLE 39.1: Immunologic changes in immunoglobulin E-mediated food allergy versus effective immunotherapy.

Immune parameters	*Food allergy*	*Effective immunotherapy*
Allergen-specific IgE	Increased	Decreased
Allergen-specific IgG4	Negligible	Increased
Allergen-specific IgA	Negligible	Increased
IgE epitope binding	Variable	Targeted binding
Mast cell and basophil activation	Increased	Decreased
Th2 cytokines	Increased	Decreased
Regulatory T-cell activity	Negligible	Increased

(IgE: immunoglobulin E; Th2: T-helper cell type 2 cell)

and the protocol including any adverse side effects or problems with the treatment.

The goal of immunotherapy is to raise the threshold dose of food protein that results in an FA reaction. Successful immunotherapy can result in the ability to eat an increased amount of the problem food without an allergic reaction. This can be lost if the problematic food is not consumed on an ongoing basis.

Table 39.1 shows a summary of the immunologic changes in allergy versus immunotherapy.

WHAT ARE THE OUTCOMES OF IMMUNOTHERAPY?

Therapeutic outcomes after food allergen immunotherapy have typically been defined using the terms desensitization and sustained unresponsiveness. **Figure 39.1** depicts the different outcomes of immunotherapy, including additional outcomes, that have been considered in clinical trials include patient-reported outcomes such as QOL and reaction severity.

- Desensitization is defined as the elimination of clinical reactivity with an increased reaction threshold to a food allergen while on active therapy.
- Sustained unresponsiveness is defined as the elimination of clinical reactivity to a food allergen that persists after a specified period of cessation. Sustained unresponsiveness has been achieved only in a subset of individuals.
- Immune tolerance, defined by the US FDA as "complete and permanent resolution of clinical response following exposure to any amount of the identified allergenic food," has not been assessed in clinical trials.
- "Field efficacy" is defined by the FDA as "the rate and/or severity of reactions to food exposures encountered outside a controlled clinical setting." This is being assessed in the ongoing multicentric Natasha oral immunotherapy (OIT) trial for milk and peanut allergies in children.

WHICH TYPES OF IMMUNOTHERAPIES ARE AVAILABLE?

During the past two decades, clinical trials in FA have focused primarily on allergen-specific immunotherapy encompassing three major forms: (1) OIT, (2) sublingual immunotherapy (SLIT), and (3) epicutaneous immunotherapy (EPIT). Each of these forms

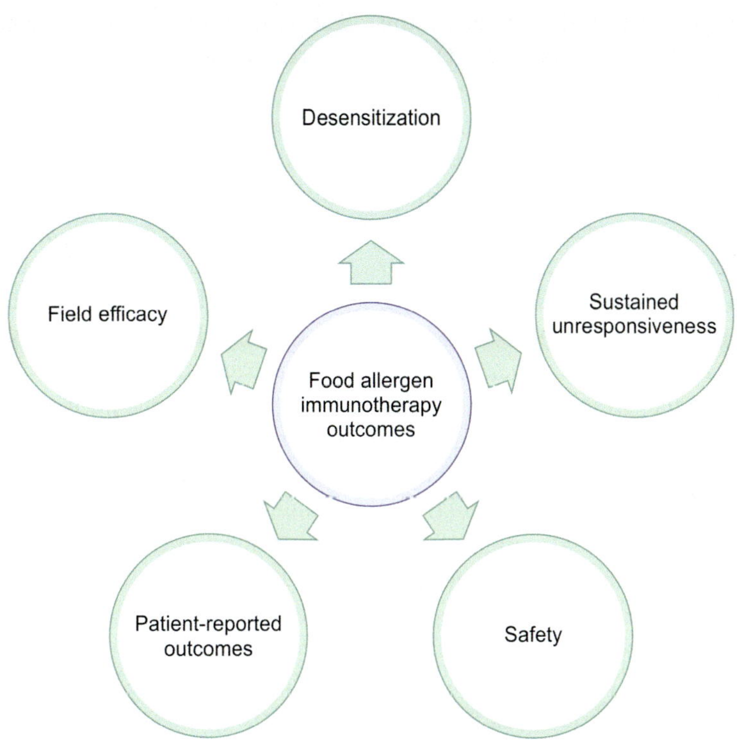

Fig. 39.1: Food allergen immunotherapy outcomes.

TABLE 39.2: Comparison of allergen-targeted immunotherapies in clinical trials

Comparison factors	***OIT***	***SLIT***	***EPIT***
Allergens	*Single allergen:* Milk, egg, and peanut (*others:* Wheat, tree nuts, and fish) multiallergen	Peanut, milk, hazelnut, and peach	Milk and peanut
Daily maintenance dose	300–4,000 mg	1–10 mg	50–500 µg
Primary side effects	Oral, gastrointestinal (systemic symptoms associated with infection, exercise, and menses)	Oropharyngeal	Skin
Desensitization	Significant effect	Moderate effect	Moderate effect
Sustained unresponsiveness	Effective in subset of patients	Ongoing investigation	Ongoing investigation
Immune modulation	Significant	Present	Present

(EPIT: epicutaneous immunotherapy; OIT: oral immunotherapy; SLIT: sublingual immunotherapy)

of immunotherapy is in a different stage of investigation, with similar immunologic targets but with clear differences in the route of administration, antigen dose, and clinical outcomes, as depicted in **Table 39.2**.

WHAT IS ORAL IMMUNOTHERAPY?

Oral immunotherapy refers to feeding an allergic individual an increasing amount of an allergen with the goal of increasing the threshold that triggers a reaction. OIT is the therapeutic approach with the largest body of evidence in clinical trials for FA to date. Multiple clinical trials involving OIT treatment for milk, egg, and peanut allergies were associated with clinical desensitization compared with placebo. The major hurdle to the success of these studies has been sustained responsiveness, which is short-lived.

In patients with peanut allergy, high-certainty evidence shows that available peanut OIT regimens considerably increase allergic and anaphylactic reactions over avoidance or placebo, despite effectively inducing desensitization. Although further long-term investigation of safety, efficacy, tolerability, and patient-prioritized outcomes is needed, these studies highlight the efficacy of OIT induction of desensitization and treatment-specific immunomodulation.

The ongoing Natasha trial, which is a 3-year multicentric randomized controlled trial involving patients between 2 and 23 years with milk and peanut allergies, reinforces the necessity of safety, desensitization, and the management of reactions due to OIT. It utilizes a more practical approach, as OIT is being performed using commonly available food products and will also measure the effect of OIT on QOL. One of the authors of this article has been fortunate to observe the trial suo moto. The results are to be released in 2027.

Omalizumab treatment before and during OIT has shown benefits in reducing side effects and shortening buildup dosing time to maintenance therapy during a trial of 11 subjects treated with milk OIT and during a trial of 13 children treated with peanut OIT. Both studies report lower overall side effect profiles during buildup and maintenance dosing. Additionally, omalizumab pretreatment in both studies reduced the time interval of OIT buildup phase to maintenance therapy by several months compared with other studies employing OIT alone.

Extensively heated foods such as OIT have been under investigation. Clinical trials performed in milk-allergic and egg-allergic children have demonstrated that approximately 70–80% of milk-allergic or egg-allergic children can safely ingest baked milk or egg products because of disruption of conformational epitopes by heating. In patients with IgE-mediated egg allergy who passed physician-supervised oral food challenges (OFCs) to extensively heated egg (e.g., muffin) and incorporated these foods into their diet, continued consumption of heated egg protein was associated with decreased skin test size, reduced egg allergen-specific immunoglobulin G4 (sIgG4) levels and increased IgG4 levels.

WHAT IS SUBLINGUAL IMMUNOTHERAPY?

Sublingual immunotherapy involves the use of smaller doses than OIT, typically starting with microgram amounts, advancing incrementally over the course of months to maintenance doses in the 1–10-mg range that are generally continued for multiple years of therapy.

Mechanistically, SLIT is thought to take advantage of tolerogenic antigen-presenting cells in the oral mucosa, with further benefit thought to be derived from exposure to the food protein in the intact form before proteins are subjected to gastric digestion. The desensitization achieved with SLIT can be equivalent to desensitization achieved with OIT, but SLIT is less likely to cause serious allergic reactions.

Conventional SLIT for peanut and milk allergy as described earlier shows moderate efficacy, favorable safety profile, and variable tolerability and is not currently the subject of broad investigation. However, a novel approach using peanut extract (PE) combined with glucopyranosyl lipid A (GLA) (SAR439794, http://www.clinicaltrials.gov NCT03463135) is underway. It is a randomized, double-blind, placebo-controlled study to assess the tolerability and safety of SAR439794 (PE SLIT adjuvanted with GLA) after repeated sublingual (SL) daily administration in peanut-allergic adult and adolescent patients.

WHAT IS EPICUTANEOUS IMMUNOTHERAPY?

Epicutaneous immunotherapy uses an allergen-containing patch to deliver antigens for uptake by the epidermal layer of skin, activating Langerhans cells that subsequently traffic to regional lymph nodes and promote regulatory immune responses. To date, this therapy is still under clinical investigation and is not yet approved by the US FDA.

SUMMARY

Food allergy is growing as an epidemic in not just the developed but also the developing countries. In the Indian scenario, it is necessary to spread awareness among the general population about the prevalence of FA, its severity, and management.

With regard to the advances in management, the availability of immunotherapy as an intervention has led to a significant paradigm shift in the management of FA. However, these therapies are not without risk, and the potential benefits must be carefully considered in the context of safety and efficacy and consideration of outcomes important to patients and caregivers, such as improved QOL, reduced anxiety about accidental ingestions and unpredicted reactions, and the constant anxiety associated with the need for dietary vigilance to prevent adverse reactions.

Continued investigation of novel therapies, as well as refinement of existing approaches, is critical to address existing knowledge gaps. It is imperative to develop protocols for immunotherapy, the use of biologics, and perform this management in well-equipped centers by recruiting trained staff.

KEY POINTS

- Definition of food allergy
  - Immune-mediated adverse reaction to food proteins
  - Distinguished from nonallergic food intolerance (e.g., lactose intolerance)
- Epidemiology
  - *Prevalence:* ~6–8% of children affected
  - *Common allergens:* Cow's milk, egg, peanut, tree nuts, wheat, soy, fish, and shellfish
  - Higher incidence in infants and young children
- Pathophysiology
  - IgE-mediated vs. non-IgE-mediated mechanisms
  - Mixed (IgE and cell-mediated) forms
  - Role of genetic predisposition, environmental factors, and early-life exposures
- Clinical manifestations
  - *Cutaneous:* Urticaria, angioedema, atopic dermatitis
  - *Gastrointestinal:* Vomiting, diarrhea, abdominal pain
  - *Respiratory:* Rhinitis, wheezing, cough
  - *Systemic:* Anaphylaxis (rapid onset, life-threatening)
- Diagnosis
  - Comprehensive history (timing, reproducibility, symptom pattern)
  - Skin prick test (SPT) and serum-specific IgE measurement
  - Oral food challenge (gold standard)
  - Differential diagnosis (e.g., food intolerance, other dermatological or GI disorders)

- Management principles
  - Strict avoidance of identified allergens
  - Education of caregivers on label reading and cross-contamination risks
  - *Emergency action plan:* Use of epinephrine autoinjectors for anaphylaxis
  - Nutritional counseling to prevent growth deficits and deficiencies
- Prevention strategies
  - Current recommendations on early introduction of allergenic foods
  - Role of breastfeeding and maternal diet
  - Prognosis
  - Many children outgrow allergies to milk, egg, wheat, and soy
  - Peanut, tree nut, fish, and shellfish allergies often persist into adulthood
- Psychosocial impact
  - Anxiety in families, social limitations, impact on quality of life
  - Support groups and psychological counseling as part of holistic care

SUGGESTED READING

1. Akdis CABI, Bahceciler N, Akdis M. Immunological mechanisms of sublingual immunotherapy. Allergy. 2006;61(Suppl. 81):11-4.
2. American Academy of Allergy, Asthma & Immunology. (2025). The Current State of Oral Immunotherapy. [online] Available from https://www.aaaai.org/tools-for-the-public/conditions-library/allergies/the-current-state-of-oral-immunotherapy. [Last accessed April, 2025].
3. Anagnostou K, Islam S, King Y, Foley L, Pasea L, Bond S, et al. Assessing the efficacy of oral immunotherapy for the desensitisation of peanut allergy in children (STOP II): a phase 2 randomised controlled trial. Lancet. 2014;383(9925):1297-304.
4. Bollinger ME, Dahlquist LM, Mudd K, Sonntag C, Dillinger L, McKenna K. The impact of food allergy on the daily activities of children and their families. Ann Allergy Asthma Immunol. 2006;96:415-21.
5. Boyce JA, Assa'ad A, Burks AW, Jones SM, Sampson HA, Wood RA, et al. Guidelines for the diagnosis and management of food allergy in the United States: report of the NIAID-sponsored expert panel. J Allergy Clin Immunol. 2010;126(6):S1-58.
6. Burks AW, Jones SM, Wood RA, Fleischer DM, Sicherer SH, Lindblad RW, et al. Oral immunotherapy for treatment of egg allergy in children. N Engl J Med. 2012;367(3):233-43.
7. Chu DK, Wood RA, French S, Fiocchi A, Jordana M, Waserman S, et al. Oral immunotherapy for peanut allergy (PACE): a systematic review and meta-analysis of efficacy and safety. Lancet. 2019;393(10187):2222-32.
8. Comstock SS, DeMera R, Vega LC, Boren EJ, Deanne S, Haapanen LAD, et al. Allergic reactions to peanuts, tree nuts, and seeds aboard commercial airliners. Ann Allergy Asthma Immunol. 2008;101:51-6.
9. Dioszeghy V, Mondoulet L, Dhelft V, Ligouis M, Puteaux E, Benhamou P-H, et al. Epicutaneous immunotherapy results in rapid allergen uptake by dendritic cells through intact skin and downregulates the allergen-specific response in sensitized mice. J Immunol. 2011;186(10):5629-37.
10. Du Toit G, Roberts G, Sayre PH, Bahnson HT, Radulovic S, Santos AF, et al. Randomized trial of peanut consumption in infants at risk for peanut allergy. New Engl J Med. 2015;372:803-13.
11. Du Toit G, Sayre PH, Roberts G, Sever ML, Lawson K, Bahnson HT, et al. Effect of avoidance on peanut allergy after early peanut consumption. N Engl J Med. 2016;374:1435-43.
12. Fleischer DM, Greenhawt M, Sussman G, Bégin P, Nowak-Wegrzyn A, Petroni D, et al. Effect of epicutaneous immunotherapy vs placebo on reaction to peanut protein ingestion among children with peanut allergy: the PEPITES randomized clinical trial. J Am Med Assoc. 2019;321(10):946-55.
13. Food Allergy Research & Education. (2025). Facts and statistics: key information to help better understand food allergy and anaphylaxis. [online] Available from www.foodallergy.org/resources/facts-and-statistics. [Last accessed April, 2025].
14. Food and Drug Administration. (2020). FDA approves first drug for treatment of peanut allergy for children. [online] Available from

https://www.fda.gov/news-events/press-announcements/fda-approves-first-drug-treatment-peanut-allergy-children. [Last accessed April, 2025].

15. Food and Drug Administration. (2022). FASTER Act video for food industry and other stakeholders. [online] Available from https://www.fda.gov/food/cfsan-constituent-updates/faster-act-video-food-industry-and-other-stakeholders. [Last accessed April, 2025].
16. Kim EH, Yang L, Ye P, Guo R, Li Q, Kulis MD, et al. Long-term sublingual immunotherapy for peanut allergy in children: clinical and immunologic evidence of desensitization. J Allergy Clin Immunol. 2019;144(5):1320-6.
17. Lemon-Mulé H, Sampson HA, Sicherer SH, Shreffler WG, Noone S, Nowak-Wegrzyn A. Immunologic changes in children with egg allergy ingesting extensively heated egg. J Allergy Clin Immunol. 2008;122(5):977-83.
18. Leonard SA, Sampson HA, Sicherer SH, Noone S, Moshier EL, Godbold J, et al. Dietary baked egg accelerates resolution of egg allergy in children. J Allergy Clin Immunol. 2012;130(2):473-80.
19. Leung DY. Pediatric Allergy, 4th edition. Amsterdam: Elsevier; 2020.
20. Mondoulet L, Dioszeghy V, Busato F, Plaquet C, Dhelft V, Bethune K, et al. Gata3 hypermethylation and Foxp3 hypomethylation are associated with sustained protection and bystander effect following epicutaneous immunotherapy in peanut-sensitized mice. Allergy. 2019;74(1):152-64.
21. Mondoulet L, Dioszeghy V, Ligouis M, Dhelft V, Dupont C, Benhamou P-H. Epicutaneous immunotherapy on intact skin using a new delivery system in a murine model of allergy. Clin Exp Allergy. 2010;40(4):659-67.
22. Nadeau KC, Schneider LC, Hoyte L, Borras I, Umetsu DT. Rapid oral desensitization in combination with omalizumab therapy in patients with cow's milk allergy. J Allergy Clin Immunol. 2011;127(6):1622-4.
23. Natasha Allergy Research Foundation. (2025). The Natasha Clinical Trial. [online] Available from https://www.narf.org.uk/the-natasha-clinical-trial-update. [Last accessed April, 2025].
24. Nowak-Wegrzyn A, Bloom KA, Sicherer SH, Shreffler WG, Noone S, Wanich N, et al. Tolerance to extensively heated milk in children with cow's milk allergy. J Allergy Clin Immunol. 2008;122(2):342-7e1-2.
25. Perkin MR, Logan K, Marrs T, Radulovic S, Craven J, Flohr C, et al. Enquiring About Tolerance (EAT) study: feasibility of an early allergenic food introduction regimen. J Allergy Clin Immunol. 2016;137(5):1477-86.e8.
26. Schneider LC, Rachid R, LeBovidge J, Blood E, Mittal M, Umetsu DT. A pilot study of omalizumab to facilitate rapid oral desensitization in high-risk peanut-allergic patients. J Allergy Clin Immunol. 2013;132(6):1368-74.
27. Skripak JM, Nash SD, Rowley H, Brereton NH, Oh S, Hamilton RG, et al. A randomized, double-blind, placebo-controlled study of milk oral immunotherapy for cow's milk allergy. J Allergy Clin Immunol. 2008;122(6):1154-60.
28. Togias A, Cooper SF, Acebal ML, Assa'ad A, Baker JR, Beck LA, et al. Addendum guidelines for the prevention of peanut allergy in the United States: report of the National Institute of Allergy and Infectious Diseases–sponsored expert panel. J Allergy Clin Immunol. 2017;39(1):29-44.
29. Tordesillas L, Mondoulet L, Blazquez AB, Benhamou P-H, Sampson HA, Berin MC. Epicutaneous immunotherapy induces gastrointestinal LAP+ regulatory T cells and prevents food-induced anaphylaxis. J Allergy Clin Immunol. 2017;139(1):189-201.e4.
30. Vickery BP, Vereda A, Casale TB, Beyer K, du Toit G, Hourihane JO, et al.; PALISADE Group of Clinical Investigators. AR101 oral immunotherapy for peanut allergy. N Engl J Med. 2018;379(21):1991-2001.
31. Wood RA, Togias A, Sicherer SH, Shreffler WG, Kim EH, Jones SM, et al. Omalizumab for the treatment of multiple food allergies. N Engl J Med. 2024;390(10):889-99.

CHAPTER 40

Vaccination in Allergic Patient

Tina N Goel

INTRODUCTION

Immunization has been a major breakthrough in mankind's fight against infectious diseases. All the vaccines under the National Immunization Schedule should be mandatorily prescribed to all children at appropriate times. The schedules can be disrupted due to many causes. One of the common causes is the history of allergies. This leads to multiple doubts in the parents' minds about the continuation of immunization as scheduled. Some healthcare providers also may either avoid or delay the administration of vaccines in such children, leaving them open to the perils of various diseases. This makes it all the more important to understand the various allergens of available vaccines and what strategies to be devised to be able to safely administer the vaccines.

An *allergy* is when the body's immune system overreacts to a normally harmless substance. The range of symptoms in an allergic reaction can be from mild discomfort to life-threatening severe anaphylactic reactions.

However, not all allergic reactions that are attributed to the vaccines are due to the vaccines themselves. It is very important to determine the relationship between an adverse event and a vaccine. This will help us identify whether the casualty of the adverse reaction can be directly traced to the vaccine or some other positive factor. This determination becomes more relevant as increasing concern about the possibility of allergic reactions following vaccination is being evaluated in light of increased allergic diseases among pediatric patients.

Reactions to the vaccine may either be immunologically mediated (hypersensitivity reactions) or they may be nonimmunological reactions (physiological or due to the irritants in the vaccine) **(Table 40.1)**.

Hypersensitivity reactions: These reactions may be due to:

- The media in which the vaccines have been grown
- The preservatives included in the vaccines
- Other substances which is used to either stabilize or maintain the form of the vaccine

Vaccine allergens : A summary of common vaccine allergens is provided in **Table 40.2**.

ALLERGIC REACTIONS FOUND WITH COMMON VACCINES

Diphtheria, Tetanus, and Pertussis Vaccine

Only two per million doses of these vaccines are known to cause allergic reactions. The reaction may occur during the administration of a booster dose due to specific IgE antibodies against the acellular

TABLE 40.1: Vaccine-related reactions.

Reaction type/severity		***Examples of symptoms***	***Timing***
Nonallergic	Local	• Rash, muscle and joint pain • Pain, redness, or swelling at the local site	Within 1–7 days after vaccination
	Systemic	Fever, chills, irritability, stomach upset, headache	Within 1–7 days after vaccination
	Vasovagal	Hypotension, pale skin, bradycardia, weakness, vomiting, giddiness	Immediate
Mild allergic		• Itchy rash such as hives • Flushing • Swelling of lips, eyes, or extremities	Within 0–72 hours after vaccination
Severe allergic (Anaphylaxis)	Skin	• Itching • Hives • Flushing • Facial swelling	Occur abruptly, from 5 minutes to within 2 hours of vaccination
	Respiratory	Shortness of breath, wheezing, severe bronchospasm, cough	
	Circulatory	Confusion, disorientation, dizziness, light-headedness, weakness, fast heart rate	
	Gastro-intestinal	Nausea, vomiting, stomach cramps, diarrhea	

TABLE 40.2: Common allergens, relevant vaccines and their adjuvants, stabilizers, mediums, and preservatives.

Common allergens	***Relevant vaccines***	***Adjuvant/stabilizer/medium/ preservative***
Oval bumin (egg)	MMR, influenza, yellow fever	Residual medium, stabilizer
Dextran	MMR, rotavirus	Medium nutrient, stabilizer
Gelatin	MMR, varicella	Stabilizer
Casein (milk)	DTaP	Medium nutrient
Neomycin	DTaP, hepatitis a, influenza, MMR, varicella	Antimicrobial
Thiomersal	Influenza, hexavalent vaccines, HPV	Preservative
Aluminum	Meningococcal, pneumococcal, Tdap	Adjuvant
Yeast	Meningococcal, pneumococcal	Medium nutrient
Latex	Meningococcal, rotavirus, Tdap, TD, yellow fever	Bottle/syringe cap
Polyethylene glycol	COVID-19	Surfactant of mRNA

(COVID-19: coronavirus disease 2019; DTaP: diphtheria, tetanus, and acellular pertussis; HPV: human papillomavirus; MMR: measles, mumps, and rubella; TD: tetanus and diphtheria; Tdap: tetanus, diphtheria, and acellular pertussis; WHO: World Health Organization) pertussis component. Diphtheria, tetanus, and pertussis (DTP) vaccines contain casein as a nutrient medium, and this may cause allergic reactions (even anaphylaxis) to occur. These reactions are very rare even in children with severe milk allergy and high levels of IgE against milk. There is no evidence to suggest that DTP vaccines contribute to the development of allergic diseases, or that atopy is a contraindication for these vaccines.

Influenza Vaccine

Influenza vaccines also contain ovalbumin, but the quantities are very low (<0.12 μg/mL), found no significant systemic reaction with this component. Several studies, such as the SNIFFLE study, found no systemic reaction. A few patients (even with a history of anaphylaxis to eggs) might experience a reaction, which, however, is self-limited and mild. The quadrivalent vaccine, recombinant subunit vaccine, and live attenuated vaccines have all been considered as being safe in individuals with preexisting asthma. According to Advisory Committee on Immunization Practices (ACIP) guidelines, it can be administered safely to patients with egg allergy, including those with severe reactions, under the supervision of a healthcare provider managing serious allergic conditions.

Measles, Mumps, and Rubella Vaccine

Measles, mumps, and rubella (MMR) vaccines have been recommended as being safe for children having egg allergy (British Society of Allergy and Clinical Immunology). Reactions, if any, are usually due to gelatin, which is used as a stabilizer in these vaccines. If there is a history of an immediate type of reaction to gelatin, then confirmation by skin test or serum-specific IgE antibody test is advisable with gelatin-containing vaccine prior to administration.

Hepatitis Vaccine

The reactions to this vaccine are rare, with an incidence of <1/100,000 administrations. The reactions to the vaccine have been attributed to residual yeast cell (*saccharomyces cerevisiae*) antigen, as the vaccine manufacturing involves the use of yeast as a nutrient medium. No confirmed cases of anaphylaxis have been confirmed (by skin test or IgE measurement) even though such reactions have been reported. If a patient has a history of reaction to Baker's or Brewers' yeast and has a positive skin test for *Saccharomyces cerevisiae*, it is recommended to test with yeast-containing vaccine before administration.

Pneumococcal Vaccine

Local redness, swelling, and pain can occur with this vaccine. Children with allergies can be safely administered the pneumococcal vaccine as reactions are extremely rare. Caregivers are instructed to inform the vaccine provider if the child has had any reaction to a vaccine containing diphtheria toxoid.

Meningococcal Vaccine

Meningococcal vaccine may cause anaphylaxis, but it is very rare.

COVID-19 Vaccine

The polyethylene glycol and polysorbate 80 components of different COVID-19 vaccines were implicated in the reactions to these vaccines. Most reactions were urticarial, and anaphylaxis was usually not seen. More studies are needed to further clarify the safety profile of these vaccines.

Yellow Fever Vaccine

Children with egg allergies should be skin tested prior to administration of the yellow fever vaccine, and if the results are negative, then the vaccine can be administered in the usual manner, but the children should be monitored for at least 30 minutes. However, in case of a positive skin test graded administration of doses is recommended along with facilities to handle reactions if they occur.

PRACTICAL APPROACH TO VACCINATION IN ALLERGIC CHILDREN

If the child to be vaccinated has a previous history of severe or life-threatening reactions to any of the components present in the vaccine, such as egg, gelatin, latex, or yeast, then the child should be tested by skin testing prior to administration of these vaccines.

Egg and yeast extracts for the skin testing are commercially available, and gelatin can be prepared by dissolving one teaspoon or 5 g of any sugar gelatin powder in 5 mL of normal saline to create a skin prick test solution. Alternatively, commercially available in vitro assays for specific IgE antibodies may be used. There are no commercially available immediate-type skin test reaction agents or specific IgG tests for neomycin or thiomersal.

If the skin test is negative: The likelihood that a patient has an IgE antibody to any vaccination component is very low if the skin test results are negative. Additionally, vaccinations can be given in the customary way. However, in a patient whose medical history points to an allergic reaction. It is advisable to administer the vaccine while under monitoring, with access to alternative therapies and epinephrine.

If the skin test is positive: The suspect vaccine (or other vaccine with common ingredients) can be given in graded doses under monitoring.

If the full vaccine dose is normally a volume of 0.5 mL, then the patient is first given 0.05 mL of 1:10 dilution. The full-strength dose of the vaccine can then be administered after a 15-minute interval in divided aliquots of 0.05 mL, 0.1 mL, 0.15 mL, and finally 0.2 mL (for a cumulative dose of 0.5 mL), 30 minutes of observation should be done at each step.

This procedure (in a presumed allergic patient) should be performed under direct medical supervision with emergency medication and resuscitative equipment immediately available to promptly treat an anaphylactic reaction should it occur.

Such challenges may be performed in an office or hospital setting with or without an intravenous line in place, depending upon the severity of the original reactions to the vaccine and the patient's medical condition.

OTHER SERIOUS ASSOCIATED ADVERSE EVENTS OF VACCINES

The vaccines are capable of causing other rare but serious reactions that might contradict the administration of future doses.

Flu vaccines may cause Guillain-Barré syndrome (one per million).

Tetanus toxoid has some potential association with Guillain-Barré syndrome and with a rare local neurological event called Brachial neuritis, which involves shoulder pain followed by weakness.

Varicella vaccine is another live immunization that can cause varicella-like lesions. It can cause the onset of fever after 7 days and rarely Febrile seizures, but without long-term sequelae.

Varicella disease can be more severe in children with atopic dermatitis; however, the varicella vaccine can be safely administered in children with atopic dermatitis without any increased risk of complication.

Pertussis vaccines have a very severe side effect of encephalopathy, that can cause permanent neurological sequelae and is an absolute contraindication to further pertussis vaccination.

Recipients of the *MMR vaccine* can also have thrombocytopenia, which can rarely cause hemorrhage.

Rubella vaccine can cause acute arthritis in approximately 15% of adult women. This might represent a direct infection of the joints by the vaccine virus, but it has a questionable association with chronic arthritis, and none of these events are contraindications to the administration of subsequent uses of MMR vaccine.

SUMMARY

Allergies are perceived as a major hindrance to immunization. It is very important to determine the relationship between an adverse event and a vaccine. This will help us identify whether the casualty of the adverse reaction can be directly traced to the vaccine or some other positive factor. This determination becomes more relevant as increasing concern about the possibility of allergic reactions following vaccination, especially in light of increased burden of allergic diseases among children. The chapter encapsulates the various allergies and allergens associated with commonly used vaccines.

KEY POINTS

- *Vaccines and allergies:* Allergic reactions to vaccines are rare, and allergies are not a contraindication for most childhood vaccinations. It is critical to distinguish between true allergic reactions to vaccines and those caused by other factors to avoid unnecessary delays in immunization.
- *Vaccine allergens:* Common allergens in vaccines include egg (ovalbumin), gelatin, casein (milk), neomycin, thiomersal, aluminum, yeast, latex, and polyethylene glycol. Awareness of these components is essential for assessing risk in allergic patients.
- *Reaction management:* If a child has a history of severe allergy to a vaccine component (e.g., egg, yeast, gelatin, latex), skin testing or specific IgE testing should be considered before administration. Negative tests allow routine vaccination, while positive tests necessitate graded dosing under close medical supervision.
- *Vaccine-specific recommendations:* Vaccines like MMR and influenza are generally safe even in children with egg allergies. Severe reactions to DTP, hepatitis B (yeast allergy), and yellow fever (egg allergy) are extremely rare, and most children can be safely vaccinated with appropriate precautions.
- *Anaphylaxis and other adverse events:* Anaphylactic reactions to vaccines are extremely uncommon. Other rare but severe adverse events, such as Guillain-Barré syndrome or encephalopathy, are noted with certain vaccines, but most are not a reason to avoid future vaccination unless explicitly contraindicated.
- *Safe vaccination practices:* Immunizations should continue as scheduled in allergic children, using monitoring, skin testing, and graded administration when warranted. The presence of allergies requires careful assessment and preparation, but should not generally interrupt routine immunization schedules.

SUGGESTED READING

1. Barış HE, Boran P, Kıykım A, Barış S, Özen A, Aydıner EK. Immunization practices in children with a history of allergies. Turk Pediatri Ars. 2020;55(3):244-50.
2. Goel T. Immunization in allergy. In: Kumar R, Mohan R, Neeraj G, Narmada A (Eds). IAP Case Based Reviews In Pediatric Allergy. New Delhi: Jaypee Brothers Medical Publishers; 2023. pp. 257-67.

3. Gupta N. Vaccination in an allergic patient. In: Gupta N, Moitra S, Nagarajan S (Eds). Comprehensive Textbook of Allergy: Striking the Right Balance, 1st edition. New Delhi: Jaypee Brothers Medical Publishers; 2024. pp. 757-61.
4. Kroger A, Bahta L, Long S, Sanchez P. General Best Practice Guidelines for Immunization. Best Practices Guidance of the Advisory Committee on Immunization Practices (ACIP). [online] Available from https://www.cdc.gov/vaccines/hcp/acip-recs/general-recs/downloads/general-recs.pdf [Last accessed June, 2025].
5. Tsai MH, Chiu CY. Allergic reactions to vaccines in children: from constituents to specific vaccines. Biomedicines. 2023; 11(2):620.

CHAPTER 41

Drug Allergy Testing

Taha Ashraf Qureshi, Muzima Jeelani, Mohammad Naveed, Afaq Jalali, Imtiyaz A Bhat, Tabasum Shafi, Ayaz Gull, Shamsa Tariq

INTRODUCTION

Testing for drug allergy is important in proper diagnosis of adverse drug reactions. Inaccurately diagnosing patients as "drug allergic" by not performing appropriate testing may result in the avoidance of effective and often first-line treatment. This not only undermine the efficacy of treatment but can also be a factor in antimicrobial resistance, especially when wider-spectrum antibiotics are employed as alternatives. Thus, clear identification and verification of drug allergies by the right kind of testing are vital for maximized, safe, and evidence-based treatment.

IMPORTANCE OF DRUG ALLERGY TESTING

Drug allergy testing is an important role for the proper diagnosis and management of patients presenting with adverse drug reactions. Inappropriately labeling a patient as drug allergic can lead to avoidances that are not necessary, denying effective and often first-line medications, with the use of less effective, more toxic, or more expensive alternatives. For antibiotics such as penicillin, such misdiagnosis can lead to or contribute to antibiotic resistance through the inappropriate use of broader-spectrum antibiotics. Hence, a drug allergy testing procedure becomes a clinically valuable tool to label or delabel the patient for a drug allergy.

INDICATIONS FOR DRUG ALLERGY TESTING

It is primarily indicated in patients with previous drug hypersensitivity reactions who must determine whether there is a possibility of future intake of a certain drug without exposure to allergic reactions. The objectives here are the identification of the offending drug and, further, the assessment of safety regarding the use of other agents of the same pharmacologic class and determination whether the allergy has been outgrown. A confirmed diagnosis helps avoid unnecessary avoidance of drugs, improves patient safety, and allows clinicians to make more informed treatment decisions.

Key Indications

- *Uncertain allergy history:* These are patients with a history of a previous reaction that is either vague or not clear; for example, someone who is labeled as "allergic to penicillin" without documented evidence.
- *Severe reactions:* Patients who have had life-threatening reactions, such as anaphylaxis, may benefit from testing to clarify the specific triggers.

- *Multiple drug allergies:* Most patients reporting multiple drug allergies are subjected to testing to elucidate true allergies from nonallergic reactions.

TESTING METHODS

Skin Testing

Skin testing is used primarily for beta-lactam antibiotics (such as penicillin) and other medications known to cause immunoglobulin E (IgE)-mediated reactions. Patch testing is used for the diagnosis of delayed non-IgE-mediated reactions.

Preparation and Patient Selection

Like with any other form of allergy testing, a careful history is required. The patient's history of exposure to drugs, nature of reactions, and any contraindications to testing are assessed. This history then picks out the suspected drug for testing. Similarly, as with skin prick testing (SPT) for aeroallergens, the patients are instructed to avoid antihistamines, corticosteroids, or other medications that may impact test results for a specified period before the test—typically 48–72 hours.

Test Preparations

The allergen is prepared in a strictly controlled dilution. Some drugs, for example, penicillin, have standardized concentrations; however, some other drugs only have the concentrations adjusted according to clinical standards **(Table 41.1)**. These standardized solutions having nonirritating concentrations of the drugs have minimal causative potential

TABLE 41.1: Nonirritating concentrations of 15 antibiotics.

Antimicrobial drug	*Full-strength concentration (mg/mL)*	*Dilution from full strength*	*Nonirritating concentration*
Azithromycin	100	10^{-4}	10 µg/mL
Cefotaxime	100	10^{-1}	10 mg/mL
Cefuroxime	100	10^{-1}	10 mg/mL
Cefazolin	330	10^{-1}	33 mg/mL
Ceftazidime	100	10^{-1}	10 mg/mL
Ceftriaxone	100	10^{-1}	10 mg/mL
Clindamycin	150	10^{-1}	15 mg/mL
Cotrimoxazole	80	10^{-2}	800 µg/mL
Erythromycin	50	10^{-3}	50 µg/mL
Gentamicin	40	10^{-1}	4 mg/mL
Levofloxacin	25	10^{-3}	25 µg/mL
Nafcillin	250	10^{-4}	25 µg/mL
Ticarcillin	200	10^{-1}	20 mg/mL
Tobramycin	80	10^{-1}	4 mg/mL
Vancomycin	50	10^{-4}	5 µg/mL

Source: Joint Task Force on Practice Parameters; American Academy of Allergy, Asthma and Immunology; American College of Allergy, Asthma and Immunology; Joint Council of Allergy, Asthma and Immunology. Drug allergy: an updated practice parameter. Ann Allergy Asthma Immunol. 2010;105(4):259-73.

for severe reaction and carry least potential to produce false-positive results on skin testing.

Control Solutions

A positive control, for example, histamine, and a negative control are valid.

Prick Tests

Skin prick testing is one of the most commonly used procedures for diagnosing drug allergies, particularly for identifying IgE-mediated (type I hypersensitivity) allergic reactions. This test involves exposing the skin to small amounts of the suspected drug allergen to observe if an allergic reaction occurs.

Skin prick testing is used to identify if a person has an immediate allergic reaction to a drug (such as penicillin, insulin, or certain chemotherapeutic agents). It is particularly useful for type I hypersensitivity reactions, which occur within minutes to a few hours after drug exposure. Common symptoms of such reactions include urticaria (hives), angioedema, bronchospasm, or anaphylaxis.

Skin Prick Testing Procedure

After obtaining written informed consent, a solution of the antigen is injected into the skin, and a needle is inserted through the solution into the skin. A general estimate is that approximately 3 μL of fluid penetrate the skin. Histamine and normal saline are used as positive and negative controls, respectively, to ensure standardization. Saline, negative control shows the initial reactivity of the skin. A histamine-positive control is used to rule out interference with any substances that inhibit skin reactivity. For skin test results to be valid, the diameter of the bleb in the negative control should be <3 mm, while the size of the bleb at the histamine prick site should be 3 mm larger than the bleb in the negative control of the place. If the bleb diameter at the histamine site is <3 mm, some intervention, such as prophylactic antihistamines, is indicated. Therefore, the patient, prior to the examination, should discontinue antihistamines and immunosuppressive medications (*the use of histamine and saline controls in skin prick testing* in *Clinical and Experimental Allergy*).

Intradermal Tests

Intradermal testing is a more sensitive method than SPT for diagnosing immediate-type drug allergies (IgE-mediated reactions). This method involves injecting a small amount of the suspected drug into the dermis (the second layer of the skin) to observe for an allergic response. Intradermal testing is typically used when skin prick tests are negative, but there is still a strong suspicion of drug allergy, particularly for certain medications such as antibiotics (e.g., beta-lactams), local anesthetics, or vaccines.

Procedure of Intradermal Testing

The procedure involves injecting a small amount of the drug into the dermis layer of the skin. The patient is then observed for signs of an allergic reaction. Intradermal testing is more invasive than SPT and carries a higher risk of inducing a systemic allergic reaction, so it must be performed under strict medical supervision. Injection of the test solution into skin uses small syringes with fine needles, usually 26–27 gauge.

Testing Site and Injection Technique

The intradermal test is usually done on the volar aspect of the forearm; however, it can be done on the upper arm or the back in some cases. The area of skin whose reaction is to be tested is cleaned with an antiseptic solution so as not to risk infection.

Inject a minute volume, typically 0.02–0.05 mL, of the diluted drug beneath the skin surface to raise a small wheal, which is approximately 3–5 mm in diameter. The injection should be superficial and only to the dermis.

Control injections: In control injections, controls both positive and negative are injected similarly, often at places a few centimeters apart from the injection sites of the test allergen.

Observation and Monitoring

- *Immediate observation:* 15–20 minutes observation for any symptom of an allergic reaction such as wheal and flare at the injection site. Measure and record the diameter of the wheal.
- *Extended observation:* There may also be delay in the responses; thus, an extended observation is conducted at the test site after 24–48 hours to identify any late-phase reactions.
- *Delayed observation:* It involves evaluating the reaction (type IV hypersensitivity), which typically occurs several hours to days after exposure to the drug, mainly 72–96 hours.

Interpretation of Results

- *Positive outcome:* A positive outcome is when there is significant enlargement of wheal (typically at least to >5 mm in diameter) combined with surrounding erythema compared to control, indicating the existence of drug-specific IgE.
- *Negative outcome:* A negative outcome here would indicate there is no significant reaction at the injection site. This does not, however, rule out an allergy completely, especially in cases of non-IgE-mediated drug reactions or delayed hypersensitivity reactions.

Safety and Precautions

- *Risk of systemic reaction:* Intradermal testing is much riskier than SPT, because it has a higher risk of causing systemic allergic reaction, including anaphylaxis. So, the test must be conducted in an environment where all treatments such as epinephrine, corticosteroids, and antihistamines can be administered easily in case of requirement.
- *Monitoring:* Patients are closely monitored during the test and for some period after the test is completed. Some patients might be expected to stay overnight at the clinic for surveillance purposes in case when there is a delayed systemic reaction.

Patch Tests

Patches that carry the drug are applied to the skin for 48 hours. This is particularly well used in the evaluation of delayed hypersensitivity reactions, which can often occur with contact dermatitis or response to medication, such as anticonvulsants or NSAIDs. The skin is assessed for a reaction, such as redness or blistering, 48 hours after the patch has been removed. It is helpful in identifying non-IgE-mediated responses that may occur days after being exposed.

IN VITRO/BLOOD TESTING

Specific Immunoglobulin E Tests

Specific immunoglobulin E tests measure the presence of drug-specific IgE antibodies in the blood. They are used very commonly whenever it is contraindicated or not possible to carry out skin testing, particularly on antibiotics and biologics. Blood samples are taken to the laboratory for analysis. IgE antibodies that might be binding specifically to the suspected drug are searched for. They are noninvasive and do not risk an allergic reaction. They are useful when skin testing carries a high risk of provoking an allergic reaction.

Basophil Activation Test

Basophil activation test (BAT) measures the degree of activation of basophils—a type of white blood cell and a key participant in the allergic reaction—in response to drug exposure in vitro. BAT is emerging as an adjunctive tool for both immediate and delayed reactions. Blood cells are incubated in the laboratory with the drug; afterward, it is examined for markers triggering basophil activation through flow cytometry. It can be very useful when topical testing is not feasible, especially for drugs that pose a higher likelihood of severe reactions, such as chemotherapeutic agents.

Lymphocyte Transformation Test

Lymphocyte transformation test assesses the drug-induced immunity mediated by T cells. It is useful particularly in the diagnosis of reactions characterized by delayed hypersensitivity, such as drugs such as anticonvulsants or antibiotics. Lymphocytes are incubated with the drug in an in vitro system, and proliferation is determined as a measure of sensitivity. It identifies non-IgE-mediated reactions and may provide useful information on some drugs, such as anticonvulsants and antibiotics.

DRUG PROVOCATION TESTS: THE GOLD STANDARD

Graded Oral Challenge

Increasing doses of the suspected drug are given to the patient in gradually increasing amounts in usually two or three steps with 30–45-minute interval between each dose and a final observation period of 1–1.5 hours after the final dose. A gold standard for confirming or excluding drug hypersensitivity, especially when the test results from skin and in vitro tests are inconclusive. The patient is monitored in escalating doses for reactions. Definite diagnosis of immediate as well as delayed drug reactions. It provides evidence that a patient can tolerate a drug if negative.

Intravenous Provocation Testing

Similar to an oral challenge but administered intravenously, usually with high-risk medications such as chemotherapy agents or biologics. Only in patients who may require these drugs for therapeutic purposes but are suspected to have allergies.

Drug provocation tests (DPTs) are administered in a controlled setting where access to emergency care is readily available immediately after the medication has been given. There is assured patient safety while testing for possible reactions to the medication that could save the patient's life. After the DPT or any sort of skin testing, a patient is further put under observation to check for possible delayed reactions that may appear some hours after the procedure.

Fitness for Graded Drug Challenge (GDC)

- No decompensated cardiac illness
- If asthmatic, should be stable and well controlled
- Spirometry should be done a day before.
- Baseline blood workup should be normal.
- Patient should be off antihistamines, beta-blockers, and angiotensin-converting enzyme (ACE) inhibitors
- 4–6-week interval from a previous drug reactions

CONTRAINDICATIONS

Drug allergy testing is often done to determine whether a patient is allergic to a certain drug.

However, there are some contraindications that make such testing inappropriate or even dangerous given as follows:

- *History of severe anaphylaxis:* The patients whose reactions to a specific drug are severe enough to kill them should not be subjected to skin testing since their risk to have another serious reaction is too high.
- *Current use of antihistamines or other medications:* Drugs that would abolish skin response, including antihistamines, tricyclic antidepressants, and some antipsychotics, may cause allergy tests to be less sensitive. These drugs may have to be discontinued for a certain period of days prior to testing, and in situations where they cannot be discontinued, testing may be contraindicated.
- *Untreated asthma:* Patients with uncontrolled asthma are at a greater risk of having an exaggerated reaction to allergy testing. Typically, it is recommended that asthma can be controlled prior to undertaking skin testing.
- *Pregnancy:* Drug hypersensitivity skin testing is generally not undertaken during pregnancy, because the risk that anaphylaxis would pose both to the mother and her fetus is significant.
- *Severe cutaneous adverse reactions (SCARs):* If the patient has had a history of SCARs, such as Stevens-Johnson syndrome or toxic epidermal necrolysis triggered by the drug, then drug allergy testing is contraindicated. These are not IgE mediated, and the risk for relapse cannot be predicted with skin testing.
- *Chronic skin conditions:* Conditions that extensively cover the patient's body surface, such as eczema and psoriasis, may be challenging to find appropriate testing sites and/or interpreting results. Controlled setting and monitoring.

LONG-TERM MANAGEMENT AND PREVENTION

Long-term management and prevention strategies include educating the patients on how to avoid taking the offending drugs and having them wear medical alert bracelets. Management plans should be documented in writing, discussing both alternative drugs to be used as well as the treatment if an accidental exposure occurs.

SUMMARY

- Drug allergy testing is important for managing and diagnosing adverse drug reactions, ensuring patients receive safe and effective medications.
- Such findings may help distinguish between allergic and nonallergic reactions, avoiding unnecessary avoidance of first-line treatments.
- Common testing methods include skin prick, intradermal, and patch tests, and each of these tests is specifically used depending on the suspected reaction type. In some cases, further confirmatory or ruling out of allergies is done through in vitro tests and DPTs.
- Testing should be performed in a controlled setting to manage adverse allergic reactions.

KEY POINTS

Drug allergy testing confirms suspected allergies to medications and helps in future treatment choices.

- *Indications:* Recommended in patients with prior drug reactions, uncertain allergy history, or suspected multiple drug allergies.
- *Testing methods:*
  - *Skin prick testing (SPT):* For IgE-mediated reactions; least invasive.
  - *Intradermal testing:* More sensitive than SPT; used if SPT is negative but suspicion remains.

- *Patch testing:* Evaluates delayed hypersensitivity reactions.
- *In vitro tests:* Measure specific IgE, basophil activation, or lymphocyte transformation.

- *Contraindications:* Includes a history of severe anaphylaxis, uncontrolled asthma, pregnancy, and severe cutaneous drug reactions.
- *Long-term management:* Patient education, drug allergy cards, and documented management plans are critical.

SUGGESTED READING

1. Borch JE, Andersen KE, Bindslev-Jensen C. The prevalence of suspected and challenge-verified penicillin allergy in a university hospital population. Basic Clin Pharmacol Toxicol. 2006;98(4):357-62.
2. Brockow K, Garvey LH, Aberer W, Atanaskovic-Markovic M, Barbaud A, Bilo MB, et al. Skin test concentrations for systemically administered drugs—an ENDA/EAACI Drug Allergy Interest Group position paper. Allergy. 2013;68(6):702-12.
3. Ciarrocca K. Cutaneous drug reactions: recognition and management. Cleveland Clin J Med. 2018;85(3):221-8.
4. Demoly P, Adkinson NF, Brockow K, Castells M, Chiriac AM, Greenberger PA, et al. International consensus on drug allergy. Allergy. 2014;69(4):420-37.
5. Edwards IR, Aronson JK. Adverse drug reactions: definitions, diagnosis, and management. Lancet. 2000;356(9237):1255-9.
6. Joint Task Force on Practice Parameters. Annals of Allergy, Asthma & Immunology. 2020.
7. Khan DA, Solensky R. Drug allergy. J Allergy Clin Immunol. 2010;125(2 Suppl 2):S126-37.
8. Pichler WJ. Drug hypersensitivity reactions: classification and mechanisms. J Allergy Clin Immunol. 2003;111(3):S560-9.
9. Schnyder B, Pichler WJ. Mechanisms of drug-induced allergy. Mayo Clin Proc. 2009;84(3): 268-72.
10. Sullivan TJ, Tilles SA. Drug allergy: immunologic principles and clinical presentation. Allergy Asthma Proc. 2001;22(3):171-6.

CHAPTER 42

Drug Desensitization

Taha Ashraf Qureshi, Muzima Jeelani, Mohammad Naveed, Hadeeqa Aejaz, Afaq Jalali, Tabasum Shafi, Ayaz Gull

INTRODUCTION

Drug desensitization is a temporary, controlled process that allows patients with established drug allergies to receive absolutely necessary drugs for which there is no alternative. It is a process of slow escalation of the drug dose in order to change the temporary immune response and make the patient tolerate the drug for the duration of therapy. This process is lifesaving in situations where there is a life-threatening infection, cancer treatment, or cardiovascular condition where the offending drug is a necessity.

DEFINITION AND IMPORTANCE OF DRUG DESENSITIZATION

Definition

Drug desensitization is a medical technique aimed at temporarily allowing a patient to tolerate a drug that previously triggered an allergic or hypersensitivity reaction. This approach is particularly beneficial when the medication is crucial for the patient's treatment and no suitable alternatives exist. The process involves administering progressively increasing doses of the drug at specific intervals, gradually allowing the patient to tolerate a full therapeutic dose without severe allergic responses.

However, desensitization does not eliminate the underlying allergy; instead, it temporarily alters the immune response, enabling safe use of the medication during that specific treatment period and hence it is also known as temporary induction of drug tolerance. It should be carried out only by the experienced healthcare professionals with expertise on drug allergy and anaphylaxis handling.

Indications and Significance

Drug desensitization is indicated when the patient should receive a medication that he or she is allergic to, but the drug is irreplaceable, because it is crucial for treatment. Indications include:

- Life-threatening conditions that require chemotherapy or biologic agents, such as cancers and autoimmune diseases.
- Infections requiring treatment with first-line antibiotics such as penicillin
- Chronic conditions, which may entail long-term use of a drug, such as aspirin for cardiovascular disease

Desensitization has to be individualized based on a risk-benefit analysis, in which the benefit of using the optimal drug overshadows the risk of possible allergic reactions. A patient with an anaphylaxis to a chemotherapy drug, for example, whose cancer shows high responsiveness to that particular drug will be a candidate for desensitization.

Contraindications

- Any patient who has had a past history of severe or life-threatening drug reactions and cannot be safely managed during the procedure.
- Severe uncontrolled asthma that also might increase the risk of severe respiratory reactions during desensitization
- Unstable cardiovascular conditions or severe cardiac arrhythmias
- Recent myocardial infarction or any other condition that would increase the risk of complications associated with desensitization
- If the allergic reaction is non-IgE mediated, in which desensitization is unlikely to ameliorate it, as in Stevens-Johnson syndrome or toxic epidermal necrolysis

Besides, in those patients for whom a suitable, safe and cost-effective drug is reasonably available to which they are not allergic, desensitization need not be considered at all.

MECHANISMS OF DRUG DESENSITIZATION

Drug desensitization primarily involves immune-mediated hypersensitivity reactions, of which IgE-mediated reactions are the most common. Desensitization may also be effective in non-IgE-mediated (non-immunological) reactions, though the precise mechanisms are less well understood. Some of the non-IgE-mediated reactions may involve T cells and cytokine release, which can be transiently suppressed by the incremental drug exposure during desensitization, too.

Cellular and Molecular Basis

Cellularly, drug desensitization is characterized by a temporary "reprogramming" of the effector cells that include mast cells, basophils, and T cells. In the process of cellular tolerance, the drug prevents an inflammatory mediator release that can occur upon antigen challenge. Mast cells and basophils are functionally inhibited temporarily, so that there is an overall reduced mediator release in spite of the presence of the drug. This could be brought about at the molecular level, which involves changes in intracellular calcium fluxes, reduction of degranulation pathways, or altered expression of surface receptors, thus reducing the chances of a full-blown allergic response.

DESENSITIZATION PROTOCOLS

Stepwise vs. Rapid Desensitization Protocols

Drug desensitization protocols are often categorized into stepwise or rapid protocols. Pharmacologic desensitization through a stepwise approach involves cardinal extension of the offending drug in gradually increased doses over some hours or even days. Stepwise protocols are very often used in patients with severe allergic reactions. There are rapid protocols for urgent cases, such as when resumption of chemotherapy is to be sooner.

Tailoring Protocols to Specific Drugs and Patients

The desensitization protocols need to be drug-specific but also tailored to the severity of the patient's hypersensitivity and the urgency of the treatment. A patient with a mild reaction to penicillin would get a far less intensive protocol compared to one who has had severe anaphylaxis to platinum-based chemotherapy. Other considerations which may weigh eventually in the choice of protocol and adjustments include individual patient variables such as age, comorbid conditions, and underlying diseases.

Monitoring During Desensitization

Continuous monitoring so as to quickly identify and manage adverse reactions would, therefore, be an extremely important part of desensitization. Patients are usually exposed to the procedure within a controlled environment where their vital signs may be closely followed, and immediate interventions taken up if need be.

PREPARATION PHASE

Predesensitization Assessment

- *Evaluate the patient's medical history:* Understand the severity of the previous allergic reaction and assess for any contraindications.
- *Baseline vitals:* Record vital signs (blood pressure, heart rate, respiratory rate, and oxygen saturation).
- *Establish intravenous (IV) access*: Place IV lines for drug administration and emergency medications.
- *Emergency drugs and equipment:* Ensure that epinephrine, antihistamines (e.g., diphenhydramine), corticosteroids, and resuscitation equipment (e.g., oxygen, defibrillator) are readily available.

Premedication

Dosage is divided into incremental steps and is administered in increments. The time intervals and dosages can vary depending on the drug and the previous reaction of the patient.

Start with a very small dose:

- *Initial dose:* Administer 1/1,000 to 1/10,000 of the final dose, e.g., if the therapeutic dose is 1 g of a drug, start with 0.1 mg (1/10,000 of the final dose).

Administration

- Each dose is administered by protocol over a 15–30 minute interval in between each dose.
- Double the dose with each step or increase it by a factor of 2–4, depending on the protocol.
- For example:
    - *Step 1:* 0.1 mg
    - *Step 2:* 0.2 mg (after 15–30 minutes if tolerated)
    - *Step 3:* 0.4 mg
    - *Step 4:* 0.8 mg
    - *Step 5:* 1.6 mg
- Continue doubling the dose until the therapeutic dose is reached cumulatively **(Table 42.1)**

Close Monitoring and Handling Mild-to-severe Reactions

- Monitor the patient's vital signs (blood pressure, heart rate, respiratory rate, and oxygen saturation), and look for signs of hypersensitivity (e.g., rash, itching, wheezing, or anaphylaxis) after each dose
    - If no reactions are observed, proceed to the next dose.
    - In case of mild reactions (e.g., skin rash or mild itching), pause the desensitization, administer antihistamines, and resume the procedure once the symptoms are resolved.
    - In the event of more severe reactions, including anaphylaxis, the procedure is immediately stopped, with emergency treatments possibly involving injections of epinephrine, oxygen, and intravenous fluids. Desensitization can be resumed following the control of the reaction, but at a lower dose and at a slower rate to minimize further risk of recurrence.

TABLE 42.1: Oral penicillin desensitization protocol.

Dose number	*Penicillin concentration (mg/mL)*	*Amount (mg/mL)*	*Dose (mg)*	*Cumulative dose (mg)*
1	0.5	0.1	0.05	0.05
2	0.5	0.2	0.1	0.15
3	0.5	0.4	0.2	0.35
4	0.5	0.8	0.4	0.75
5	0.5	1.6	0.8	1.55
6	0.5	3.2	1.6	3.15
7	0.5	6.4	3.2	6.35
8	5.0	1.2	6.0	12.35
9	5.0	2.4	12.0	24.35
10	5.0	5.0	25.0	49.35
11	50	1.0	50.0	100.0
12	50	2.0	100.0	200.0
13	50	4.0	200.0	400.0
14	50	8.0	400.0	800.0

Source: With permission from Kathuria PC, Rai M. Skin testing and drug allergy;2023.

Time Intervals

The desensitization procedure usually lasts 4–8 hours, depending on the drug and the patient's response.

Postdesensitization Phase

Completion of Desensitization

Once the full therapeutic dose is given and tolerated by the patient without any adverse reactions, the desensitization procedure is considered successful.

Ongoing Drug Therapy

To maintain desensitization, the patient must be kept under treatment at regular intervals, usually 24–48 hours.

Note: If the drug is stopped for >48 hours, the patient can lose the state of being desensitized. Therefore, it may be required to repeat the process all over again.

Observation Period

- After administering the last dose, the patient should be closely observed for at least 6 hours in case of delayed hypersensitivity reactions.
- Monitor the patient's vital signs and watch for signs of a late allergic reaction.

Postdesensitization Care and Follow-up

Monitoring for Delayed Reactions

Following drug desensitization, the patient requires monitoring for delayed reactions—those occurring hours to days following the procedure. The severity of delayed reactions is often less than in immediate reactions, but can include fever, rash, or mild gastrointestinal complaints. Clinic monitoring for several hours postdesensitization is generally recommended, followed by home monitoring by the patient.

Long-term Management and Repeat Desensitization

Desensitization merely confers temporary tolerance, and if the drug is stopped for an extended period of time, the allergy may recur. The patient may have to undergo desensitization again if he/she needs the medication. Long-term follow-up often involves periodic check-ups with the allergist for further desensitization needs or the use of alternative therapies. Some are maintained on long-term, low-dose maintenance therapy to keep the patient in a desensitized state.

SUMMARY

- A life-saving procedure, drug desensitization is used to allow a patient to tolerate a known allergic medication (for that patient) if no suitable alternative is available.
- This approach includes administering incremental dosing of the drug.
- Desensitization protocols can be stepwise or rapid, depending upon the severity of treatment urgency, and will need to be tailored to individual patients.
- There should be continuous monitoring during the procedure to manage adverse potential reactions that may arise during the procedure.
- Effects of desensitization are short-lived, and treatment has to be repeated in case the drug is required again, when treatment is stopped.

KEY POINTS

- *Definition:* Temporary induction of drug tolerance by administering increasing doses of the allergenic drug.
- *Indications:*
  - Life-threatening diseases needing chemotherapy or biologics.
  - Severe infections requiring first-line antibiotics like penicillin.
  - Chronic conditions (e.g., aspirin for heart disease).
- *Contraindications:* Severe uncontrolled asthma, unstable cardiac status, history of life-threatening non-IgE mediated reactions.
- *Protocols:*
  - *Stepwise or rapid:* Based on urgency and severity.
  - *Tailored:* Individualized according to drug, patient history, and reaction severity.
  - *Monitoring:* Continuous observation for adverse reactions during and after desensitization is mandatory.
  - *Postdesensitization:* Effects are short-lived—interruption in drug therapy may require repeating the process.

SUGGESTED READING

1. Adkinson NF, Bochner BS, Busse WW, Holgate ST, Lemanske RF, Simons FER. "Chapter 65 - Adverse Reactions to Foods: Respiratory Food Hypersensitivity Reactions." Middleton's Allergy Principles & Practice, Elsevier; 2008.
2. Brewer RJ, Waldman JP. Severe anaphylaxis and drug desensitization. In: Grammer LC, Greenberger PA, (Eds). Patterson's Allergic Diseases, 8th edition. Philadelphia (PA): Lippincott Williams & Wilkins; 2018.
3. Brockow K, Garvey LH, Aberer W, Atanaskovic-Markovic M, Barbaud A, Bilo MB, et al. Skin test concentrations for systemically administered drugs - an ENDA/EAACI Drug Allergy Interest Group position paper. Allergy. 2013;68(6):702-12.
4. Carter DM, Desai N. Cellular mechanisms of drug desensitization. Immunol Allergy Clin North Am. 2019;39(4):739-52.
5. Castells MC, Phillips EJ, Pichler WJ, Wong JT, Coop CA, Schatz M, et al. Drug hypersensitivity and anaphylaxis: mechanisms and management. J Allergy Clin Immunol. 2019;143(3):854-9.
6. Cox L, Nelson H, Lockey R, Calabria C, Chacko T, Finegold I, et al. Allergen immunotherapy: a practice parameter third update. 2011;127(1 Suppl):S1-55.

7. Cox L, Sicherer S, Borish L, El-Qutob M, Khan D, Lang D, et al. Drug desensitization protocols: guidelines and practice. J Allergy Clin Immunol Pract. 2020;8 (5):1204-11.
8. Khan DA, Solensky R. Drug allergy: a practice parameter update. Ann Allergy Asthma Immunol. 2010;105(4):273-80.
9. Lang DM, Daul AG. Drug desensitization for allergy. J Allergy Clin Immunol. 2009; 124(6):1255-64.
10. O'Leary CA, Feldweg AM. Drug desensitization. Immunol Allergy Clin North Am. 2020;40(1):123-36.
11. Pichler WJ, Adam J, Watkins S, Wuillemin N, Yun J, Yerly D. Drug Hypersensitivity: How Drugs Stimulate T Cells via Pharmacological Interaction with Immune Receptors. Int Arch Allergy Immunol. 2015;168(1): 13-24.
12. Pichler WJ. Drug hypersensitivity: classification and clinical features. J Allergy Clin Immunol. 2014;133(3):610-6.
13. Solensky R, Khan DA. Drug allergy: an updated practice parameter. Ann Allergy Asthma Immunol. 2010;105(4):259-73.

CHAPTER 43

Insect Venom Hypersensitivity

Narmada S

INTRODUCTION

Insect stings are a common cause of allergic reactions, much researched in Western countries. In India, apart from very few studies on the same, not much research has been done on the same. However, with rising interest and training in allergic disorders among the Indian medical community, there is bound to be a need to understand the topic from a better perspective. This improved understanding of the condition will provide the basic framework for evaluation, management, and prevention of anaphylaxis for the affected individuals. Historically, there have been several reports of anaphylaxis to insect venom in the literature. However, it was from 1902 that anaphylaxis to insect stings was recognized by the scientific community, and in 1911, there were reports of using immunotherapy for the management of the same. Though the insect sting allergy can occur at any age, the potential to cause a systemic reaction is less in children. Many insects have been implicated in anaphylaxis; however, the antibodies to the Hymenoptera are the most common reason for the same and are well studied in the literature. When evaluating insect allergy, it is imperative to understand that prior sensitization to inhalant allergen and the cross-sensitization with pollens, while a positive family history can also predispose an individual to venom hypersensitivity.

HOW SERIOUS IS THE ISSUE IN INDIA?

While understanding the serious nature of the venom hypersensitivity, it is imperative to understand the basic difference between sensitization and allergy. While sensitization refers to the immunological presence of IgE antibodies to insect venom, the allergic reaction is the clinical manifestation of the hypersensitivity. The Western population has a sensitization rate of 56.5–94.5% and an estimated mortality of 0.03–0.45 per one million inhabitants. There is also a significant difference in the nature of the insects causing allergic reactions depending on the geographical area and ethnic groups. Yellow jackets and honeybees are commonly implicated in Central Europe, paper wasp has been implicated in Southern Europe. In the USA, however, ants have been implicated as the prevalent cause of anaphylaxis. In India, many nonhymenopteran insects, such as cockroaches, have been implicated in inhalant allergens and mosquitoes in skin reactions, but the sensitization pattern in hypersensitivity and anaphylaxis has not been evaluated. The first such study on the same has come from West Bengal by Laha et al. who evaluated 450 patients reporting to the specialized allergy center with symptoms suggestive of various allergic manifestations due to insect bites and venom and found that sensitization was highest for common black ant (87.6%), fire ant (84.5%), honeybee (67.02%), and common wasp (30.27%). They also found that there was significant sensitivity to nonhymenopteran such as mosquitoes (66%), American cockroach (33.41%), housefly, and grasshopper. In spite of the high sensitization, this study had not investigated the clinical properties of the persons who participated in the study and the incidence of anaphylaxis in the same. However, this study was the first in India to understand the sensitization pattern among the East Indian population. If there are further studies done across India, we would be able to get the sensitization pattern pan India as this may help us understand if the nonhymenopteran species sensitization is a major cause for morbidity unlike the West.

Interestingly, two studies from the Himalayan region done to look at the prevalence of acute kidney injury quoted that wasp bite-induced non-IgE-mediated reaction was one of the major causes of acute kidney injury among those who had the same.

Hence, in summary, there is a high degree of sensitization among our population, and non-IgE-mediated severe reactions are also possible in our population. Future research will help us understand the same in a better perspective.

PRACTICE POINTS

Common cause of concern with regard to insect bites: Generally, practitioners in India are worried about papular urticarial rash and hyperpigmentation arising due to insect bites. Also, one of the reasons for urticaria in children is due to insect bites. Generally, papular urticaria is not discussed under insect venom hypersensitivity as the tendency to lead on to systemic anaphylaxis is rare in such cases. However, urticaria can be a part of the systemic manifestation of insect venom hypersensitivity and would need careful evaluation.

The four classes of medically important insects are the Chilopods (centipedes), Diplopods (millipedes), Insecta (Hymenoptera, mosquitoes, bedbugs, fleas, kissing bugs, etc.), and Arachnids (spiders, scorpions, mites, and ticks).

The insects belonging to the class Insecta are responsible predominantly for the papular urticaria, and the Hymenoptera order in the same is responsible for the insect venom hypersensitivity—the cutaneous and systemic manifestations, which are discussed in detail in this chapter.

Papular urticaria due to insect bite: It is the result of type I hypersensitivity reaction to arthropods—mosquitoes, gnats, fleas, and bedbugs. The reaction is generally due to hematogenously disseminated antigen deposited on a previously sensitized patient. The antigen is, however, unknown. Each papule has a central punctum, and new lesions can provoke reactivation of old ones. Generally, the spots remain for a few days to months and can leave behind hyperpigmentation. Further, it can resolve spontaneously. Treatment is generally supportive.

Urticaria due to insect bites: It can be a part of the systemic manifestation of the insect venom hypersensitivity.

Insect venom hypersensitivity generally refers to the allergic sensitization occurring in adults and children and capable of causing fatal reactions. The discussion of the same will be the main point of concern in this chapter.

Etiology: Stinging insects belong to the order Hymenoptera. Generally, Apidae, Vespidae, and Formicidae are the three main families in this order. There is a significant cross-reactivity among the families and is a cause of concern while the management options are discussed.

The Apidae family mainly encompasses the Apis (honeybees), Bombus (bumble bees), and the Xylocopa (carpenter bees). Apis dorsata (giant honeybee) is the largest and most aggressive bees that have been implicated in several countries, but not in India. The predominant incidents due to honeybees occur in India due to stings encountered when the beehive is disturbed by human activity, or that which happens in areas where the domesticated honeybees are cultured for commercial purposes. As they attack in large numbers, the large amount of venom injected can cause toxic reactions. Usually, the honeybees are nonaggressive and attack only when provoked, and leave behind barbed stings, which help in the identification of the insect. Bumble bees are not commonly seen in India, and carpenter bees are solitary and very rare. Case reports of fatal anaphylaxis have been reported across the globe.

The most common insect venom hypersensitivity, according to the limited Indian studies, appears to be from the Vespidae family. The yellow jackets, hornets, and wasps are ubiquitously present and are usually found near garbage cans, leftover foods, and in areas of outdoor events. Their nests, unlike honeybees, are on the grounds and easily encountered when children play around. The wasps are usually aggressive and bite even when unprovoked. *Ropalidia marginata* is the most common wasp in India, while *Vespa basalis* is commonly seen in northern, eastern, and northeastern India. *Vespa crabro* (European hornet) is present across Asia.

Formicidae has a true sting apparatus and can cause multiple stings. The fire ants are the most common species capable of producing anaphylactic reaction. Most of the studies have come from the USA, Iran, Australia, and Brazil. They are very aggressive species and also produce pustules in the area of bite that helps us in identification.

VENOM CHARACTERISTICS OF THE HYMENOPTERA

The techniques in bioinformatics have helped us to understand the most bio-active compounds that are the peptides and proteins. Generally, the venoms have vasoactive amines that are dopamine, histamine and norepinephrine, acetylcholine, and kinins. These chemicals can cause itching and an intense burning sensation at the site of the sting. Some of the compounds can cause toxic reactions when injected in large quantities, including rhabdomyolysis. However, the major allergenic components from Hymenoptera belong to three groups—Group 1A1—phospholipases, Group 1A2 phospholipases, and Group 2—hyaluronidases, Group 3—acid phosphatases. Phosphatases cause inhibition of platelet aggregation, and hyaluronidase helps in the spread of the venom allergen. Though the basic compounds appear to be the same, they are being tagged with other peptides and proteins that contribute to unique allergens in each of the insects, which helps us in identification. The proteins also show homology with proteins involved in mammalian reproduction. The minor allergens include proteins of unknown functions and show homology to plant proteins.

Interestingly, the salivary allergens of the fleas, mosquitoes, and horseflies contain allergens, which are the apyrases, an enzyme that catalyzes the breakdown of ATP to release phosphatase that acts as a platelet aggregation agonist, hyaluronidase, and lipocalins.

Clinical Features

Insect stings can cause local or systemic reactions. They can also be immediate or late onset. The reactions that are contiguous to the sting site are the local reaction. Those that are above 20 cm or involving whole limbs are called large local reactions (LLRs). There is usually an initial mild reaction and then followed by large reactions, both of which are IgE dependent. Systemic reactions can cause reactions involving multiple systems and are often IgE-mediated. The onset is usually in minutes. The following table explains in detail about the symptoms involving various systems that can occur in a systemic reaction **(Table 43.1)**.

Massive envenomation can result in rhabdomyolysis, renal failure, respiratory distress, and encephalopathy. In rare cases, seizures have also occurred, especially in the fire ant.

In some cases, delayed reaction due to unknown causes has resulted in Guillain-Barré syndrome, renal failure, cranial neuropathies, and myocarditis.

TABLE 43.1: Systemic reaction occurring in insect venom hypersensitivity.

System	*Reaction*	*Frequency*
Cutaneous	Generalized urticaria	Common
	Angioedema	Sole manifestation in 15% of adults and 85% in children
	Flushing	
	Pruritus	
Respiratory symptoms	Throat changes Dysphagia Dyspnea Stridor or dysphonia Wheezing	Common
Cardio-vascular	Dizziness	Common
	Hypotension	
	Shock	
Gastro-intestinal	Cramps Diarrhea Vomiting	Less common

Management of Insect Bite

Table 43.2 describes the management in case of an insect bite. Depending on the reaction, the treatment is generally supportive.

TABLE 43.2: Management of insect bite.

Type of reaction	*Treatment*
Local reaction—small	Supportive care—ice compression and antihistamines if itchy
Local reaction—large	• Head and neck—high-dose steroids • Those involving the limbs—moderate-dose steroids and ice compression • If presenting after 48 hours may require only ice compression and supportive care. No need for antibiotics
Systemic reaction	• Urgent intervention and close monitoring • Urticaria—antihistamines • Anaphylaxis—epinephrine injections—0.3–0.5 mg of 1 in 1000 dilution intramuscular • Hypotension—fluids, supportive care • Respiratory distress—oxygen, nebulizers • Injectable steroids

Diagnosis of Insect Venom Hypersensitivity

A detailed history after the episode is mandatory as evaluation of the presence of IgE antibodies is to be done only in people who have had anaphylaxis and in those who have a risk of life-threatening reaction. The evaluation is to be done only by people trained in allergy.

History

It helps in the identification of the culprit insect, nature and timing of the sting reactions, concurrent medications, and treatment given.

Skin Tests

Once the history is confirmative of a systemic onset reaction, then all efforts to be made to find the culprit insect using skin testing. Skin testing can be done intradermally or epicutaneously. Intradermal tests are done at a concentration of 0.001–1 µg/mL and epicutaneous tests from 1 to 100 µg/mL. The epicutaneous tests should be the first to be done and should be done in increasing concentrations. However, even if the patient with a definitive history does not react at 100 µg/mL, then it has to be followed by intradermal tests. Skin tests are generally positive when the history is very clear. However, in case, if the testing is done within 4–6 weeks of the systemic manifestation, it could be due to anergy or, in some cases, could be non-IgE mediated. Commercial venom extracts are available and usually are venom products except in the case of fire ants, where whole-body extract is used. Many patients may test positive for multiple venoms. This could be due to cross-reactivity, which is extensive among members of the same family and will require further evaluation.

In Vitro Tests

Serum specific IgE is done in conditions when skin prick tests cannot be done due to skin conditions. Improved methods have led to improved diagnostic accuracies. The correlation between skin tests and serum tests is imperfect.

Component resolved diagnosis (CRD) with recombinant allergens can improve the specificity and prognostic value of serologic testing. The CRD can find out cross-reactive carbohydrate determinants, which are thought to be responsible for double positivity reaction to honeybee and yellow jacket.

Activated basophil test can help in conditions where history is suggestive and results of serum-specific IgE are negative.

Predictors of Risk for Severe Sting Reaction

- Age—it is more common in adults compared to children
- A previous history of systemic reaction cannot predict the severity of future reactions, as well as LLRs. The eventual anaphylaxis in LLR is only 5–10%
- Male gender
- No urticaria or angioedema
- Multiple stings
- Medications (ACE inhibitors)
- *Systemic mastocytosis*: The levels of serum tryptase during and after the acute episode help to identify the systemic mastocytosis and also in predicting the risk of future reactions.

Further Management of Insect Venom Hypersensitivity

- Prescription of epinephrine and instruction on proper usage
- Finding the culprit insect and ruling out cross-reactivity
- *Venom immunotherapy* in case of systemic sting reaction and positive skin test or in vitro response—treatment of choice in prevention of future episodes. There are

no adverse events related to the same. It is known to be 95–97% efficacious. The mechanism of protection has been elucidated only partly; however, there is a suppression of venom-specific IgE antibodies and an increase in IgG levels. The venom therapy is started at the lowest possible dose, and a maintenance dose of 100 µg/mL is reached. However, in some individuals, 200 µg/mL may be needed. The schedules can vary according to the needs of the patient. The maintenance dose can be reached in days in rush and ultra rush, and in weeks as far as conventional immunotherapy is concerned. The maintenance dose is generally preferred for 3–5 years; however, when there is a constant risk of exposure and in those patients with systemic mastocytosis, the duration may be prolonged.

SUMMARY

- Insect venom hypersensitivity is a less researched topic, but as the awareness increases, there is a growing need of knowledge on the same.
- Predominantly Hymenoptera order—Apidae, Vespidae, and Formicidae are the most common causes of IgE-mediated hypersensitivity reactions.
- However, there are allergenic reactions caused due to salivary proteins of mosquitoes, flies, and bugs that can cause skin reactions.
- It is essential to evaluate any person who has had a systemic reaction to the insect venoms.
- Skin testing and in vitro testing are helpful in the identification and further follow-up of the patients
- Venom immunotherapy is very effective in controlling the future risk of anaphylaxis in patients who are at risk for the same.

KEY POINTS

- *Prevalence and Indian perspective:* Insect venom hypersensitivity is under-researched in India, but limited studies show high sensitization rates, especially to black ants, fire ants, honeybees, and wasps. Nonhymenopteran species (mosquitoes, cockroaches, flies) may also play a significant role in allergic diseases in the Indian population.
- *Important insects:* Clinically significant stings are mostly from insects in the order Hymenoptera (honeybees, wasps, hornets, ants). These can cause both IgE-mediated allergic reactions and non-IgE-mediated toxic envenomation, sometimes leading to systemic complications such as acute kidney injury.
- *Venom composition:* Hymenoptera venoms contain vasoactive amines, peptides, and allergenic enzymes (phospholipases, hyaluronidases, acid phosphatases). These contribute to local toxic effects, systemic hypersensitivity, and cross-reactivity between species.
- *Clinical features:* Reactions may be local (small or large, with swelling >20 cm) or systemic (cutaneous, respiratory, cardiovascular, gastrointestinal). Severe systemic manifestations include anaphylaxis, hypotension, respiratory distress, and rarely neurologic or renal complications.
- *Diagnosis:* A detailed history is essential. Skin testing (epicutaneous or intradermal) and serum specific IgE testing are key diagnostic tools. Component-resolved diagnostics help detect cross-reactivity. In some cases, basophil activation tests may aid diagnosis.
- *Management and prevention:* Local reactions are treated supportively (ice packs, antihistamines, steroids for severe swelling). Systemic reactions require urgent epinephrine injection, supportive care, and monitoring. Venom immunotherapy (VIT) is the treatment of choice in patients with systemic reactions, preventing recurrence in up to 95–97% of cases.

SUGGESTED READING

1. Blank S, Haemmerle S, Jaeger T, Russkamp D, Ring J, Schmidt-Weber CB, et al. Prevalence of Hymenoptera venom allergy

and sensitization in the population-representative. German KORA cohort. Allergo J Int. 2019;28(6):183-91.

2. Golden DBK, Demain J, Freeman T, Graft D, Tankersley M, Tracy J, et al. Stinging insect hypersensitivity. Ann Allergy Asthma Immunol. 2017;118(1):28-54.
3. Golden DBK. Insect allergy. In: Burks AW, Adkinson NF Jr, Bochner BS, Busse WW, Holgate ST, Lemanske RF Jr, O'Hehir RE, (Eds). Middleton's Allergy: Principles and Practice, 8th edition. Philadelphia: Elsevier's Saunders; 2014. pp. 1260-74.
4. Laha A, Sarkar T, Dey D, Mondal P, Bhattacharya S, Moitra S, et al. Assessment of Hymenoptera and non-hymenoptera insect bite and sting allergy among patients of tropical region of West Bengal, India. J Med Entomol. 2020;57(1):1-7.
5. Powers J, McDowell RH. Insect Bites. StatPearls. Treasure Island (FL): StatPearls Publishing; 2024.
6. Stewart G, Richardson J, Zhang Z, Robinson C. The structure and function of allergens. In: Burks AW, Adkinson NF Jr, Bochner BS, Busse WW, Holgate ST, Lemanske RF Jr, O'Hehir RE, (Eds). Middleton's Allergies: Principles and Practice, 8th edition. Philadelphia: Elsevier's Saunders; 2014. pp. 398-426.
7. Sturm GJ, Boni E, Antolín-Amérigo D, Bilò MB, Breynaert C, Fassio F, et al. Allergy to stings and bites from rare or locally important arthropods: Worldwide distribution, available diagnostics and treatment. Allergy. 2023;78(8):2089-108.
8. Vikrant S, Jaryal A, Parashar A. Mortality due to mass hymenoptera attacks: a serious but underrecognized public health problem in a mountainous state of india. Ind J Public Health. 2019;63(2):154.

CHAPTER

Prescribing Biologicals in Pediatric Asthma: Practice Points

Andrew Bush, Kushalinii Hillson

INTRODUCTION

Asthma biologicals have revolutionized the treatment of severe asthma, and rarely if ever do we now see a child on regular or alternate-day oral corticosteroids (OCSs). However, biologicals are expensive and need to be given by regular injections; hence, they should only be used when conventional therapies have failed. Licensing indications may vary across the globe, and local requirements should be checked before prescribing.

Who should, and who should not, be treated with biologicals?

Most children with asthma respond very well to low-dose inhaled corticosteroids (ICSs), sometimes with an additional long-acting β2 agonist (LABA) if administered regularly with an appropriate delivery device. The most common causes of failure to respond are (1) incorrect diagnosis—the child does not have asthma at all or (2) the child is not being given the treatment correctly. The right response is not to prescribe ever more treatment, but to determine in the first instance why the child is not responding. We recently presented data on >400 children assessed for biological therapy at the Royal Brompton Hospital, but only around 10% actually went on to be prescribed one of these treatments. Details of the multidisciplinary assessment of these children have been published elsewhere. Those who went on to biologicals either had true, severe resistant asthma, or refractory difficult asthma, meaning flaws in basic management, usually poor adherence, had been identified but could not be corrected despite multiple efforts by the team.

RELEVANT PATHOLOGY OF ASTHMA

In summary, school-age asthma is usually driven by type 2 (TH-2) inflammation, driven by the signature type 2 cytokines interleukin (IL)-4, -5, and -13, leading to eosinophilic airway inflammation, and other than tezepelumab, currently available biologics exclusively target the type 2 pathway **(Fig. 44.1)**. Biomarkers for this pathway include peripheral blood eosinophil count and fractional exhaled nitric oxide (FeNO). A small subset of asthmatic children has TH-2 low asthma, the pathways of which are ill understood, and they do not have raised TH-2 biomarkers. This distinction is important when planning treatment with biologicals, because obviously if TH-2 inflammation is not a factor, targeting it is an expensive waste of time.

What are the options for treating children with severe asthma?

In this section, the indications for the five biologics licensed for children are discussed and summarized in **Table 44.1**. With the exception of omalizumab, the data for these

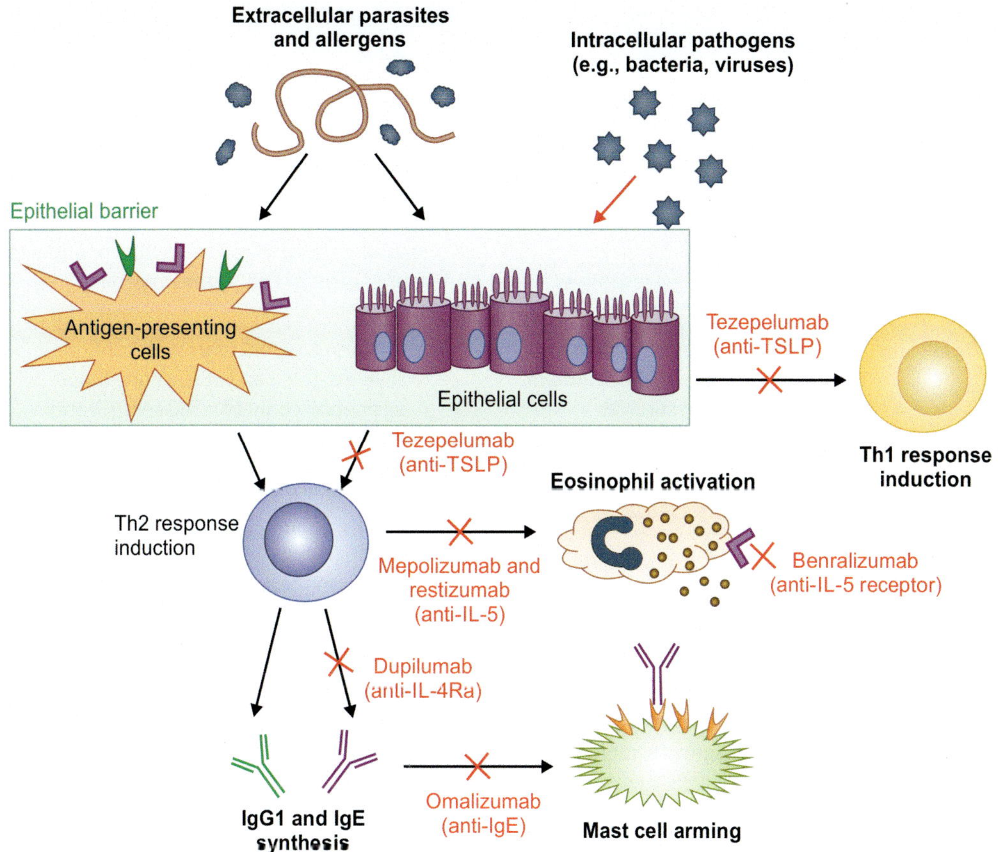

Fig. 44.1: Outline of the pathophysiology of asthma and the mode of action of the biologics. (IgE: immunoglobulin E; IL-5: interleukin-5; Th2: T helper 2; TSLP: thymic stromal lymphopoietin)

agents in children are much more limited than in adults. There are no published comparisons between these agents, although there is an ongoing randomized controlled comparison between mepolizumab and omalizumab, the TREAT trial.

The peripheral blood eosinophil count is most used for direct treatment. There are important issues in children opposed to adults. First, the normal range for blood eosinophils is significantly higher in children, yet we base recommendations on adult eosinophil levels. Second, there are developmental roles for eosinophils, and there may be unexpected consequences if numbers are reduced too drastically. It should also be noted that most data on the indications for, and safety of, biologicals have been in high-income settings with a low parasite burden, and this needs to be rectified. All TH-2 biologicals, or only benralizumab, associated with increased parasite infections are currently unclear. It is essential that normal blood eosinophil levels are determined in high parasitic burden settings. Furthermore, eosinophils have a role in response to nonparasitic infections, and too drastic a reduction in a high infection burden setting may render the child vulnerable.

All the below agents are given by injection. Traditionally, this was in the hospital, with a

TABLE 44.1: Summary of currently available biologics.

Biologics	*Action*	*Indication*
Omalizumab	• Binds circulating IgE preventing binding to FcεRI and FcεRII (CD23) receptors on mast cells and basophils • Downregulates the high-affinity receptors • Boosts antiviral responses	Children aged ≥6 years with confirmed severe asthma, serum IgE between 30 and 1,500 IU/mL, and evidence of sensitization to at least one perennial aeroallergen, regardless of eosinophil count, adherent to standard therapy, and more than or equal to four courses of OCS in the preceding 12 months
Mepolizumab	Binds circulating IL-5, reducing eosinophil growth, recruitment, activation, and survival	• Children aged ≥6 years with confirmed severe asthma and at least one blood eosinophil count of ≥300 cells/μλ and *either* at least four asthma attacks requiring OCS treatment or prednisolone equivalent 5 mg/day for ≥6 months • Children aged ≥6 years with confirmed severe asthma and at least one blood eosinophil count ≥400 cells/μλ with more than three attacks requiring OCS in the previous year
Reslizumab	As for mepolizumab	Not licensed in children
Benralizumab	Binds to IL-5 receptor (IL-5Rα) reducing eosinophil growth, recruitment, activation, and survival	• Children aged ≥6 years with confirmed severe asthma and at least one blood eosinophil count of ≥300 cells/μλ and *either* at least four asthma attacks requiring OCS treatment or prednisolone equivalent 5 mg/day for ≥6 months • Children aged ≥6 years with confirmed severe refractory eosinophilic asthma and at least one blood eosinophil count ≥400 cells/μλ with more than three attacks requiring OCS in the previous year
Dupilumab	Binds to IL-4/-13 receptor (IL-4Rα) leading to multiple anti-inflammatory effects	Children aged ≥6 years with confirmed severe asthma with either blood eosinophil count ≥150 cells/μL or FeNO ≥25 ppb and poorly controlled asthma defined as more than or equal to four asthma attacks in the preceding 12 months
Tezepelumab	Binds circulating TSLP leading to multiple anti-inflammatory effects	• Children aged ≥16 years with severe asthma defined as more than or equal to three attacks in the previous year or requiring maintenance OCS • No biomarker threshold

(FeNO: fractional exhaled nitric oxide; IgE: immunoglobulin E; IL-5: interleukin-5; OCS: oral corticosteroid; TSLP: thymic stromal lymphopoietin)

2-hour observation period afterward to detect adverse reactions. We have now moved to home administration after the carer has been trained and provided three injections have been given safely in the hospital. Injections are given with real-time video monitoring by the specialist nurse to check adherence and troubleshoot any problems. There is no evidence that this has compromised the quality of care, and it is preferred by families.

Omalizumab: There is most pediatric experience with this monoclonal antibody. Omalizumab binds to circulating immunoglobulin E (IgE), which prevents its binding to the high-affinity receptors FcεRI and FcεRII (CD23) on mast cells and basophils. Inhibition of binding leads to reduction of inflammatory mediator release, thus reducing tissue inflammatory cell infiltration and also downregulation of the receptors themselves. There is also evidence of antiviral effects.

In the United Kingdom, omalizumab is approved for subcutaneous use in children aged 6 years and older with confirmed severe, persistent, IgE-mediated allergic asthma. They are mandated to have required four or more courses of OCS in the previous year or be taking daily or alternate-day OCS. IgE must be in the range of 30–1,500 IU/mL, and there must be sensitization to at least one aeroallergen. They must also be adherent to standard therapy. These three last criteria are illogical given as follows:

1. If a child has had an asthma attack, and a detailed review has failed to prevent a subsequent attack, then there is no logic to waiting for two more attacks before instituting therapy, since the strongest predictor of a future asthma attack is a previous attack.
2. Adults with a raised IgE and no aeroallergen sensitization respond to omalizumab.
3. A child should not be penalized for not offering omalizumab just because the family will not give standard treatment. Something has to be done to keep the child alive.

Dosing depends on baseline serum IgE and body weight; many children with severe asthma are ineligible because their IgE is >1,500 IU/mL. There are no data in children on which biomarkers predict response. In adults, high TH-2 markers (FeNO, blood eosinophils, periostin) were predictive of a better response, but this was not confirmed in a subsequent study. We give a 16-week initial trial, continuing if there are improved asthma outcomes. Omalizumab is very safe, but side effects include a serum sickness-like reaction, thrombocytopenia, and eosinophilic granulomatosis with polyangiitis (Churg-Strauss syndrome); this last may be due to the underlying disease being unmasked by the reduction of OCS.

Mepolizumab: This was the second monoclonal antibody licensed in children. Mepolizumab binds circulating IL-5, thus preventing binding to its receptor, IL-5Rα, and reducing eosinophil growth, recruitment, activation, and survival. In the United Kingdom, no other TH-2 biologic can be prescribed until mepolizumab has been tried and failed. This is not logical because the results in younger children in the MUPPITS-2 study were (1) substantially inferior to those in adult studies, e.g., DREAM and (2) substantially inferior to dupilumab (VOYAGE and EXCURSION studies below). The poor response to mepolizumab in children compared to adults was unexpected. The reason is not clear, but possibilities include that the children came from a heavily polluted area, and some of their symptoms were not allergy driven; also mechanisms of severe asthma, in particular the importance of IL-5, may differ over the life course. This further emphasizes the need not to extrapolate uncritically from adult data to children.

Mepolizumab is licensed for children aged 6 years and older. The criteria include (1) at least one blood eosinophil count of ≥300 cells/μλ and *either* at least four asthma attacks requiring OCS treatment or prednisolone equivalent 5 mg/day for ≥6 months or (2) blood eosinophil count ≥400 cells/μλ with more than three attacks requiring OCS in the previous year. Of note, the blood eosinophil count falls when the child takes OCS, and the test should be repeated after cessation of this therapy if possible. The same comments as to attack frequency and adherence as were made for omalizumab (above) apply to mepolizumab. Mepolizumab is given subcutaneously every 4 weeks, in doses of 40 mg for children aged 6–11 years and 100 mg in those ≥12 years. Treatment is reviewed after a year and continued if there has been at least a 50% reduction in asthma attacks or the ability to wean daily OCS. Side effects are rare and include abdominal and back pain, fever, eczema, headache, hypersensitivity reactions, increased infection risk, and nasal congestion.

Other biologics blocking the interleukin-5 axis: Reslizumab is a monoclonal antibody which, such as mepolizumab, binds circulating IL-5. There are no big studies in children, and in the United Kingdom, it is not licensed. Benralizumab binds to IL-5Rα. There are no efficacy data in children, but it has been licensed in the United Kingdom on the basis of a safety and pharmacokinetic study. Indications are the same as for mepolizumab (above). The side effect profile is greater than mepolizumab, with increased susceptibility to infection related to a greater fall in eosinophil counts is much greater. This needs to be remembered in areas where there is a high parasite burden. Neither reslizumab nor benralizumab is used in our pediatric practice.

Dupilumab: IL-4 and IL-13 are structurally similar cytokines with a shared receptor, IL-4Rα. Signaling through this receptor plays a key role in many facets of the inflammatory pathway. Among other effects, IL-4 and IL-13 increase airway nitric oxide synthesis by inducible nitric oxide synthase (iNOS); hence, FeNO is a useful biomarker of response to dupilumab. Dupilumab binds to this receptor, thus reducing type 2 inflammation. Initially, dupilumab was used for children with severe atopic eczema, and it remains a good choice for asthmatic children who also have eczema. It is now licensed in the United Kingdom, with the indications being (1) a failed trial of mepolizumab, a requirement which is illogical given the superior effect of dupilumab in VOYAGE and EXCURSION compared with MUPPITS-2 and (2) either or both of blood eosinophil count ≥150 cells/μL and FeNO ≥25 ppb plus more than or equal to four asthma attacks requiring OCS in the previous year. Dosing depends on age and body weight; children over 12 years, body weight 15–59 kg, receive a single initial dose of 400 mg, administered subcutaneously as two separate 200 mg injections at different sites, followed by 200 mg every 2 weeks. If body weight is ≥60 kg, the corresponding doses are 600 mg initial injection and 300 mg maintenance. Children aged 6–11 years receive 300 mg on day 1, day 15, and then every 4 weeks if weight is between 15 and 59 kg. If they weigh >60 kg, then the initial dose is 600 mg in two injections, followed by 300 mg every 2 weeks. It is recommended to assess response after 16 weeks of treatment. Side effects are rare and include arthralgia, hypersensitivity reactions, ocular side effects, increased risk of upper respiratory tract infections (URTIs), transient hypereosinophilia, and eosinophilic granulomatosis with polyangiitis (Churg-Strauss syndrome), again usually associated with the reduction of OCSs.

Tezepelumab: Excitingly, tezepelumab is a monoclonal antibody that is active in children with severe asthma without TH-2 inflammation. Thymic stromal lymphopoietin (TSLP) is an alarmin secreted by epithelial cells, the first point of contact of allergens and other noxious stimuli with the airway. TSLP is upstream in the inflammatory cascade and has multiple proinflammatory actions, which are blocked when it is bound to tezepelumab. Tezepelumab is licensed in the United Kingdom for children aged ≥12 years who have severe uncontrolled asthma, defined as more than or equal to three asthma attacks requiring OCS in the preceding year, or be prescribed continuous OCS, despite treatment with high-dose ICS and at least one additional medication [LABA, leukotriene receptor antagonist (LTRA), and theophylline—this last being little used currently]. There is no threshold requirement for FeNO or blood eosinophil count, although the higher these markers, the greater the efficacy in the clinical trials. Dosing is 210 mg every 4 weeks given subcutaneously. Treatment is reviewed after a year in the first instance, and success is defined as a 50% reduction in OCS requirement and/or attack rate. Side effects are rare and include arthralgia, rashes, headache, increased risk of URTIs, hypersensitivity reactions, and back pain.

Asthma biologicals are expensive, but transformative treatments, but are not needed by many children, for whom excellent outcomes, can be obtained by using cheap, standard therapies if regularly and correctly administered. Hence, a detailed reassessment of all aspects of diagnosis and management is mandatory before committing the child to biologicals. For the small minority of children with true severe, therapy-resistant asthma or refractory nonadherence to treatment despite multiple attempts to support them, biologicals may be lifesaving. We still have much to learn about how best to use biologicals in children, especially in high-infection settings. Finally, the major barrier to treatment in many settings remains cost.

SUMMARY

Asthma biologics are expensive and require multiple injections and should only be used after a detailed evaluation of the child to ensure the basics have been got right; most children referred can be managed successfully without biologics. Biologics are indicated in those with true, therapy-resistant asthma and also those with refractory difficult asthma, usually the result of persistent poor adherence. Omalizumab, mepolizumab, benralizumab, dupilumab, and tezepelumab are licensed in children, and all target type 2 inflammation; only tezepelumab is effective in children with type 2 low asthma. Indications are largely based on adult values of blood eosinophil counts, but adult normal ranges are much lower than in children. More work is needed to determine the biomarkers for response, especially in low- and middle-income settings.

KEY POINTS

- *Role of biologics:* Biologics in asthma have transformed care in severe pediatric asthma, but they are costly, require injections, and should only be considered after ensuring correct diagnosis, adherence, and proper use of conventional therapies.
- *Indications and assessment:* Only a small proportion of children evaluated for biologics truly require them; careful multidisciplinary assessment is essential to exclude misdiagnosis and poor adherence before starting treatment.

- *Pathophysiology and biomarkers:* Most school-age asthma is driven by type 2 (TH-2) inflammation mediated by IL-4, IL-5, and IL-13. Biomarkers include blood eosinophils and FeNO, but normal eosinophil ranges are higher in children than in adults, complicating cut-offs.
- *Available biologics in children:* Omalizumab, mepolizumab, benralizumab, dupilumab, and tezepelumab are licensed for pediatric use with varying age restrictions and biomarker requirements; reslizumab is not licensed in children.
- *Special considerations:* Safety and efficacy data are limited in children compared to adults. Biologics that suppress eosinophils may increase infection risk, especially in high-parasite or high-infection-burden settings, highlighting the need for local data.
- *Practical use and follow-up:* Treatment initiation requires careful eligibility assessment, often a trial period (e.g., 16 weeks), and regular review for response (typically ≥50% reduction in attacks or OCS requirement). Home administration with remote monitoring is increasingly feasible and family-preferred.

SUGGESTED READING

1. Bacharier LB, Maspero JF, Katelaris CH, Fiocchi AG, Gagnon R, de Mir I, et al. Assessment of long-term safety and efficacy of dupilumab in children with asthma (LIBERTY ASTHMA EXCURSION): an open-label extension study. Lancet Respir Med. 2024;12:45-54.
2. Bush A, Saglani S, Fleming L. Severe asthma: looking beyond the amount of medication. Lancet Respir Med. 2017;5:844-6.
3. Cook J, Beresford F, Fainardi V, Hall P, Housley G, Jamalzadeh A, et al. Managing the paediatric patient with refractory asthma: a multidisciplinary approach. J Asthma Allergy. 2017;10:123-30.
4. Corren J, Menzies-Gow A, Chupp G, Israel E, Korn S, Cook B, et al. Efficacy of tezepelumab in severe, uncontrolled asthma: pooled analysis of the PATHWAY and NAVIGATOR clinical trials. Am J Respir Crit Care Med. 2023;208:13-24.
5. Hillson K, Saglani S, Bush A. The new biologic drugs: which children with asthma should get what? Pediatr Pulmonol. 2024;59:3057-74.
6. Jackson DJ, Bacharier LB, Gergen PJ, Gagalis L, Calatroni A, Wellford S, et al. Mepolizumab for urban children with exacerbation-prone eosinophilic asthma in the USA (MUPPITS-2): a randomised, double-blind, placebo-controlled, parallel-group trial. Lancet. 2022;400:502-11.

CHAPTER 45

Genomic Interventions in Allergy

Sheena P Kochumon

INTRODUCTION

Allergy is an odd complex immunological response to normally harmless substances in genetically susceptible individuals. Antibodies are produced by immune cells mainly immunoglobulin E (IgE) antibodies, leading to mast cell stimulation with histamine release and type 2 helper T-cell-induced mucosal inflammation. It is the pathophysiology behind all the adverse allergic responses. Allergic diseases, including allergic asthma, allergic rhinitis, atopic dermatitis, and food allergy, affect millions of individuals worldwide. It has been documented that around 500 and 300 millions of people have allergic rhinitis and allergic asthma, respectively. Many complex factors contribute to the pathogenesis of allergic disorders, including maternofetal environment, environmental conditions, gut microbiota, drug intake, genetics, epigenetics, and immune system and are characterized by an overreaction of the immune system. Genomic interventions aim to target the genetic, epigenetic, and other omics technologies contributing to the management and long-term cure for allergic diseases.

GENETICS OF ALLERGY

Multiple genes linked to allergic diseases have been identified by high throughput sequencing and genomics studies. Genome-Wide Association Studies (GWAS) have elucidated associations of nearly 200 asthma genes/loci and multiple genes/loci for allergic rhinitis, atopic dermatitis, and food allergies. The key genes are *IL-4*, *IL-13*, and *ADAM33* for allergic rhinitis; filaggrin (*FLG*) for atopic dermatitis; and *HLA-DQ* and *TLR4* for food allergies **(Table 45.1)**.

GENETIC COUNSELING

Genetic counseling is a psychoeducational task to convey information about the risk of occurrence or recurrence of a genetic disease by a geneticist or a genetic counselor. They would explain the diagnosis, its natural course, treatment and its outcome, risk of recurrence or occurrence, and ways to prevent it and prenatal diagnosis.

Objectives of Genetic Counseling in Allergy

- Risk assessment depends on individuals or families increased risk for developing allergies by correlating with family history, genetic testing reports, and recent understanding of genetic factors.
- Clinical updation on how genetic factors contribute to allergies, including the role of specific genes, inheritance patterns, and gene-environment interactions.

TABLE 45.1: Key genes in allergic diseases.

Genes	*Role*	*Mutation*
IL-4	Stimulates the differentiation of CD4+ T cells into Th2 cells and IgE production	Increased susceptibility to Th2-driven allergic conditions
IL-13	Cytokine involved in IgE class and induces chemotaxis and activation of eosinophils	Causing inflammation in eczema and airway hyperresponsiveness in allergic asthma
FCER1A	High-affinity IgE receptor on mast cells and basophils stimulates the Ag-IgE interaction and induces allergic responses	Allergic asthma, anaphylaxis, and mast cell leukemia
ADAM33	Promotes airway fibroblast and smooth muscle proliferation, airway remodeling, and inflammation	Impact on early lung function and bronchial hyperresponsiveness in asthma
TNF	Induces systemic inflammation	Mutation causes airway hyperresponsiveness in asthma and inflammation in eczema
• *HLA* • *HLA-DRB1* in allergic asthma • *HLA-DQB1* in occupational asthma • *HLA-DPB1* in aspirin-sensitive asthma *HLA-G*	Exhibits viral or bacterial protein to immune system, bronchial hyperresponsiveness, and elevated IgE levels	Atopy, occupational asthma, and aspirin-sensitive asthma
GATA3	Transcription factor for Th2 cell differentiation and cytokine production	Allergic asthma and eczema
TSLP	Cytokine that activates dendritic cells and promotes Th2 responses	Asthma, atopic dermatitis, eosinophilic esophagitis, and ocular allergies
STAT6	Transcription factor activated by IL-4 and IL-13 plays a crucial role in cell growth and apoptosis	Infantile-onset multisystem autoimmune disease and hyperimmunoglobulin E syndrome
Filaggrin (FLG)	Encodes FLG protein plays a crucial role in skin barrier function	Ichthyosis vulgaris, atopic dermatitis, and risk for asthma
TLR4, VDR, DPP10, PHF11, GPR154	Promotes inflammation and Th2 responses	Allergic asthma
ORMDL3	Involved in the regulation of airway inflammation, remodeling, and hyperreactivity	Variants associated with asthma susceptibility

(HLA: human leukocyte antigen; IgE: immunoglobulin E; IL-4: interleukin-4; Th2: T helper 2; TNF: tumor necrosis factor; TSLP: thymic stromal lymphopoietin)

- Pregenetic test counseling would convey the benefits, limitations, and potential outcomes of testing and assures individuals decision for genetic testing.
- Postgenetic test counseling would offer management and prevention strategies such as lifestyle modifications and early intervention strategies.
- Emotional and psychosocial support must be given to entire family.
- Prenatal diagnosis is possible and can offer options for family planning after explaining the recurrence in future generations.

GENETIC TESTINGS IN ALLERGIC DISEASES

Genetic testings are essential for diagnosis. Risk assessment and management also aids in designing novel therapeutic strategies such as personalized therapies. All individuals with genetic risk factors are not at same risk, as epigenetic factors play a pivotal role in the pathophysiology of allergic diseases **(Table 45.2)**.

CURRENT TREATMENT STRATEGY

Traditional treatments for allergic disorders are antihistamines, corticosteroids, and immunotherapy. These cannot offer permanent cure. They can only mitigate the symptoms. Role of monoclonal antibodies have been implicated in refractory conditions. Antitumor necrosis factor (TNF)-alpha therapy may improve the quality of life, lung function, airway hyperresponsiveness, and a reduction in exacerbation frequency in asthma patients. Omalizumab targets IgE in treating allergic asthma and chronic urticaria. Omalizumab binds with IgE and blocks its interaction with allergens, reducing allergic inflammation. Dupilumab, a monoclonal antibody, targets IL-4 and IL-13, key cytokines causing allergic inflammation in severe asthma and atopic dermatitis, respectively. It helps in mitigating the severity of symptoms and provides good quality of life.

FUTURE TREATMENT STRATEGIES

Gene Therapy

Recent research has illustrated that a single dose of AAV vector gene therapy can effectively induce tolerance to food allergens in a preclinical mouse model, suggesting a novel and revolutionary approach for offering a durable relief in allergies. Future researches are mandatory to confirm these findings in clinical trials and elucidate the therapy's safety and efficacy in humans.

Gene Editing Clustered Regularly Interspaced Short Palindromic Repeats-Cas9 Technology

The clustered regularly interspaced short palindromic repeats (*CRISPR*) gene editing has been employed with precision to make gene knockouts for knowing the functions of genes, alter genes, to know the outcome of gene editing, and identify new genes that cause allergic disorders.

Clustered regularly interspaced short palindromic repeats/Cas9 has got two key components: (1) A single guide RNA (sgRNA) that detects the specific sequence in the genome and (2) the Cas9 enzyme that binds to the sgRNA and cleaves the DNA at the target DNA sequence. CRISPR-Cas9 technology is a revolutionary tool for targeted modification of the genome. CRISPR technology has been used to edit genes related to T helper 2 (Th2) cell differentiation and IgE production

TABLE 45.2: Genetic testings in allergic diseases and its implications.

Testing type	***Aim***	***Associated conditions***	***Example***
Single-gene testing	Identifies specific mutations or variants in single genes associated with allergy	Atopic dermatitis, asthma, and specific IgE-related allergies	Mutations in *FLG, IL-4, IL-13, FCER1A, ORMDL3, ADAM33, HLA*, and *DQ*
Genetic panel testing	Assess multiple genes for various allergic conditions	Multiple allergies, asthma, and atopic dermatitis	Panels that include multiple genes such as *IL-4, IL-13, FCER1A, ORMDL3, ADAM33, HLA*, and *DQ*
Whole-exome sequencing (WES)	Analysis all coding regions of genes to identify variants associated with allergic diseases	Rare and complex allergic conditions	Comprehensive analysis of exons of 22,000 genes
Whole-genome sequencing (WGS)	Analyzes the entire genome to detect genetic variations	Broad spectrum of allergic conditions and potential rare genetic variants	Includes both coding and noncoding regions of all genes
Genome-wide association studies (GWAS)	Identify genetic variants associated with increased risk of allergies through large-scale studies	Common allergies (e.g., asthma, allergic rhinitis)	Identifies SNPs in genes such as *IL-4* and *IL-13*
Pharmacogenomic testing	Assesses how genetic variations affect responses to allergy medications	Personalized medicine for allergy treatments	Testing for genes influencing drug metabolism
Biomarker testing	Evaluates genetic or epigenetic biomarkers	Assess allergy risk and treatment efficacy	Epigenetic markers and gene expression profiles
Genotyping	Detect genetic markers associated with specific allergies	SNPs related to peanut allergy or pollen sensitivity	SNP genotyping for allergy
Copy number variation (CNV) analysis	Identify copy number changes	CNVs related to severe eczema or complex allergy syndromes	Copy number variants in atopic diseases
Gene expression profiling	Explores differential gene expression related to allergic responses and disease severity	Expression changes in asthma and allergic rhinitis	Gene expression profiling in asthma and allergic rhinitis

(FLG: filaggrin; IL-4: interleukin-4; SNPs: single nucleotide polymorphisms) that helps to mitigate the severity of allergic reactions. CRISPR-Cas 9 can make targeted modifications to specific genes and, thus, open up new possibilities for treating genetic disorders. The production of allergic proteins can be halted by the gene modification of common allergen genes.

Recent research has utilized CRISPR-Cas9 to target and disrupt the expression of the IL-4 gene, a key cytokine involved in allergic inflammation. This research has demonstrated that CRISPR-mediated gene editing could effectively reduce the production of Th2 cytokines and alleviate allergy symptoms in preclinical models. CRISPR-mediated removal of *CRAC* genes such as *STIM1* and *ORAI1* enables to know its role in calcium signaling and immune responses, and how dysregulated calcium signaling contributes to asthma and other allergic disorders.

This approach in CRISPR/Cas-9 brings out precise modifications to DNA by editing at targeted site, which, in turn, aids in correcting genetic mutations. Altering immune responses would modify the immune cell function, thus mitigating allergic reactions. Robusting the function or number of regulatory T cells (Tregs) using CRISPR help to sustain immune tolerance and reduce allergic responses. Targeting allergen genes by gene editing CRISPR-Cas9 technology would modify the production or function of allergens.

Challenges in Clustered Regularly Interspaced Short Palindromic Repeats-Cas9 Gene Editing

Viral and nonviral vectors such as lipid nanoparticles or direct injection are being used in delivering CRISPR components effectively to the target cells or tissues.

Advances in CRISPR technology aim to improve its precision and reduce off-target effects.

Immune responses to CRISPR components are big concern in therapeutic approach. Ethical and regulatory issues ensure safety and efficacy.

Current Research

Preclinical studies have been conducted in animal models for various allergies evaluating its efficacy and safety. Clinical trials are exploring the use of CRISPR for specific allergic conditions, such as asthma and food allergies. These trials will utilize the feasibility and efficacy of CRISPR-based therapies in humans. Recent development in CRISPR/Cas9 has enabled researchers to explore novel approaches for treating allergies in preclinical trial. While still in the preclinical trial stages, the continued researches in the field of CRISPR techniques would elucidate allergy treatments and offer long-term cure for allergies. Recent studies have elucidated the roles of *AAV* gene therapy and gene editing CRISPR-Cas9 in treating refractory cases of allergy manifestations.

OMICS: THE FUTURE DIRECTION

Omics technologies—such as genomics, epigenomics, transcriptomics, proteomics, metabolomics, and immunomics—are revolutionizing the perception about allergies by providing precise insights into the molecular basis of these conditions. Each omic approach offers novel insights into the mechanisms of allergy and prospective direction for management of allergy in future.

Omics technologies are exploring the immunology and pathophysiology of allergies by deciphering the molecular basis of these conditions. These high-throughput revolutionary technologies have unraveled the intricacy of allergic disorders by exploring the complex link with genetic and environmental factors.

Genomics

Genomics is the study of the entire genetic material of cells/organisms and its functions. Genomics studies the genome in its entirety, while epigenomics studies how the genome gets modified. Genomics identifies the genetic variants associated with susceptibility to allergic diseases. It aids in understanding the genetic basis of disease mechanisms. GWAS identify many risk alleles and loci causing allergies. GWAS scan entire genome for single nucleotide polymorphisms (SNPs) associated with specific traits disorders, such as asthma, eczema, rhinitis, and food allergies. Variants in interleukin-10 (IL-10) and thymic stromal lymphopoietin (TSLP) are linked to allergic rhinitis. Chromosome 17q21 encompasses several genes, including *ORMDL3*, which have been linked to asthma risk. Chromosome 5q31-33 encompasses genes involved in immune response and inflammation such as IL-4, IL-13, and IL-5. Allergic disorders have complex etiologies involving both genetic and environmental factors. GWAS also aid in identifying the disease-associated genes that encode specific proteins targeted by specific drugs. It can be utilized for validating existing targets and unravel novel drug targets. GWAS have identified genes such as filaggrin (*FLG*) associated with eczema. FLG mutations lead to impaired skin barrier function, which increases susceptibility to eczema.

Metagenomics

Metagenomics is the study of all genomes of the microbiota. Microbiota covers all the microorganisms—bacteria, archaea, viruses, fungi, and protozoans. It enables to study a mixture of DNA simultaneously such as the genetic material identified from multiple organisms such as viruses, viroids, and free DNA. Metagenomics research has focused on the association of allergies and microbiota. The change in microbiome number and its function have got a crucial link in the occurrence of allergic responses. Metagenomic research studies have identified the association of alteration in skin microbiome composition and flaring up of atopic dermatitis. Another study has demonstrated the association of asthma exacerbation with the alteration of respiratory tract microbiome composition. Many research studies have revealed the implication of metagenomics to decipher the intricate mechanism behind the association between microbiota and allergies such as atopic dermatitis, allergic rhinitis, asthma, and food allergy. Analysis of metagenome in the gut, skin, or respiratory tract can unravel the interaction of microbiota and its impact on allergic responses.

Epigenomics

Epigenomics is the study of epigenetic changes that affect gene expression without altering the DNA sequence. Epigenetic changes directly influence gene expressions whether to turn on or turn off the functions of gene. It means the accessibility of DNA for transcription has been modified by several post-translational modifications (PTMs) such as methylation, histone modification, and miRNA regulation. These all have an impact on gene expression. This field explores how environmental factors and genetic predispositions influence PTMs. Recent research has elucidated the impact of epigenetics on the development and progression in allergy. Potential target therapy can be designed based on these mechanisms in near future **(Table 45.3)**.

TABLE 45.3: Omics technologies in allergic research.

Omics technology	*Definition*	*Role in allergy research*	*Implications*
Genomics	Study of the entire genetic material of cells/organisms and its functions	Identify genetic variants associated with allergic diseases and susceptibility loci by GWAS	To know genetic predispositions, to discover biomarkers, and to design novel targeted therapies
Epigenomics	Study of epigenetic modifications such as DNA methylation, histone modification, and miRNA regulation	Analysis how epigenetic changes influence gene expression	To explore environmental impacts on gene expression and its role in epigenetic-based therapies
Transcriptomics	Study of the transcriptome, which is the complete set of ribonucleic acid molecules in a cell	Analysis gene expression profiles, pathway analysis, and identify biomarkers	To explore gene expression changes during allergic reactions and identification of potential therapeutic targets
Proteomics	Study of all molecular forms of a protein arising from a specific gene	Profiling proteins, post-translational modifications, and protein–protein interactions	To discover new allergy-related proteins and diagnostic tools
Metabolomics	Study of all metabolites, including microbiota-derived small molecules together with microenvironment	Assesses metabolite profiles and metabolic pathways alterations and biomarker discovery	To explore metabolic pathways disrupted in allergies and novel therapeutic approaches
Metagenomics	Study of structure and functions of microbiota	Assesses the role of gut and skin microbiota in allergies	To identify microbiota-related factors and potential probiotic or prebiotic interventions in allergies
Immunomics	Study of immune system regulation and response to pathogens	Analysis immune system profiles to understand immune responses in allergies	Facilitates the identification of immune markers and helps develop personalized immunotherapies

(GWAS: Genome-Wide Association Studies)

SUMMARY

Genomic studies are mandatory for diagnosis, identifying rare variants, assessment of allergy risk and treatment efficacy, gene expression, targeted gene therapies, and novel drug developments such as personalized therapy.

Genetic counseling and prenatal diagnosis must be offered to individuals with inherited allergic diseases.

Future research is imperative to confirm findings from preclinical to clinical trials and elucidate the therapy's safety and efficacy in humans.

Gene therapy and gene editing—CRISPR-Cas9 are the future revolutionary tools for a long-term cure in allergic diseases.

KEY POINTS

- Insect venom hypersensitivity is a less researched topic in Indian scenario but a few studies show it may be a huge problem in our region also
- It is essential to understand the medically important insects in Indian scenario, venom hypersensitivity pattern and management
- Essential to increase the availability of allergens and immunotherapy for Insect venom hypersensitivity in India

SUGGESTED READING

1. Cardenas A, Fadadu RP, Koppelman GH. Epigenome-wide association studies of allergic disease and the environment. J Allergy Clin Immunol. 2023;152:582-90.
2. Ezechukwu HC, Adegboye OA, Okunowo WO, Emeto TI. Targeting IgE and Th2-cytokines in allergy: brief updates on monoclonal antibodies and antibody gene therapy. Allergies. 2023;3:90-104.
3. Falcon RMG, Caoili SEC. Immunologic, genetic, and ecological interplay of factors involved in allergic diseases. Front Allergy. 2023;4:1215616.
4. Morii W, Kasai K, Nakamura T, Hayashi D, Hara M, Naito T, et al. A genome-wide association study for allergen component sensitizations identifies allergen component-specific and allergen protein group-specific associations. J Allergy Clin Immunol Glob. 2023;2(6):100086.
5. Radzikowska U, Baerenfaller K, Cornejo-Garcia JA, Karaaslan C, Barletta E, Sarac BE, et al. Omics technologies in allergy and asthma research: an EAACI position paper. Allergy. 2022;77:2888-908.
6. Wang M, Schedel M, Gelfand EW. Gene editing in allergic diseases: identification of novel pathways and impact of deleting allergen genes. J Allergy Clin Immunol. 2024; 154:51-8.

CHAPTER 46

Ethical and Medicolegal Aspects in Allergy Practice

Dhanesh Volvoikar

INTRODUCTION

Allergy practice in India is evolving rapidly, with increasing awareness, growing patient needs, and expanding therapeutic options. Alongside this progress, ethical responsibilities and medicolegal considerations play a crucial role in ensuring safe, transparent, and accountable clinical practice. Physicians must be aware of the regulatory framework laid down by the Medical Council of India/National Medical Commission, the guidelines for professional conduct, and the legal implications of procedures such as diagnostic testing and allergen immunotherapy. This chapter highlights the key ethical principles, medicolegal challenges, and consent-related issues that every practitioner should understand to deliver high-quality, evidence-based, and legally sound allergy care.

MEDICAL ETHICS

Medical ethics, for all practical purposes, may be defined as a code of conduct accepted voluntarily by medical practitioners within the profession. Medical ethics implies the obligations of the physician toward the patient as well as the same obligations toward physicians.

MEDICAL COUNCIL OF INDIA CODE OF ETHICS

Every practicing doctor in any field of modern medicine should have complete knowledge of the professional code of ethics given by the Medical Council of India (MCI)/National Medical Commission (NMC). One signs a declaration at the time of registration that he has read and agreed to abide by this code. If one is found violating the same, one can be punished by the state council or NMC after a thorough investigation. The aggrieved person can appeal in the High Court. The code of ethics is being reviewed by the NMC, which has now replaced the erstwhile MCI. The newer version of the "NMC Registered Medical Practitioner (Professional Conduct) Regulation, 2023 was published in the Gazette of Government of India on August 2, 2023." But it was subsequently withdrawn with a gazette notification dated August 23, 2024. Once revised and published, these new regulations will be applicable.

MEDICOLEGAL ISSUES FOR ALLERGY PRACTICE

In this chapter, we will look into medicolegal issues applicable specifically to allergy practice in India.

Q1. Who can practice allergy in India?

Ans. We need to look into following the existing MCI Code of Ethics of 2002.

Code no. 7.20: A physician shall not claim to be a specialist unless he has special qualifications in that branch. (The caveat in this code is not mentioning of word "recognized" before the special qualification.)

If someone has MCI/NMC recognized qualification in allergy, then there is no issue. MCI had started a process to give recognition to allergy and clinical immunology as a specialized qualification. A diploma in allergy and clinical immunology was listed but no medical college or any other recognized institute has taken up this diploma.

Now, in the absence of this, we need to look into the following.

A specialist is defined as one who learns more about less and less. The Supreme Court, in its various other judgments, has made it clear that medical practitioners should practice within the scope of their qualifications and skills.

So, what is available today in India is a 1-year part-time diploma and fellowship, which is a special qualification. Authenticity of the same is based on the curriculum, teachers, institute, and the Director of Program. One will also need to keep all other proof of obtaining special knowledge of allergy through all other courses, workshops, trainings, etc. Medical Council accredited programs will give more weightage. Even after the NMC-recognized postgraduate (PG) degree and diploma holders come out in clinical practice, all other abovementioned courses will still hold good since they were achieved before such recognized PG qualifications were available in India. In case asked by any authorities or court for proof, it is better to keep records of all of your credentials including paper presentations and articles in journals. As of now, no foreign qualification is recognized by NMC in allergy. The same above mentioned clarification applies to them if the authenticity of training and knowledge is questioned.

Q2. How to display these allergy qualifications?

Ans. The answer is based on the MCI code of ethics no. 1.4.2, which states that "Physician shall display to their names only recognized medical degrees or such certificates/diplomas and membership/honors, which confer professional knowledge or recognize any exemplary qualification/achievements."

Definition of the word recognized is not specified anywhere in the draft of the code of ethics. But the code belongs to MCI and recognized qualification is defined in its act, and they are mentioned in different schedules of the MCI Act 1956. Hence, it is advisable not to add any unrecognized qualification immediately after your main qualifications such as MBBS, MD, DCH, or DNB. One can add in a separate line all of your other credentials in full form and from which institute or university one has obtained them.

Q3. Can one call himself a consultant allergist?

Ans. The answer lies in the gray zone in the absence of NMC-recognized qualification. In the absence of the same, to be on the safer side, one can write as allergy clinic or allergy and immunotherapy clinic, etc., or else one needs to prove himself as a specialist based on all explanations given in answer to Q1 and Q2.

Q4. What about quacks or how to tackle quackery?

Ans. The answer lies in following the rule of the NMC Act of 2019.

Rule no. 34(1): No person other than a person who is enrolled in the state register or the national register, as the case may be, shall:

- Be allowed to practice medicine as a qualified medical practitioner
- Hold office as a physician or surgeon or any other office, by whatever name called, which is meant to be held by a physician or surgeon

(2): Any person who contravenes any of the provisions of this section shall be punished with imprisonment for a term, which may extend to 1 year or with a fine, which may extend to 5 lakh rupees or with both.

Q5. What is the role of guidelines and standard recommendations in routine allergy practice?

Ans. It is always advisable to practice within the broad ambit of known guidelines. In India, the following two guidelines have been framed:

1. Guidelines for practice of Allergen Immunotherapy in India 2017: Indian Journal of Allergy, Asthma and Immunology volume 31, issue 1. Developed by the Indian College of Allergy, Asthma, and Applied Immunology.
2. Indian Guidelines on Allergic Rhinitis formulated by the Association of Otolaryngologists of India (AOI).

Indian Academy of Pediatrics (IAP) Guidelines for Rational Allergy Practice in India is in the process of developing and once published will be of immense help for Allergy Practice in children. All other important international guidelines and recommendations such as those of the World Allergy Organization (WAO) and European Academy of Allergy and Clinical Immunology (EAACI), etc. will be "added" guide to your clinical practice.

The Medical Council of India code of ethics 1.2.1 is self-explanatory and states that "Physicians should try continuously to improve medical knowledge and skills and should make available to their patients and colleagues the benefits of their professional attainments. Physicians should practice the method of healing founded on scientific basis and should not associate professionally with anyone who violates this principle."

Q6. Are there any issues with available antigens in India?

What about legal issues with standardized antigens for testing and immunotherapy?

What about imported antigens?

Ans. Standardized allergens are ones where you know the content of major and minor allergens. There is no batch-to-batch variation, and one can get consistent results with the skin prick test (SPT). The result of both the SPT and the effect of immunotherapy is better with standardized antigens. It is advisable to use standardized allergen extracts of known potency with good shelf-life for immunotherapy to ensure consistency and reproducibility of the efficacy and safety of the product in the management of allergic diseases. Standardized sublingual immunotherapy (SLIT) tablets are currently available in India only for house dust mite allergens and not for other such as grass pollen. Similarly, standardized allergens for skin prick testing are also lacking. As a result, to a large extent, allergy practice in India still relies on indigenously available products for both diagnostic testing and immunotherapy.

Both antigen products for testing and immunotherapy are manufactured and licensed for human use as per pharmacopeia guidelines. Such products are manufactured and available in India (Indian Pharmacopeia 2018, volume III). In recent years, a lot of knowledge has been generated in India on the characterization of major/minor allergens of pollen, fungi, food, and insect sources. However, the purified proteins (major allergens) and monoclonal/polyclonal antibodies are not available for characterization based on major allergen content. Under these circumstances, allergen extracts are standardized based on weight/

volume and protein estimation by modified Lowry's, bicinchoninic acid assay, or micro-Kjeldahl methods. In India, as of date, manufactured and available antigens are labeled as weight/volume (weight in grams per volume in milliliters) or protein nitrogen unit (PNU). Such extracts have a legal basis for usage but may have a wide variability of biological potency, and the final results will be variable.

Allergen extracts vary from one manufacturer to another; hence, it is suggested that diagnostic and therapeutic allergen extracts should be procured from the same allergen manufacturer. The drug controller of India/state units regulates the allergen manufacture in the country. Currently, the emphasis is on good manufacturing practices to be implemented in these drug antigen units. However, the coordinated efforts of authorities are required to upgrade the quality control of allergen extracts following standard WHO/IUIS/EMA protocols. There is a need to develop allergen certification centers in the country such as the Food and Drug Administration (FDA), the Centre for Biologics Evaluation and Research in the United States, and Paul Ehrlich in Europe.

Diagnostic and therapeutic allergens should be used on patients under the supervision of medical professionals trained in allergy and immunotherapy. The manufacturer should dispense therapeutic vaccines only after obtaining the SPT results of the patient (Indian Pharmacopeia).

Some centers in India are procuring standardized allergens for their patients from the United States or Europe under import licenses. Hope in the near future, they can be available in the open market or Indian manufacturers raise their level and standardized antigens will be openly available in India.

Q7. What is the status of sublingual immunotherapy (SLIT) in India?

Ans. Standardized sublingual immunotherapy (SLIT) tablets are currently available in India only for house dust mite (HDM). With the availability of standardized HDM SLIT tablet for allergic rhinitis above 12 years and for asthma above 18 years it is now perfectly legal to use this product. It is approved for 5 years onwards in 20 countries with very good robust data. But for this age group if required it will be off label in India until a required licence is issued by appropriate authorities.

There are several indigenously manufactured products in India used for both diagnostic testing and for allergen immunotherapy, but they lack adequate standardization.

Immunotherapy is tailor-made for individual patients. From available immunotherapy material from authorized licensed Indian manufacturers, allergy consultants can use it for their patients as SLIT based on their expertise and competency as off-label medication taking due precaution and appropriate consent. Indian drug rules permit a doctor to prescribe, compound, dispense, or dilute FDA-approved products for his patients but cannot sell or commercialize.

Q8. Do you need separate consent for testing and immunotherapy?

Ans. Proper informed consent is a must for every procedure that carries some risk. Hence, written consent is required to be taken in every procedure of testing from SPT, drug test, or exercise challenge test, mentioning the type of procedure and risk involved. The risk involved may be negligible in routine SPTs to very high in exercise challenge tests or any other test done after severe reaction or anaphylaxis. Also, separate consent is required before initiating immunotherapy. SLIT may have minimal risk compared to subcutaneous immunotherapy. More important is to equip your clinic to tackle any untoward reaction, which can happen on rare occasions. Also, mention that utmost care should be taken during the concerned procedure, and if at all, in rare occasions any untoward reaction does occur, the clinic or hospital is well-equipped to tackle it. All other routine matter concerned with consent has to be followed such as using the same pen and taking the signature of the witness along with the patient or guardian, and avoid taking blanket consent, which has no legal validity, as they do not mention any specific procedure or its possible complications.

SUMMARY

Every medical practitioner practicing medicine in today's world should be aware of their limitations and should practice their subject within the ambit of what is permissible. It is always better to regularly update your knowledge, and proof of the same should be produced if asked. Always take separate written consent for different procedures and treatments and do not forget to take all required precautions and keep your clinic well-equipped to tackle any emergency.

KEY POINTS

- Practitioners must adhere strictly to the MCI/NMC Code of Ethics and practice within the scope of their qualifications and training.
- Display of qualifications must follow ethical norms: only recognized medical degrees should be placed after the name, while other training credentials may be listed separately with full details.
- Informed consent is mandatory for every diagnostic test and immunotherapy procedure. Separate, specific, and detailed consents should be obtained, avoiding blanket consents that lack legal validity.
- Practicing within the ambit of evidence-based guidelines (Indian and international) ensures patient safety, reduces medicolegal risks, and strengthens the scientific basis of allergy practice in India.

Consent Form for Immunotherapy

Name of patient: ______________________________ Age: ________ Sex: ______

Address: ____

Date: ______________________Time: _________________________

I undersigned Mr./Mrs./Ms. ____________________________ father/mother of ________________ age____ years, from____________ have been explained about immunotherapy in detail in a language understood by me. I have been advised to stay in the clinic for 30 minutes after the dose. I have been informed that the antigen to which the patient is sensitive is being given in diluted form and gradually increasing the strength over a long period. The positive effect may take up to 6 months to 1 year, and further, it has to be continued for 3–5 years. Chances of improvement of medical condition and untoward effects if any are also explained. I have been advised to get medical help instantly if any untoward effects arise. I will take all the precautions explained by my doctor during immunotherapy. I/we have been advised to stay in the clinic/hospital for 30 minutes after every dose of injectable immunotherapy or during the first dose of sublingual immunotherapy for observation. The chances of adverse effects are extremely rare, and in case they occur, this clinic/hospital is well-equipped to handle the emergency. I have opted for sublingual immunotherapy as against subcutaneous or injectable immunotherapy, given all the pros and cons such as a visit to the doctor's clinic for each dose and a lesser chance of severe reaction. I have understood the aforesaid, and I am giving my consent willingly with a sound mental state without any coercion, undue influence, fraud, misrepresentation, or mistake of facts.

______________________ ______________________

Patient/guardian Doctor

______________________ ______________________

Witness 1 Witness 2

____

Consent for Skin Prick Test

Name of patient: ______________________________ Age: ________ Sex: ______

Address: ____

Date: ______________________________ Time: ______________________________

I undersigned Mr./Mrs./Ms. ____________________ father/mother/guardian of ____________ ________________________ age____ years, from____________ give my consent for myself/ my ward to conduct allergy testing by various antigens through skin prick testing. The allergen will be placed as drops on the forearm or back region. These drops will be introduced just below the upper layer of skin by a needle/lancet. Allergic response will be noted by red raised itchy hives within 15–20 minutes. I/we have been advised to stay in the clinic for 30 minutes after the last prick. I have been explained the procedure and risks involved, if any, in a language understood by me. The chances of adverse effects or risk are extremely rare, but in any case, if any risk occurs, this clinic/hospital is well-equipped to handle the emergency. I have understood the aforesaid, and I am giving my consent willingly with a sound mental state without any coercion, undue influence, fraud, misrepresentation, or mistake of facts.

______________________________ ______________________________

Patient/guardian Doctor

______________________________ ______________________________

Witness 1 Witness 2

____

SUGGESTED READING

1. Bijli KM, Singh BP, Sridhara S, Gaur SN, Arora N. Effect of various stabilizing agents on *Imperata cylindrica* grass pollen allergen extract. Clin Exp Allergy. 2003;33:65-71.
2. Code of Medical Ethics Regulations, 2002. MCI Code of Ethics 2002 updated up to October 8, 2016. [online] Available form https://www.nmc.org.in/rules-regulations/code-of-medical-ethics-regulations-2002/ [Last accessed June, 2025].
3. Gaur SN, Raj K, Singh AB, Agarwal MK, Naveen A. Guidelines for the practice of allergen immunotherapy in India. Indian J Allergy Asthma Immunol. 2017;31(1).
4. Gupta R, Singh BP, Sridgara S, Gaur SN, Chaudhari VK, Arora N. Allergen of *Curvalaria lunata* during cultivation in different media. J Allergy Clin Immunol. 1999;104:857-62.
5. Park K. Park's Textbook of Preventive and Social Medicine, 18th edition. Jabalpur: Banarsidas Bhanot; 2005. pp. 508-11.
6. Singh BP, Gangal SV. Defined allergen extracts: need for efficient diagnosis of allergy and immunotherapy. Indian J Allergy Appl Immunol. 2001;15:67-72.
7. Singh BP, Kukreja N, Arora N. Clinically relevant allergens from fungi imperfecti and yeast. In: Kurup VP (Ed). Mold Allergy, Biology and Pathogenesis. Trivandrum, India: Research Signpost; 2005. pp. 77-92.
8. Singh BP, Sridhara S, Arora N, Gangal SV. Evaluation of protein assay method for pollen & fungal spore extracts. Biochem Int. 1992;27:477-84.
9. Singh BP, Verma J, Arora N, Sridhara S. Status of allergen standardization in India. Arbeiten aus dem Paul Ehrlich Institute Band 93, 9th International Paul-Ehrlich Seminar (1999). Dermstadt: GIT Verlag; 2000. pp. 41-5.
10. Thangam SV, Arora N, Sridhara S, Gaur SN, Singh BP. Biopotency and identification of allergenic proteins in *Periplaneta americana* extract for clinical applications. Biologicals. 2007;35:131-7.
11. The Association of Otolaryngologists of India. Indian Guidelines on Allergic Rhinitis. [online] Available from https://www.aoidelhi.org/picture/150224092818AOI-AR-Guidelines.pdf. [Last accessed April, 2025].
12. Tiwari S, Baldwa M, Tiwari M, Kuthe A. Textbook of Medicolegal Issues: Related to Various Medical Specialties, 1st edition. New Delhi: Jaypee Brothers Medical Publishers (P) Ltd; p. 162.

CHAPTER 47

Setting Up an Allergy Clinic

Krishna Mohan R, Narayan Prasad Modi

INTRODUCTION

The incidence and prevalence of allergic diseases in children are increasing rapidly worldwide, reaching epidemic proportions. The impact of allergies is profoundly distressing, not only for the affected children but also for their entire families. The spectrum of allergic diseases is broad and varied, ranging from allergic rhinitis to life-threatening anaphylaxis.

While pediatric allergy is a highly sought-after specialty in the Western world, it remains in its nascent stages in developing countries such as India. Therefore, it is crucial for doctors trained in allergy to practice the specialty professionally to benefit a growing number of patients.

Establishing a well-equipped allergy clinic is essential to ensure accurate diagnosis, safe management, and effective patient education. This chapter provides a practical guide to setting up such a center. These include registration with local health authorities, enrollment under the Clinical Establishments Act, approval from the Pollution Control Board for biomedical waste disposal, a fire safety license, and professional indemnity insurance, all of which are mandatory before starting a center.

BASIC LAYOUT OF A PEDIATRIC ALLERGY CLINIC

First and foremost, an ideal location to start the clinic should be decided upon. The basic layout of an allergy clinic **(Fig. 47.1)** should be discussed with the engineer/architect before planning the infrastructure. Depending upon the place, affordability, and patient load, some improvisations may be made.

BASIC REQUIREMENTS OF AN ALLERGY CENTER

Staff Requirement

A hospital's success is fundamentally dependent on having well-trained, dedicated, and hardworking staff. The number of personnel needed can vary based on the patient load and the complexity of the facility **(Box 47.1)**.

Display of Services Available

The hospital name and address are available in adjoining areas of the hospital/main roads/highways, etc. There should be sufficient signage boards in English and local language. The doctor's name, availability, timings of outpatient department (OPD), and other services should be displayed clearly. The layout of the hospital is displayed at least in one prominent area. There should be sufficient signage boards in English and local language.

Reception and Registration Area

A carefully designed reception area is essential and can enhance the patient experience.

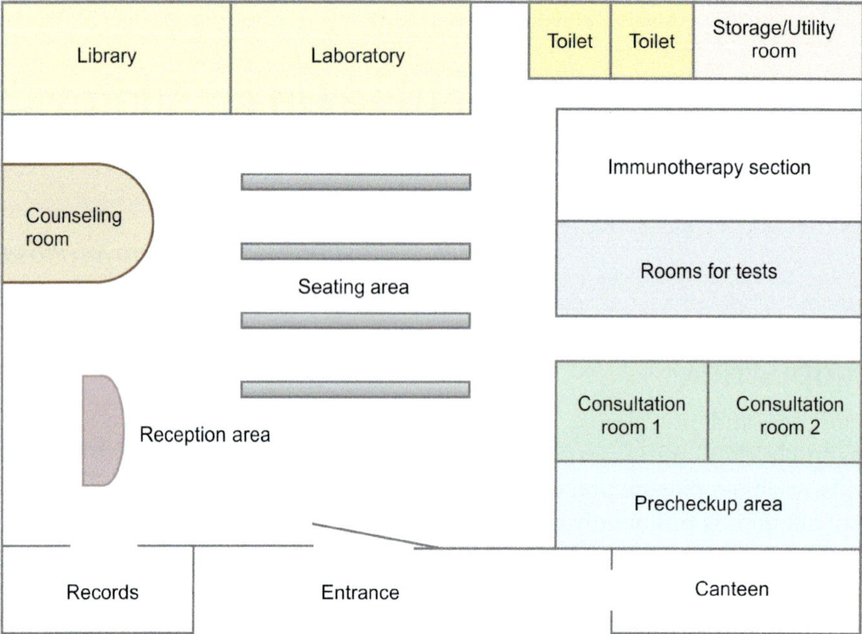

Fig. 47.1: Basic layout of an allergy clinic.

BOX 47.1: Staff requirements of an allergy center.

Staff required:
- Reception and administrative staff
- Nursing staff
- Laboratory technicians
- Counselors trained in the field of allergy
- Security staff and cleaning staff
- Respiratory technicians (optional)
- Research assistants (optional)

There should be facilities to welcome the patient and help in registration. A dedicated section will help in the patient flow and movement smoothly. An OPD register with the OPD number, name, and age should be maintained.

Waiting Area

The waiting area should be spacious with adequate number of chairs, as pediatric patients will usually be accompanied by parents and siblings too. There should be a secondary waiting area if the primary waiting area is not sufficient. The waiting area should have audiovisuals, patient education leaflets, posters, etc., for information, education, and communication (IEC) activities. There should be proper lights and fans. Safe drinking water should be freely available. Adequate number of toilets should be there.

A breastfeeding area with privacy for mothers should be arranged.

Precheckup Area

Trained staff should examine the patients and document basic parameters such as height, weight, pulse, blood pressure, peak flow rate, and oxygen saturation. There should be a stadiometer for height measurement and a scale for weight measurement. Those patients who need immediate care should be triaged and given early care. Adequate resuscitative facilities should be available here as well.

All children should also be assessed for their immunization status.

Consultation Rooms

The rooms should be well-ventilated. Adequate seating facilities should be available. There should be an examination table, preferably covered with disposable sheets. Other basic requirements in the consultation room include stethoscope, torch, thermometer, tongue depressor, nasal speculum, magnifying glasses, pulse oximeter, otoscope, and ophthalmoscope.

Emergency Management Room and Observation Area

There should be a separate area for managing emergencies, fully furnished with necessary equipment and medications. Though rare, life-threatening emergencies such as anaphylaxis can occur during the various in vivo tests, challenge tests, and immunotherapy. Staff in this area should be sufficiently trained to handle emergencies. This room can also be used for nebulization and observing patients after skin prick tests (SPTs), immunotherapy, etc. The must-have list of equipment and medications in the emergency room is shown in **Box 47.2**.

BOX 47.2

Emergency equipments required:
- Stethoscope
- BP apparatus (with adult and pediatric cuff sizes)
- Syringes and needles of different sizes
- IV catheters and IV drip sets
- Ambu bags (pediatric and adult)
- Face masks (pediatric and adult)
- Oxygen supply
- Nebulizer
- Laryngoscopes
- Endotracheal tubes (pediatric and adult)
- Pulse oximeter with pediatric and adult probes
- Nasopharyngeal and oropharyngeal airways
- Suction machine and suction catheters
- Automated external defibrillator

Emergency medicines required:
- Injection adrenaline (1:1,000)
- IV fluids-normal saline, Ringer's lactate, and dextrose
- Injection chlorpheniramine maleate and injection cetirizine
- Injection hydrocortisone and injection methylprednisolone
- Injection glucagon
- Salbutamol/levosalbutamol solutions for nebulization
- Injection dopamine
- Injection ondansetron

(BP: blood pressure; IV: intravenous)

Diagnostic Services

Allergy practice requires investigations both for diagnosis and follow-up. There are tests for cause identification (triggers), tests for functional and structural assessment, and supportive tests. There are both in vivo and in vitro tests.

In Vivo Tests: Skin Prick Test Section

Skin prick test, which is considered as the gold standard for diagnosis of immunoglobulin E (IgE) mediated allergic diseases, is one of the unavoidable components of any allergy clinic. It should be performed only at a place well-equipped with resuscitation facilities.

Ideally, the doctor/counselor should explain the procedure of SPT before doing it. An informed consent should be taken, mentioning the possible side effects. Each patient should have an allergy skin test recording sheet, which contains the information as follows: patient's name, age, sex, address, contact information, clinic registration number, date, time of start of SPT, time SPT is read, signature/name of the person performing the skin testing, antigen name, concentration, manufacturer, and batch number.

Essential requirements in skin prick test room:

- Make the patient seated comfortably or make the patient lie down
- Trolley stool to keep the allergen extracts while performing the SPT and to discard the lancets
- Standardized allergen extracts are to be used for SPT. Studies have shown that Indian-manufactured allergen extracts of dermatophagoides pteronyssinus (DP) and dermatophagoides farina (DF) were less potent than US Food and Drug Administration (USFDA)-approved allergen extracts. So, there is an urgent need for the standardization of allergens by the concerned statutory bodies. Many of the food extracts lose their potency fast. Hence, especially for fruits and vegetables, pricking the uncooked food and then pricking the patient's skin (prick and prick technique) may be used.
- *Refrigerator:* The allergen extracts should be stored at 2–8°C in a refrigerator.
- Allergy prick lancets with 1 mm tips
- A transparent measuring scale for measuring the wheal diameter
- Emergency drugs should be kept ready, including epinephrine.

Precautions to be taken while performing skin prick test: Skin tests should be performed only in the presence of a qualified doctor who is competent enough to treat systemic reactions, if any. The staff should be trained to recognize early symptoms and treat reactions in a setting equipped with emergency medicines.

Please see the medications the patient is already on. It is necessary to withhold certain medicines such as antihistamines for a specific time period before doing SPT. SPT should not be done during an acute attack of asthma.

The stability and date of expiry of the allergenic extracts should be doubly checked.

Wherever possible, use standardized allergen extracts only.

A positive and a negative control solution should be included.

SPT should be performed in a normal skin area. So, avoid it in patients with severe eczema and dermatographism.

The wheal responses should be measured at the appropriate time (15–20 minutes after SPT).

Challenge tests: Allergen challenge tests involve directly exposing a patient to an allergen to find out if he/she is allergic to it. Those staff who assist with the challenge tests should be well-versed in recognizing and treating anaphylaxis. All challenge tests should be performed only in the presence of a trained allergy specialist, capable of handling emergencies. All challenge tests should be documented in the patient's medical record, along with the reason for performing the challenge. Explain the procedures in detail before performing the test and take an informed consent.

Food challenge test: The challenge is usually performed over 90 minutes. The total amount of food protein to be administered is 4 g for children ≤4 years of age and 8 g for those ≥5 years of age. Each dose is administered at 15-minute intervals. The first dose is started with 5% of the total dose and increased by 5% increments with each subsequent dose, with the final two doses being 25% of the total amount to administer. The child should be closely monitored for any reaction during the procedure. Weighing scale with the ability to measure up to four digits, microwave oven for food preparation, and measurement cups are some of the common requirements in a challenge test room. If there is a high likelihood of a reaction to the food item chosen, food challenges should better be avoided. Recent history of anaphylaxis, high levels of food-specific IgE and/or SPT wheal size, unstable cardiovascular disease, pregnancy, treatment with β blockers, uncontrolled eczema, allergic rhinitis or asthma, concurrent illnesses, fever, and active respiratory symptoms are some reasons to postpone open food challenge.

Bronchial challenge test: Rarely done in routine pediatric allergy practice. This is done more to rule out the diagnosis of asthma due to its high sensitivity and high negative predictive value. Methacholine is the most common drug used during the bronchial challenge test. The amount is delivered through a nebulizer or by a dosimeter. Spirometry equipment is necessary to measure pulmonary function before and after methacholine administration. The staff should be aware of when to abort the test and should be well-trained in handling emergencies.

Nasal challenge test: This is not done routinely and is more of a research tool. Allergen is introduced by inhalation, and monitoring is done for the symptoms and signs of allergic rhinitis. The assessment of nasal block can be done either by rhinomanometry or by peak nasal inspiratory flow meter (PNIF).

Drug provocation test (DPT): DPT is the gold standard for the identification of the drug eliciting a drug allergy. It can confirm or exclude a drug allergy or demonstrate tolerance to a less likely eliciting drug. The oral route is preferred whenever possible. DPTs are contraindicated in noncontrollable and/or severe life-threatening drug hypersensitivity reactions such as severe cutaneous reactions [e.g., Stevens–Johnson syndrome (SJS), toxic epidermal necrolysis (TEN), drug reaction with eosinophilia and systemic symptoms (DRESS), vasculitis, and acute generalized exanthematous pustulosis (AGEP)], systemic reactions (e.g., DRESS), hematologic reactions, internal organ involvement, and if there is a risk of severe life-threatening reactions.

Drug provocation tests are not indicated when:

- The offending drug is unlikely to be needed and several structurally unrelated alternatives exist
- Severe concurrent illness.

Drug provocation tests should be performed under safe conditions with trained staff and emergency resuscitation equipment.

Other Laboratory Services Including In Vitro Allergy Tests

Basic equipment for routine blood tests should be made available. A place should be identified for the collection of blood samples. Equipment for in vitro allergy testing may be procured (e.g., ImmunoCAP test and Phadia 250 machine). If the same is not available in the center, samples may be collected and transported to the nearest lab with the same facility as per the specifications for blood collection and transport. Periodic maintenance of all laboratory equipment is important, and there should be a system for regular quality assessment. Make sure that all laboratory staff are using adequate personal protective equipment. Color-coded bins should be available in the blood collection area as per the biomedical waste management rules. Details of all available tests and their tariffs should be displayed outside the laboratory.

Caveats while using in vitro specific immunoglobulin E allergy tests:

- Due to the use of extracts containing different allergen compositions, interassay variation between manufacturers will be there. Hence, the results from one assay cannot be compared to those from another analytical system.

- In patients with very high total IgE, there is a chance for false-positive results (due to nonspecific binding of patient's IgE).
- In vitro tests should be ordered only on the basis of a detailed history and clinical examination. Doing a large panel of tests without an adequate clinical history is not recommended.

Spirometry

Spirometry is a very important component of any comprehensive allergy center. There are different choices available to select a spirometer for your clinic. There are portable ones and those that can be connected to laptops or personal computers (PCs). The decision to choose a spirometer should be based on the patient load and the setup of your office. Regular calibration should be done as per the manufacturer's recommendation.

Advanced techniques such as *impulse oscillometry and fractional exhaled nitric oxide (FENO) measurement* may also be procured, especially in research and academic centers with a high patient turnover.

Rhinolaryngoscopy Section

The flexible fiberoptic rhinoscope helps in examining the upper airways with minimal discomfort to the patient. The procedure is relatively easy to perform with good knowledge about the upper airway anatomy and physiology. The examinations may be recorded for permanent record keeping, and recordings may be played to the patients to make them understand their problems better. A flexible fiberoptic rhinoscope, examining chair with an adjustable headrest, topical decongestant (oxymetazoline), and lidocaine/xylocaine (for nasal anesthesia) are the minimum requirements.

Immunotherapy Section

As per the World Allergy Organization Statement, risk and safety requirements for diagnostic and therapeutic procedures in allergology include: Any center doing immunotherapy should have an allergy specialist—a doctor who has received specialized training in allergy; pulmonologists/physicians/pediatricians/ENT surgeons/dermatologists trained in allergy; resuscitative equipment and medicines; and adequate number of trained staff able to handle emergencies.

Strict aseptic precautions should be followed in the preparation as well as administration of immunotherapy. As allergen extracts vary from one manufacturer to another, it is suggested that diagnostic and therapeutic allergen extracts should be procured from the same allergen manufacturer.

Each patient is to be evaluated every time and confirmed that none of the contraindications of immunotherapy are present. Label the prepared immunotherapy vials with patients' name, antigens mixed, dose in the preparation, and the date of expiry. Always document the immunotherapy visits. One copy of the immunotherapy prescription form is kept in the file, and the second copy should be given to the patient. All vials (build-up and maintenance vials) should be color-coded uniformly and are to be numbered. The numbering system should be used in such a way that the highest concentration should be labeled "1" and the next 10-fold dilution would be labeled as "2," and so on. The allergen extracts/vaccines should be stored at 2–8°C in a refrigerator. In case of withdrawal of more antigens from the vaccine vial, it should not be injected back into a vial to avoid contamination. In case of electricity failure for >2 hours, keep the vaccine in an ice box or any other cooling device/pack. Transportation of the antigen should be done using a cooling container.

Counseling Area

Counseling and patient education are extremely important parts of both primary and secondary prevention of allergy. A trained nurse or a counselor should be present in the room. Pamphlets printed in local language with attractive pics detailing different allergic diseases, diagnostic methods, preventive measures, details of immunotherapy, etc., will be helpful. This room should also serve as an area to demonstrate to the patients the various devices used in allergy management such as aerosol devices, intranasal sprays, and epinephrine injectors. Checklists for the correct usage of devices can be used to train the patients. Videos in local language about various allergic diseases are to be played regularly during the allergy center's working hours. Questionnaires on allergic diseases may be given to the patients and parents so that they can fill them before going to the doctor's room. The various consent forms can also be filled after proper counseling. The counseling room, if sufficiently large, can be used for conducting awareness classes for the patients as well as the nearby doctors, especially the general practitioners.

Records Section

Medical records form a permanent account of a patient's illness. The clarity and accuracy of medical records play a cardinal role in effective communication between healthcare professionals and patients. The records should be maintained in a separate record room if available. It is preferable to store records year wise or diagnosis wise. A good quality hospital management software may be used, which will help in giving appointments to patients, registration, prescription making, as well as record keeping. Such software can also send reminders and notifications (email/SMS) in local languages to the patients regularly.

The incidence and prevalence of allergic diseases among children are escalating each day. Unfortunately, there remains a lack of awareness regarding the accurate diagnosis and management of allergic disorders, even among pediatricians. Pediatric allergy is a relatively new subspecialty, and there is an urgent need to integrate allergy management into pediatric practice. Establishing dedicated allergy treatment centers, equipped with diagnostic and therapeutic facilities, as well as providing comprehensive counseling and patient education, will significantly enhance the management of allergies in our country.

SUMMARY

Allergic diseases in children are rapidly increasing worldwide, posing significant health, social, and economic burdens. In India and other developing countries, pediatric allergy is still in its early stages, making it crucial to establish well-equipped and professionally run Pediatric Allergy Clinics. This chapter provides a step-by-step guide to setting up such a clinic, covering essential legal requirements, infrastructure design, staffing, and patient-friendly services. It outlines the facilities needed for reception, waiting areas, consultation rooms, emergency care, and record keeping. Special emphasis is placed on diagnostic services like skin prick testing, food and drug challenge tests, in vitro testing, and spirometry, along with advanced tools such as rhinolaryngoscopy and exhaled nitric oxide measurement. The chapter also details requirements for immunotherapy services, patient counseling, and structured record maintenance. By integrating diagnostic, therapeutic, and educational components, dedicated Pediatric Allergy Clinics can significantly improve the quality of allergy care and patient outcomes.

KEY POINTS

- Pediatric allergy is an emerging subspecialty in India, and dedicated allergy clinics are vital to meet the rising burden of childhood allergic diseases.
- Establishing a clinic requires mandatory registrations, permits, insurance, and strict adherence to biomedical waste and safety regulations.
- Essential infrastructure includes reception and waiting areas, consultation rooms, emergency facilities, diagnostic laboratories, and counseling spaces.
- Core diagnostic services comprise skin prick testing, food/drug challenge tests, spirometry, and in vitro IgE assays, supported by standardized protocols and safety measures.
- Immunotherapy must be conducted under trained specialists with aseptic techniques, proper storage of allergen extracts, and readiness for managing emergencies.
- Patient education, counseling, and meticulous record-keeping are central to effective allergy management and long-term care delivery.

SUGGESTED READING

1. Boyce JA, Assa'ad A, Burks AW, Jones SM, Sampson HA, Wood RA, et al. Guidelines for the diagnosis and management of food allergy in the United States: report of the NIAID-sponsored expert panel. J Allergy Clin Immunol. 2010;126:S1-58.
2. Diwakar L, Cummins C, Lilford R, Roberts T. Systematic review of pathways for the delivery of allergy services. BMJ Open. 2017;7:e012647.
3. Gaur SN, Kumar R, Singh AB, Agarwal MK, Arora N. Guidelines for practice of allergen immunotherapy in India: 2017—an update. Indian J Allergy Asthma Immunol. 2017;31:3-33.
4. Gupta N, Agarwal P, Sachdev A, Gupta D. Allergy testing—an overview. Indian Pediatr. 2019;56(11):951-7.
5. Kaliner MA, Giacco SD, Crisci CD, Frew AJ, Liu G, Maspero J, et al. Requirements for physician competencies in allergy: key clinical competencies appropriate for the care of patients with allergic or immunologic diseases. A Position Statement of the World Allergy Organization. World Allergy Organ J. 2008;1(2):42-6.
6. Kowalski ML, Ansotegui I, Aberer W, Al-Ahmad M, Akdis M, Ballmer-Weber BK, et al. Risk and safety requirements for diagnostic and therapeutic procedures in allergology: World Allergy Organization Statement. World Allergy Organ J. 2016;9(1):1-42.
7. Rancé F, Deschildre A, Villard-Truc F, Gomez SA, Paty E, Santos C, et al. Oral food challenge in children: an expert review. Eur Ann Allergy Clin Immunol. 2009;41(2):35-49.

Index

Page numbers followed by *b* refer to box, *f* refer to figure, *fc* refer to flowchart and *t* refer to table.

A

B

C

D

G

H

I

J

K

L

M